Contents

Advisory board

Contributors and consultants

Darlene Nebel Cantu, RNC, MSN
Director, Faculty; Baptist Health System School of Nursing; San Antonio
(Tex.) College Nursing Department

Joyce Clement, MSN, ANP, FNP-BC
Adult and Family Nurse Practitioner; Freeman Hospital; Joplin, Mo.;
Faculty; University of Missouri at Kansas City

Carol Deresz, RNC, MSN
Clinical Instructor, University of Texas Health Science Center at San Antonio
School of Nursing, RN – Labor & Delivery, Southwest Texas Methodist
Hospital, San Antonio

Sylvia R. Doyle RN, MSN
Lead Instructor Maternal-Neonatal Health Nursing; Carolinas College
of Health Sciences School of Nursing; Charlotte, N.C.

Elizabeth C. Elkind, RNC, MSN, MBA
Faculty — Instructor, Thomas Jefferson University College of Health
Professions, Philadelphia

Julia A. Greenawalt, RNC, MA, MSN
Clinical Instructor, University of Pittsburgh

Shelton M. Hisley, RNC, PhD, WHNP
Assistant Professor and Graduate Clinical Coordinator; School of Nursing;
The University of North Carolina at Wilmington

Holly K. Kailani, RN, MS
Assistant Professor of Nursing, Hawaii Pacific University, Kaneohe

Pamela M. Mammano, RN, MS
Director of ADN Program; Instructor — Maternal-Child Nursing;
Illinois Valley Community College; Oglesby, Ill.

Nan C. Riedé, RN, MSN
Assistant Professor, Baptist College of Health Sciences, Memphis

Ronni H. Rothman, BSN, MSN, MPH, CNM
Certified Nurse Midwife; Lankenau Hospital; Wynnewood, Pa.

How to use this book

Straight A's is a multivolume study guide series developed especially for nursing students. Each volume provides essential course material in a unique two-column design. The easy-to-read interior outline format offers a succinct review of key facts as presented in leading textbooks on the subject. The bulleted exterior columns provide only the most crucial information, allowing for quick, efficient review right before an important quiz or test.

Special features appear in every chapter to make information accessible and easy to remember. **Learning objectives** encourage the student to evaluate knowledge before and after study. **Chapter overview** highlights the chapter's major concepts. Within the outlined text, color is used to highlight critical information and key points. Key points may include cardinal signs and symptoms, current theories, important steps in a nursing procedure, critical assessment findings, crucial nursing interventions, or successful therapies and treatments. **NCLEX Checks** at the end of each chapter offer additional opportunities to review material and assess knowledge gained before moving on to new information.

Other features appear throughout the book to facilitate learning. **Time-out for teaching** highlights key areas to address when teaching patients. **Go with the flow** charts promote critical thinking. Finally, a brand-new Windows-based software program (see CD-ROM on inside back cover) poses more than 250 multiple-choice and alternate-format NCLEX-style questions in random or sequential order to assess your knowledge.

The Straight A's volumes are designed as learning tools, not as primary information sources. When read conscientiously as a supplement to class attendance and textbook reading, Straight A's can enhance understanding and help improve test scores and final grades.

Foreword

One summer evening, I returned from my break to find a young patient complaining of abdominal discomfort. She was 34 weeks pregnant and had pregnancy-induced hypertension (PIH). Going through a mental list of possibilities, I remembered that PIH produces vasoconstriction and sometimes leads to clotting disturbances; therefore, the pain could be caused by bleeding in the liver or kidneys, organ ischemia, separation of the placenta from the uterine wall, or the onset of labor due to impaired circulation to the uterus.

Each of these possible concerns required a different nursing assessment. I checked laboratory data for liver, kidney, and clotting status; evaluated her urine; and palpated for uterine tenderness and rigidity that could indicate placental separation. Her discomfort increased, and I felt uterine contractions through the abdominal wall. I applied the electronic fetal monitor and found a normal fetal heart rate. A vaginal examination revealed that she was 5 cm dilated. I notified the obstetrician and intensive care nursery and prepared to support and monitor the patient through a high-risk delivery. After an intense 2-hour labor, she delivered a healthy preterm boy. I walked to my car that night remembering his tiny ruddy face and dark hair and feeling grateful that I had been able to respond to my patient's high-risk physiologic needs while supporting her as she gave birth to her first child.

Maternal-newborn nursing has many happy endings and occasional sad ones. It's a thrilling specialty because a nurse can influence the first moments a family spends together. If I hadn't known the biophysical processes of PIH, hadn't been prepared to assess new developments, and didn't bring in the care my patient needed, the outcome might have been less positive. Now I teach maternal-neonatal nursing in an academic setting, and I draw from experiences such as this one to portray the complex pathophysiology and fast-paced events that nurses encounter in this area of practice.

Straight A's in Maternal-Neonatal Nursing will help you develop mental lists of physiology to remember and parameters to assess. This handy review book starts with the social and ethical context of maternal-neonatal nursing, reviewing the anatomy and physiology of reproduction and prenatal development and then discussing the normal processes and high-risk conditions in pregnancy, labor, the postpartum recovery period, and neonatal life. It concludes with chapters on infertility, genetics, and family planning.

Each chapter follows the learning process used by novices and experts: after reviewing the normal anatomy and physiology and the social context of a health condition, you'll learn what is different or abnormal in this condition or situation, how to assess the symptoms and behaviors that arise from that change, and how to think through the nursing actions that address these symptoms and their causes.

The simple outline format streamlines your learning by providing the important information without fillers or distractions. It gets better, though! When you're short on time or just looking for a concise review of the essentials, the outer columns offer what you need. It's as if the authors have whittled down your class notes and readings to the main points you need to remember for exams and clinical practice. Each chapter even includes a list of the top things you need to study for each subject. In addition, key points and learning tips are highlighted in tables, diagrams, and sidebars.

Most important, the 200 practice questions in this book and the more than 250 questions on the enclosed CD-ROM are similar to those on the National Council Licensure Examination (NCLEX). Take them seriously! Bring together your learning from your main textbook, the classroom, this review, and your clinical experiences, and apply the full scope of your knowledge as you visualize the situation in each question. Think through why your answer is correct and why the others are incorrect. Then check your answer against the correct answer, review the rationale for the correct answer, and learn why the other answers are incorrect. That's how I teach, and it works!

Whether you see maternal-neonatal nursing in your future or you simply want to do your very best in a course or on an exam, look for a topic here that catches your interest, find clinical examples, and read everything you can find on it. When you invest your energy, the content stays with you. Find a way to make each clinical situation come alive for you! I wish you success in your academic pursuits, on your NCLEX exam, and in your future in nursing.

Margaret H. Kearney, PhD, RNC, FAAN
Associate Editor; *Journal of Obstetric, Gynecologic, and Neonatal Nursing;*
Associate Professor and Chair of Maternal-Child Nursing;
William F. Connell School of Nursing; Boston College; Chestnut Hill, Mass.

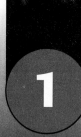

Overview of maternal-neonatal nursing

LEARNING OBJECTIVES

After studying this chapter, you should be able to:

- Define the goals of maternal-neonatal nursing.
- Describe the various roles for maternal-neonatal nurses.
- Describe the structures of different family types and the basic functions of the family in present-day society.
- Discuss current legal and ethical issues in maternal-neonatal nursing.

CHAPTER OVERVIEW

Maternal-neonatal nurses assume various roles and functions in caring for a pregnant patient and her family. In certain instances, the functions performed depend on the nurse's level of education. An understanding of the makeup and functioning of the family plays a vital role in helping the nurse deliver family-centered care. Even though the structure of the family has changed and technological advances have affected this area over the years, nurses working in this field are responsible for providing comprehensive, ethical, and legal care to the pregnant patient, her fetus, and her family.

Three periods of pregnancy

- Antepartum – conception to onset of labor
- Intrapartum – onset of contractions to 1 to 4 hours after birth
- Postpartum – birth to 6 weeks after birth

Family-centered enhancements

- Alternative settings, such as LDR and LDRP units, allow more family involvement in birth.
- Support people remain in room during birth.
- Patient remains in same room for recovery.

Maternal-neonatal nursing roles

- Care provider
- Educator
- Advocate
- Counselor

INTRODUCTION TO MATERNAL-NEONATAL NURSING

● **General information**
  - The goal of maternal-neonatal nursing is to provide comprehensive, family-centered care to the pregnant patient and her fetus or neonate during the antepartum, intrapartum, and postpartum periods
    – Antepartum period — the period from conception to the onset of labor
    – Intrapartum period — the period from the onset of contractions that cause cervical dilation to the first 1 to 4 hours after the birth of the neonate and the placenta
    – Postpartum period (also known as the *puerperium*) — the 6-week period after delivery of the neonate and the placenta, which ends when the reproductive organs return to the nonpregnant state
  - Hospitals have listened to consumer demands to provide more re-laxed, family-friendly environments for the birthing process
    – Alternative settings provide a holistic, family-centered approach to maternal and neonatal health care by permitting more family in-volvement in the birthing experience
    – Called labor, deliver, and recovery (LDR) or labor, delivery, recov-ery, and postpartum (LDRP), these units are found in most hospi-tals
    – Partners, family members, and other support people may remain in the room while the patient labors and gives birth
    – The patient remains in the same room throughout the recovery and postpartum period
  - Maternal-neonatal nurses practice in various settings
    – Community-based health centers
    – Private physicians' offices
    – Hospital clinics
    – Acute-care hospitals
    – Maternity hospitals
    – Birthing centers
    – Private homes

● **Nursing roles and functions**
  - Nurses involved in maternal-neonatal nursing assume various roles
    – Care provider
    – Educator
    – Advocate
    – Counselor

- The functions involved for each role depend on the nurse's level of education
- Registered nurse (RN)
  - Is a graduate of an accredited nursing program
  - Has passed the NCLEX-RN examination
  - Is licensed by the state
  - Plays a vital role in providing direct patient care, educating the patient and her family, and functioning as an advocate and a counselor
- Clinical nurse specialist (CNS)
  - Is an RN who has received education at the master's level
  - Focuses on providing direct patient care, promoting health, educating the patient and her family, and performing research activities
  - Serves as a role model and teacher of quality nursing care
  - May serve as a consultant to RNs working in the maternal-neonatal field
  - May be trained in neonatal care and provide care in neonatal intensive care units (NICUs)
  - As a childbirth educator, teaches the patient and her family about normal childbirth, provides them with care, and helps prepare them for the process
  - As a breast-feeding consultant, provides care to the patient as she's learning about breast-feeding and provides support to her while she's breast-feeding
- Certified nurse midwife (CNM)
  - Is an RN who has received advanced education at the master's level or has been certified
  - Independently cares for the low-risk obstetric patient throughout her pregnancy
  - Is licensed to deliver infants
- Women's health nurse practitioner (WHNP)
  - Plays a vital role in educating the patient about her body and about preventive medicine
  - Cares for the patient with a sexually transmitted disease and counsels her about reproductive life planning
  - Helps the patient remain healthy so she can have a healthy pregnancy and a healthy life
- Family nurse practitioner (FNP)
  - Provides care to all patients throughout the life cycle
  - Provides prenatal care for the low-risk obstetric patient
  - Performs physical examinations, prepares pregnancy histories, orders and performs diagnostic and obstetric examinations, and

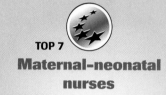

TOP 7

Maternal-neonatal nurses

1. Registered nurse
2. Clinical nurse specialist
3. Certified nurse midwife
4. Women's health nurse practitioner
5. Family nurse practitioner
6. Neonatal nurse practitioner
7. Pediatric nurse practitioner

Spotlight on CNMs

- RNs with master's degree or certification
- Can independently care for low-risk patients throughout their pregnancies
- Are licensed to deliver infants

TOP 9

Maternal-neonatal nursing functions

1. Delivery
2. Discharge planning
3. Education (about childbirth, the body, preventive medicine)
4. High-risk patient follow-up
5. Neonatal assessment and examination
6. Patient care
7. Physical examination
8. Pregnancy history
9. Care plans

Characteristics of a family

- Two or more people
- Same or different household
- Emotional bond
- Interrelated social tasks

plans care for the patient during her pregnancy and for the family after birth
– Promotes health and wellness and optimal family functioning
- Neonatal nurse practitioner (NNP)
  – Is skilled in the care of neonates and can work in levels I, II, and III nurseries
  – Can also work in NICUs and neonatal follow-up clinics
  – Performs normal neonatal assessment and physical examination as well as high-risk follow-up and discharge planning
- Pediatric nurse practitioner (PNP)
  – Performs well-baby counseling and care as well as physical assessment and detailed history interviews
  – Serves as a primary health caregiver or as the sole health care professional that the parents and child see at all visits
  – Can order diagnostic tests and prescribe appropriate drugs for therapy (prescribing privileges depend on individual state regulations)
  – May collaborate with a pediatrician to determine appropriate care if the PNP determines that the child has a major illness, such as heart disease

FAMILY-CENTERED CARE

- **General information**
  - Definition of family
    – Two or more people who may live in the same household, share an emotional bond, and perform certain interrelated social tasks
    – Group of people who may be united by blood, marriage, or adoption and have a common residence for part of their lives
  - Family dynamics
    – Families can profoundly influence individual family members
    – A new family member alters the family structure
    – Family roles must be flexible enough to adjust to the changes that a pregnancy and a neonate bring
    – If a family member is ill or is going through a rough developmental period, this puts a tremendous strain on the family
    – Family-centered care examines individual circumstances from a family or community standpoint
    – Family-centered care has become a focus of modern nursing practice
  - Family types
    – Have evolved from the traditional nuclear family

– May change over the life cycle of the family because of work, birth, death, or divorce
– May differ based on the family roles, generational issues, means of family support, and sociocultural issues
– Include nuclear family; cohabitation family; extended, or multi-generational, family; single-parent family; blended family; communal family; gay or lesbian family; foster family; and adoptive family

  • Nuclear family
    - The traditional family, with a wife, a husband, and children
    - Members feel affection for each other
    - Members provide each other with support; however, when family crisis arises, such as illness, fewer family members means fewer people to share the burden
    - Can change as a result of divorce, separation, single parenthood, remarriage, or alternative lifestyles
  • Cohabitation family
    - A heterosexual couple that lives together but isn't married
    - May be together for the short-term or the long-term
    - Offers psychological and financial support like the nuclear family
  • Extended, or multigenerational, family
    - Nuclear family plus other family members, such as grandparents, aunts, uncles, cousins, and grandchildren
    - Support person and primary caregiver may not be the spouse or the parent but another member of the family
    - May experience financial problems because income is stretched to accommodate additional family members
  • Single-parent family
    - Makes up 50% to 60% of families with school-age children
    - Single parent may be the mother or the father
    - Can result from divorce, death of a spouse, or a parent raising a child outside of marriage
    - Lacks the support of a nuclear family in times of family crisis such as illness
    - May suffer from financial problems
    - Has no backup support for child care
    - May have difficulty fulfilling all the necessary role models
  • Blended family
    - Has combined because of remarriage
    - Can foster feelings of yours, mine, and ours among members

Family dynamics

- Families profoundly influence individual members
- New family member alters structure
- Roles must be flexible to adjust to the changes
- Illness and pregnancy strain the family

Family-centered care

- Examines individual circumstances from a family or community standpoint
- Focus of modern nursing practice

Family types

- Nuclear
- Cohabitation
- Extended or multigenerational
- Single-parent
- Blended
- Communal
- Gay or lesbian
- Foster
- Adoptive

Spotlight on gay and lesbian families

- May include children
- Children can be products of previous heterosexual relationships or adopted from surrogate mothers
- Artificial insemination can also be used

Spotlight on adoptions

- Any type of family can adopt.
- There are many reasons for adopting.
- Adoption challenges the family unit.
- Many sources for adoptions exist, including private and international agencies.

- Rivalry and jealousy may develop when children are exposed to new parenting methods
  - Helps children become more adaptable to new situations
- Communal family
  - Group of people who have chosen to live together but may not be related by marriage
  - May be related by social or religious values
  - May not adhere to traditional health care procedures but may be proactive in participating in this care
  - Is highly receptive to teaching
- Gay or lesbian family
  - May choose to include children in the family
  - Children may be adopted from surrogate mothers or from previous heterosexual relationships, or one member of a female couple may be artificially inseminated
- Foster family
  - Provides care for children whose biological parents can no longer care for them
  - Usually a temporary arrangement until the biological parents can resume care
  - Foster parents may have children of their own
- Adoptive family
  - Any type of family can become an adoptive family
  - May result from an inability to have biological children—for example, because of medical reasons or because the couple is gay or lesbian
  - May adopt foster children whose parents can no longer provide care
  - May adopt the biological siblings or a family relative of the parent
  - Poses many challenges to the family unit, especially if the family also includes biological children
  - Adoptions can be through agencies, or they can be private; they can also be international
- Functions of a family
  - A healthy family typically has eight functions to ensure its success as a working unit as well as the success of its individual members
    - Distribute resources
      - Including financial wealth, material goods, affection, and space
      - Determining which family needs are met and prioritizing those needs
    - Socialize family members

- Preparing children to interact with people outside the family and live in the community
- May be challenging, especially if the family culture is different from the community culture

· Divide the labor
  - Determining who fulfills the various family roles
  - Roles include family provider, child care provider, and home manager

· Provide for basic physical needs
  - Providing food, shelter, clothing, and health care
  - Ensuring the family has ample resources to meet these needs

· Maintain order
  - Ensuring effective communication among family members
  - Establishing family values
  - Enforcing common rules for family members

· Reproduce, release, and recruit family members
  - Determining who lives in the family
  - Determining when conceptions and adoptions occur
  - Adapting when children leave home
  - Caring for elderly parents in the home

· Place family members into society
  - Selecting community activities
  - Selecting religious affiliation
  - Selecting a school
  - Selecting political group
  - Selecting a birth setting

· Maintain motivation and morale
  - Instilling a sense of pride among family members
  - Supporting each other during crises

Family influences on pregnancy

• Influencing factors
  – Factors can influence the family's response to the pregnancy
    · Maternal age
      - Mother may be nearing menopause
        ·· Adult children may view mother's pregnancy unfavorably
        ·· Spouse may resent the pregnancy and his revisiting of the father role
      - Mother may be a teenager who isn't married
        ·· Family members may fear that the mother won't be able to provide for her baby or that she won't finish her schooling
        ·· Family members may be concerned about how their own roles will change as a result of the pregnancy

Family functions

- Distribution of resources
- Socialization
- Division of labor
- Physical maintenance
- Maintenance of order
- Reproduction, release, and recruitment
- Placement
- Maintenance of motivation and morale

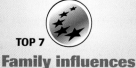

TOP 7

Family influences on pregnancy

1. Maternal age
2. Cultural beliefs and practices
3. Planning or not planning pregnancy
4. Family dynamics
5. Social and economic resources
6. Age and health status of others in the family
7. Maternal medical and obstetric history

Spotlight
on cultural views

- Cultural norms impact course of pregnancy
- Pregnancy may be shared with others
  OR
  Pregnancy may be kept secret until certain point in gestation
- Men may participate
  OR
  Women may be primary participants

Spotlight
on family dynamics

- Family structure and functioning
- Affects how pregnancy is perceived
- Family members are influenced by their changing roles
- Physical and emotional changes experienced by pregnant woman affect family
- Some family members accept pregnancy as a part of family growth; others view it as a stressor and view the new member as an intruder
- Pregnancy causes career and lifestyle changes

- - Family members may fear that they will become full-time caregivers for the child
  - - Family's religious beliefs may lead them to view the pregnancy as unacceptable or sinful
  - - Family may reject the mother and the child she's carrying
- Cultural beliefs and practices related to pregnancy
  - Some view childbearing as something to be shared with others as soon as the pregnancy is known
  - Others shy away from being public about pregnancy until after a certain gestational period
  - Cultural norms impact family roles, behaviors, and expectations
    - - In some cultures, men participate in the pregnancy and childbirth
    - - In other cultures, women are the primary participants
- Whether pregnancy is planned or not
  - Some women view pregnancy as a natural and desired outcome of marriage
  - Other women are ambivalent about pregnancy
  - Some families feel that they don't have enough experience around children
  - Some pregnancies may be unplanned and result from sexual experimentation or lack of knowledge about birth control
  - Some unplanned pregnancies are accepted and welcomed despite being unplanned
- Family dynamics
  - Includes family structure and how it functions
  - Affects how a new pregnancy is perceived
  - Family members are influenced by their changing roles
  - Family is influenced by the physical and emotional changes that the pregnant woman experiences
  - Some family members accept pregnancy as a part of the family's growth
  - Other family members view pregnancy as a stressor and consider the new member an intruder
  - Pregnancy causes career and lifestyle changes
- Social and economic resources
  - Economic status can affect how a family responds to pregnancy
  - A pregnant woman may delay prenatal care or choose not to take prenatal vitamins because of financial issues
  - Pregnancy may reduce the family income if mother can't work
- Age and health status of other family members

- Presence of ill family member may influence how the family accepts the pregnancy
- Sibling reaction depends on the age of the sibling
  ·· Toddlers may regress
  ·· Preschoolers and school-age children may show interest in the pregnancy
  ·· Adolescents may be embarrassed by the pregnancy
  ·· Sibling rivalry may be an issue
- · Maternal medical and obstetric history
  - Family members may be concerned that pregnancy could jeopardize the mother's health, especially if she has an obstetric history that includes difficult labors or births
- Implications for nursing
  – Assessment of each family member's roles and functions
  – Effect of each of these roles and functions on other family members
  – Assessment of health beliefs, practices, and resources
  – Impact of factors on childbearing and family
  – Priority and goal setting to provide individualized care based on the family's needs

ETHICAL AND LEGAL ISSUES

General information
- Great advances have been made in reproductive technology and genetic research
- These advances have created ethical and legal issues
  – Prenatal testing can provide information about gender, congenital abnormalities, and chromosomal defects and can help the parents and health care team prepare for the infant
  – However, some fear that this knowledge may be used incorrectly
    · What if the mother decides to terminate the pregnancy because she's displeased with the fetus's sex?
    · Will genetic engineering lead to the creation of only "desirable" individuals?
- The maternal-neonatal nurse must be familiar with the issues, explore her own beliefs, and remain nonjudgmental

Standards of care
- Guidelines are based on scientific principles and offer direction when providing health care
- Guidelines are set by an accrediting agency (such as the Joint Commission on Accreditation of Healthcare Organizations) and based on the scope of practice as defined by the state's nurse practice act

Nursing implications
- Assess each family member's role and function and how the pregnancy affects these roles and functions.
- Assess health beliefs, practices, and resources and how they impact childbearing and family.
- Prioritize and set goals to provide individualized care based on family needs.

Standards of care
- Guidelines that offer direction when providing health care
- Set by an accrediting agency and based on the scope of practice as defined by state nurse practice act
- Maternal-neonatal nursing organizations provide standards of care and guidelines for RNs and APNs in this specialty
- Facilities must meet the accrediting agency's minimum standards
- Nurses must observe at least the minimum standard of care

Patient's rights

- A pregnant patient has the right to participate in decisions involving her health and the health of her fetus.
- The American Hospital Association's "Patient's Bill of Rights" explains the rights of all patients.
- "The Pregnant Patient's Bill of Rights" explains rights specific to pregnant patients.

Spotlight on informed consent

- Patient must be informed of reasons for treatment or procedure as well as possible adverse effects and alternative treatments.
- Patient must sign consent form.
- Nurse must ensure that signed consent form is in the patient's chart before the procedure.

Spotlight on prenatal screening

- Can detect inherited and congenital abnormalities
- Risk to fetus creates conflict between rights of the fetus and parents' right to know the fetus's health status
- Pretest and posttest counseling are essential parts of prenatal screening

- Maternal-neonatal nursing organizations provide standards of care and guidelines for registered and advanced practice nurses for this specialty area
  - Association of Women's Health Obstetrics and Neonatal Nurses (AWHONN)
  - National Association of Neonatal Nurses (NANN)
  - National Association of Nurse Practitioners in Women's Health (NPWH)
- Facilities must meet the accrediting agency's minimum standards
- Nurses must observe at least the minimum standard of care

● **Patient's rights**
- A pregnant patient has the right to actively participate in decisions involving her health and the health of her fetus, unless a medical emergency prevents her from doing so
- The American Hospital Association's "Patient's Bill of Rights" explains the rights of all patients; "The Pregnant Patient's Bill of Rights," the specific rights of the pregnant patient

● **Ethical and legal issues**
- Informed consent
  - Before treatment, diagnostic procedures, or experimental therapy, a patient must be informed of the reasons for the treatment as well as possible adverse effects and alternative treatments
  - The physician must obtain signed consent
  - The nurse must ensure that signed consent is in the patient's chart before the procedure is performed
- Prenatal screening
  - Can detect inherited and congenital abnormalities long before birth
  - Early diagnosis may allow repair of an abnormality in utero
  - May force a patient to choose between having an abortion and assuming the emotional and financial burden of raising a severely disabled child
  - Some feel that the risk it poses to the fetus creates a conflict between the rights of the fetus and the parents' right to know the fetus's health status
  - Helps the patient fully understand the procedure
  - Pretest and posttest counseling are essential parts of an ethical prenatal-screening program
- Abortion
  - Although legal, abortion remains an emotionally charged topic
  - An obstetric nurse must explore her own beliefs and remain nonjudgmental

- In vitro fertilization (IVF)
  - With IVF, the ovum is fertilized outside the body and then implanted into the uterus
  - Between 15 and 20 embryos may result from a single fertilization effort
  - Only 3 to 5 of these embryos are implanted in the woman's uterus
  - Ethical questions arise as to what to do with remaining embryos
  - Although the procedure has allowed infertile couples to have children, some are concerned that it's unnatural
- Surrogacy
  - A surrogate mother carries a fetus for another couple, with the expectation that the couple will adopt the neonate after he's born
  - Questions have evolved over the surrogate mother's legal rights to the infant
- Fetal tissue research
  - Fetal tissue has facilitated scientific research for Parkinson's disease, Alzheimer's disease, diabetes, and other degenerative disorders
  - Transplanted fetal nerve cells help to generate new cells in the patient that somehow reduce symptoms
  - Immaturity of the fetal immune system reduces the chances of the recipient rejecting the tissue
  - Some are concerned whether the number of abortions will increase in response to the need for tissue and whether this is an ethical use of human tissue
- Eugenics and gene manipulation
  - Gene therapy can help prevent and manage different disorders
  - Researchers can learn the sex of the fetus and whether it suffers from certain serious medical conditions
  - Questions arise surrounding the ability to create designer babies, leading to a perfect population
  - Genetic testing facilitates the identification of fetuses with such disorders as Down syndrome and Tay-Sachs disease
  - The screening of neonates for phenylketonuria is legally required in most states
  - Gene therapy using deoxyribonucleic acid (DNA) can be used to increase or decrease the activity of a gene in the body or to introduce a new gene into the body
- Preterm and high-risk neonate treatment
  - Medical advances have improved survival rates for high-risk neonates
  - Some are concerned about the physical, psychosocial, and economic costs

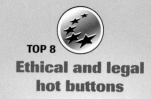

TOP 8

Ethical and legal hot buttons

1. Informed consent
2. Prenatal screening
3. Abortion
4. In vitro fertilization
5. Surrogacy
6. Fetal tissue research
7. Eugenics and gene manipulation
8. Treatment of preterm and high-risk neonates

Spotlight on eugenics and gene manipulation

- Can be used to increase or decrease the activity of a gene in the body or to introduce a new gene into the body
- Can help prevent and manage different disorders
- Can detect sex of fetus and presence of certain serious medical conditions
- Ethical dilemma related to ability to create "designer babies"
- Screening for phenylketonuria legally required in most states

– The nurse must present all available options in a compassionate, unbiased manner using simple terms

– The nurse must help family members consider the pros and cons of both initiating and withholding treatment

● **Professional development**

• The maternal-neonatal nurse must have a continued awareness of developments in maternal-neonatal nursing

– Attending continuing education programs

– Reading professional peer-reviewed literature

– Maintaining membership in professional organizations

– Obtaining certification through national nursing organizations

TOP 7

Items to study for your next maternal-neonatal nursing test

1. The goal of maternal-neonatal nursing

2. The four primary roles for maternal-neonatal nurses

3. The various functions of maternal-neonatal nurses

4. The nine types of families

5. The eight functions of a family

6. The seven family influences on pregnancy

7. The seven ethical-legal issues affecting maternal-neonatal nursing today

NCLEX CHECKS

It's never too soon to begin your NCLEX preparation. Now that you've reviewed this chapter, carefully read each of the following questions and choose the best answer. Then compare your responses to the correct answers.

1. Which of the following nurses is licensed to deliver a neonate?
- ☐ **A.** CNM
- ☐ **B.** CNS
- ☐ **C.** RN with a bachelor's degree
- ☐ **D.** APN

2. What is the benefit of using fetal tissue in the treatment of degenerative disorders?
- ☐ **A.** It allows inherited and congenital abnormalities to be detected.
- ☐ **B.** Immaturity of the fetal immune system reduces the chances of the recipient rejecting the tissue.
- ☐ **C.** Early diagnosis may allow repair of an abnormality in utero.
- ☐ **D.** It can be used to increase or decrease the activity of a gene in the body.

3. In which setting would a maternal-neonatal nurse practice?
- ☐ **A.** Long-term care
- ☐ **B.** Rehabilitation center
- ☐ **C.** Female prison
- ☐ **D.** Free-standing birthing center

4. What is the role of a maternal-neonatal nurse when dealing with an ethical issue?
- ☐ **A.** To provide advice
- ☐ **B.** To be nonjudgmental
- ☐ **C.** To provide ethical counsel
- ☐ **D.** To help the patient make decisions

5. Which organization provides standards of care and guidelines for registered and advanced practice nurses?

    ☐ **A.** ACOG

    ☐ **B.** AWHONN

    ☐ **C.** AAP

    ☐ **D.** APA

6. Which factors influence a family's response to pregnancy? Select all that apply.

    ☐ **A.** Age of grandparents

    ☐ **B.** Family structure and functioning

    ☐ **C.** Planning or not planning pregnancy

    ☐ **D.** Cultural beliefs and practices

    ☐ **E.** Social and economic resources

ANSWERS AND RATIONALES

1. CORRECT ANSWER: A

CNMs are licensed to deliver neonates. Although CNSs, RNs with bachelor's degrees, and APNs may care for laboring patients, they aren't licensed to deliver neonates.

2. CORRECT ANSWER: B

Fetal tissue research has discovered that the immaturity of the fetal immune system reduces the chances of the recipient rejecting the tissue. Prenatal testing can detect inherited and congenital abnormalities long before birth as well as allow for early diagnosis that may allow repair of an abnormality in utero. Gene therapy using deoxyribonucleic acid (DNA) can be used to increase or decrease the activity of a gene in the body or to introduce a new gene into the body.

3. CORRECT ANSWER: D

Maternal-neonatal nurses practice in various settings, including freestanding birthing centers, community-based health centers, private physicians' offices, hospital clinics, acute-care hospitals, maternity hospitals, and private homes.

4. CORRECT ANSWER: C

A maternal-neonatal nurse must be familiar with the issues, explore her own beliefs, and remain nonjudgmental.

5. CORRECT ANSWER: B

AWHONN stands for the Association of Women's Health Obstetrics and Neonatal Nurses and provides standards of care and guidelines for RNs and APNs. ACOG stands for the American College of Obstetricians and Gynecologists, AAP stands for the American Academy of Pediatrics, and APA stands for the American Psychiatric Association.

6. CORRECT ANSWERS: B, C, D, AND E

Factors that can influence the family's response to pregnancy include family structure and functioning, planning or not planning pregnancy, cultural beliefs and practices, maternal age, social and economic resources, maternal medical and obstetric history, and the presence, age, and health status of other family members. The age of the parents, not the grandparents, influences the family's response to pregnancy.

2

Structure and function of the reproductive organs

LEARNING OBJECTIVES

After studying this chapter, you should be able to:

- Describe the structure and function of the female and male reproductive organs.
- Identify the function of the male and female organs within the reproductive process.
- Describe the role played by accessory sex gland secretions in the reproductive cycle.
- State the hormonal and uterine changes that occur during the menstrual cycle.

CHAPTER OVERVIEW

Knowledge of the structure and function of the female and male reproductive systems is essential for understanding the processes involved with childbearing. Hormones circulating throughout the female reproductive cycle prepare the uterus for pregnancy. Male and female accessory glands also play a key role in this area.

FEMALE REPRODUCTIVE SYSTEM

● External genitalia

- Mons pubis
  - Provides an adipose cushion over the anterior symphysis pubis
  - Protects the pelvic bones
  - Contributes to rounded contour of the female body
- Labia majora
  - Consist of two folds of adipose tissue that converge at the mons pubis and extend down to the posterior commissure
  - Positioned lateral top of the labia minora
  - Covered by pubic hair
  - Consist of connective tissue, elastic fibers, veins, and sebaceous glands
  - Protect the external genitalia and the distal urethra and vagina
  - Fused anteriorly but separated posteriorly
- Labia minora
  - Located posterior to the mons pubis, within the labia majora
  - Consist of hairless folds of connective tissue, sebaceous and sweat glands, nonstriated muscle fibers, nerve endings, and blood vessels
  - Unite to form the fourchette, the vaginal vestibule
  - Lubricate the vulva, adding to sexual enjoyment and providing bactericidal protection
  - Are fairly small before menarche, are firm and full by childbearing age, and atrophied and smaller after menopause
- Clitoris
  - 1 to 2 cm in size
  - Located in the anterior portion of the vulva, just above the urethral opening
  - Covered by a fold of skin called the *prepuce*
  - Made up of erectile tissue, nerves, and blood vessels
  - Consists of the glans, body, and two crura
  - Homologous to the penis
  - Provides sexual pleasure
- Vaginal vestibule
  - Flattened smooth surface inside the labia
  - Is the tissue extending from the clitoris to the posterior fourchette
  - Openings to the bladder (the urethra) and the uterus (the vagina) both arise from the vestibule
  - Consists of the vaginal orifice, the hymen, the fourchette, Skene's glands, and Bartholin's glands
    - The hymen is a thin but tough, vascularized mucous membrane

---

Quick guide to external female genitalia

- **Bartholin's glands** – bean-shaped glands on either side of the vagina that provide lubrication during intercourse
- **Clitoris** – erectile tissue, nerves, and blood vessels located just above urethral opening; homologous to the penis
- **Fourchette** – ridge of tissue formed by the posterior joining of the two labia majora and labia minora that's sometimes cut during vaginal birth
- **Hymen** – thin, vascularized mucous membrane located at the vaginal orifice
- **Labia majora** – folds of adipose tissue that protect external genitalia and distal urethra and vagina
- **Labia minora** – lubricate vulva, adding to sexual enjoyment and providing bactericidal protection
- **Mons pubis** – cushions anterior symphysis pubis
- **Skene's glands** – glands located on each side of the urinary meatus that lubricate the external genitalia during intercourse

- Located at the vaginal orifice at childhood
- Perforated during intercourse, though with the use of tampons it may be perforated before the first pelvic examination
- May need to be surgically opened to permit the flow of menstruation (rare)
  - The fourchette is the ridge of tissue formed by the posterior joining of the two labia majora and labia minora
    - Sometimes cut during vaginal birth (episiotomy) to enlarge the vaginal opening
  - Skene's glands (paraurethral glands) are located just lateral to the urinary meatus, on either side
    - The ducts open into the urethra
    - Help to lubricate the external genitalia during intercourse, along with Bartholin's glands
    - May become infected and produce a discharge and pain
  - Bartholin's glands (vulvovaginal glands) are two bean-shaped glands on either side of the vagina
    - Secrete mucus along with Skene's glands during sexual stimulation
    - Alkaline pH of Skene's and Bartholin's glands help improve sperm survival in the vagina
    - May become infected and produce a discharge and pain
- Perineal body, or perineal muscle
  - Posterior to the fourchette
  - Easily stretched during childbirth to allow enlargement of the vagina and passage of the fetal head
  - Kegel exercises are aimed at this area
    - To strengthen, stretch, and relax the muscle
    - To prepare the muscle to expand during birth so that it doesn't tear
- Urethral meatus
  - Located 1 to 2.5 cm below the clitoris
- Vulvar blood supply
  - Mainly from the pudendal artery and a portion of the inferior rectus artery
  - The pudendal vein is responsible for venous return
  - Pressure of the fetal head on the pudendal vein may result in extensive back pressure and the development of varicosities in the labia majora
  - The labia majora are prone to hematoma due to their rich blood supply but also heals quickly because of the rich blood supply
- Vulvar nerve supply
  - Attained anteriorly by the ilioinguinal and genitofemoral nerves

Ways Kegel exercises benefit the perineum

- Strengthen, stretch, and relax perineal muscle
- Improve perineal tone to make the muscle more supple for birth
- Help prevent perineal tears during birth

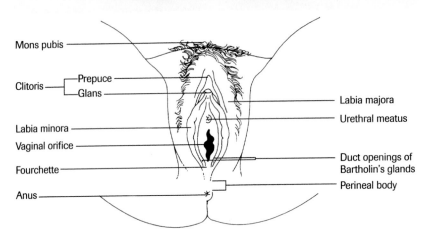

Female external genitalia

Mons pubis

Clitoris — Prepuce / Glans

Labia minora

Vaginal orifice

Fourchette

Anus

Labia majora

Urethral meatus

Duct openings of Bartholin's glands

Perineal body

Quick guide to internal female genitalia

- **Cervix** – lowest portion of the uterus
- **Fallopian tubes** – long channels that transport the ovum from the ovary to the uterus
- **Fundus** – portion of the uterus between the points of attachment of the fallopian tubes
- **Ovary** – almond-shaped glandular structure on either side of the uterus that produces, matures, and discharges ova
- **Uterus** – hollow, pear-shaped muscular organ in the lower pelvis that provides a place for fertilized ovum to implant and houses growing fetus
- **Vagina** – vascularized musculomembranous tube that extends from the external genitals to the uterus and is the organ of intercourse

– The pudendal nerve supplies the posterior portion of the vulva and vagina, making the area sensitive to touch, pain, pressure, and temperature
– Normal stretching of the perineum during childbirth results in a temporary loss of sensation to the area
– Local anesthesia for childbirth may be administered (pudendal block)

(See also *Female external genitalia.*)

● Internal genitalia

- Uterus
  - A hollow, pear-shaped muscular organ
  - Located in the lower pelvis posterior to the bladder and anterior to the rectum
  - Receives support from broad, round, uterosacral ligaments
  - During childhood it's the size of an olive (whereas the cervix is the largest portion of the organ), its proportions being the opposite of what they are later on
  - At age 8 it begins to increase in size, with maximum increase at age 17 (may explain why babies born to adolescents younger than age 17 typically have low birth weights)
  - Never returns to its prepregnancy size
  - Serves various functions
    - To receive the ovum from the fallopian tube
    - To provide a place for the ovum to implant
    - To offer nourishment and protection to the growing fetus
    - To expel the fetus from the mother's body when mature

– Consists of the body, or corpus; the fundus; the isthmus; and the cervix

- Body of the uterus
  - Uppermost portion of the uterus
  - Forms the bulk of the uterus
  - Its lining is continuous with that of the fallopian tubes
  - Expands to contain the growing fetus
- Fundus
  - Located between the points of attachment of the fallopian tubes
  - Can be palpated abdominally to determine the amount of uterine growth
- Isthmus
  - Short segment between the body of the uterus and the cervix
  - In nonpregnant women, is about 1 to 2 mm in length
  - Cut during a cesarean birth
- Cervix
  - Lowest portion of the uterus
  - Is about one-third the total size of the uterus
  - 2 to 5 cm long
  - Half lies above the vagina and half extends into the vagina
    ·· The cavity is the cervical canal
    ·· The junction of the canal at the isthmus is the internal cervical os
    ·· The distal opening into the vagina is the external cervical os

– Uterine layers

- Endometrium
  - Inner mucous membrane layer of the uterus — basal portion (closest to the uterine wall) is unaffected by hormones; inner, or glandular, portion is influenced by estrogen and progesterone
    ·· The inner portion grows and is capable of supporting pregnancy
    ·· If pregnancy doesn't occur, it's shed during menstruation
  - The endocervix continues from the endometrium and is also influenced by hormones
    ·· Secretes an alkaline mucus, which provides a lubricating surface for spermatozoa to pass through the cervix and decreases the acidic pH of the upper vagina, aiding in sperm survival
    ·· Is closed with a mucus plug during pregnancy to seal out ascending infections

Functions of the uterus

- Receives the ovum from the fallopian tube
- Provides a place for the ovum to implant
- Provides nourishment and protection for the growing fetus
- Expels the fetus from the mother's body when mature

Four parts of the uterus

- Body, or corpus — uppermost portion; bulk of uterus; expands to accommodate fetus
- Fundus — between points of attachment of the fallopian tubes
- Isthmus — short segment between corpus and cervix
- Cervix — lowest part; one-third of total size

Female internal genitalia and related structures

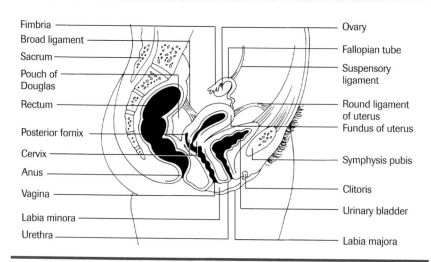

Fimbria — Broad ligament — Sacrum — Pouch of Douglas — Rectum — Posterior fornix — Cervix — Anus — Vagina — Labia minora — Urethra — Ovary — Fallopian tube — Suspensory ligament — Round ligament of uterus — Fundus of uterus — Symphysis pubis — Clitoris — Urinary bladder — Labia majora

Uterine layers

- Endometrium – inner mucous membrane layer of the uterus that's shed during menstruation
- Myometrium – three interwoven layers of smooth muscle that give the uterus its strength
- Perimetrium – outer layer that covers the body of the uterus and part of the cervix

Uterine nerve and blood supply

- Sensory and motor nerves present
- Location of sensory nerve registration allows epidural analgesia to be used during labor without stopping contractions
- Uterus receives blood from uterine arteries and ovarian arteries
- Arteries unwind and stretch to maintain adequate blood supply as uterus grows

- Myometrium
  - Consists of three interwoven layers of smooth muscle, arranged in longitudinal, transverse, and oblique directions
  - Gives extreme strength to the uterus
  - Constricts the tubal junctions and prevents regurgitation of the menstrual flow into the fallopian tubes
  - Holds the internal cervical os closed during pregnancy to prevent a preterm birth
- Perimetrium
  - Outer serosal layer
  - Covers the body of the uterus and part of the cervix

(See also *Female internal genitalia and related structures.*)

– Uterine nerve supply
  - Both afferent (sensory) and efferent (motor) nerves supply the uterus
  - Sensory innervation from the uterus registers lower in the spinal column than does motor control, which is why epidural solution can be injected near the spinal column to stop the pain of uterine contractions but not stop motor control and contractions

– Uterine blood supply
  - The ascending abdominal aorta divides into the two iliac arteries, which further divide into the hypogastric arteries, which divide into the uterine arteries
  - The uterus also receives blood from the ovarian arteries, so it always has an abundant supply of blood

... ...d supply

...y of blood from various structures.

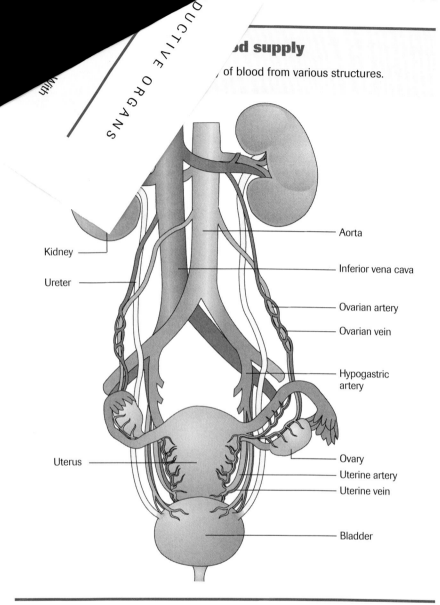

Kidney

Ureter

Uterus

Aorta

Inferior vena cava

Ovarian artery

Ovarian vein

Hypogastric artery

Ovary

Uterine artery

Uterine vein

Bladder

- These arteries are tortuous and lay against the sides of the uterine body in a nonpregnant woman
- As the uterus enlarges, the arteries unwind and can stretch to maintain an adequate blood supply as the uterus grows

(See also *Uterine blood supply*.)

– Uterine support
  • Because the uterus isn't in a fixed position, it can enlarge without discomfort during pregnancy
  • If supports become overstretched, they may not hold the bladder afterward and may herniate into the anterior vagina, resulting in a cystocele

Cystocele and rectocele

With a cystocele, the bladder herniates into the anterior wall of the vagina.
a rectocele, the posterior wall of the vagina herniates and the rectum protrudes
into the vagina.

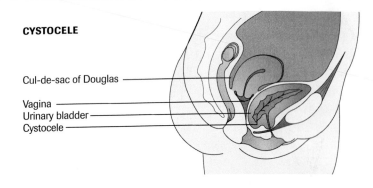

CYSTOCELE

Cul-de-sac of Douglas

Vagina
Urinary bladder
Cystocele

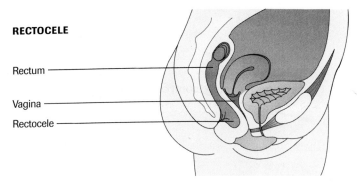

RECTOCELE

Rectum

Vagina

Rectocele

TOP 4

Ways the female body adapts to pregnancy

1. Uterus — enlarges without discomfort
2. Ovarian arteries — unwind and stretch to supply the uterus with blood
3. Pelvic cavity — prevents sudden pressure changes during delivery
4. Vagina — expands to allow the full-term neonate to pass through

- If the rectum pouches toward the vaginal wall, a rectocele may develop
(See also *Cystocele and rectocele.*)
- The broad ligaments are two folds of peritoneum that cover the front and back of the uterus and extend to the pelvic sides
- The round ligaments are two fibrous muscular cords that pass from the body of the uterus near the attachments of the fallopian tubes
  - They pass through the broad ligament into the inguinal canal and insert into the fascia of the vulva
  - They steady the uterus
– Uterine deviations
  - Deviations in the size and shape of the uterus can lead to fertility problems
    - In the fetus, the uterus first forms with a septum, which separates it longitudinally

Types of uterine deviations

When the septum that is present during fetal maturation in utero does not atrophy, the resulting uterine deviations may leave less area in which the placenta can implant. Several types of deviations are illustrated below.

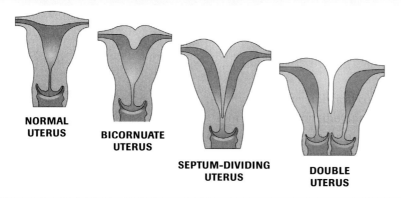

NORMAL UTERUS   **BICORNUATE UTERUS**   **SEPTUM-DIVIDING UTERUS**   **DOUBLE UTERUS**

Deviations in uterine position

- Anteversion: fundus tips forward
- Retroversion: fundus tips backward
- Anteflexion: body of uterus bends sharply forward at the junction with the cervix
- Retroflexion: body of uterus bends slightly backward

- The septum gradually deteriorates as the fetus matures so that no septum remains at birth
- In some cases, the septum never atrophies, and the uterus remains as two separate compartments
- In others, half of the septum remains
- Still others may have oddly shaped horns at the junctions of the fallopian tubes, creating a bicornuate uterus

(See also *Types of uterine deviations*.)

- Deviations in the position of the uterus may also exist
  - The body of the uterus usually tips slightly forward
  - With anteversion, the fundus is tipped forward
  - With retroversion, the fundus is tipped backward
  - With anteflexion, the body of the uterus is bent sharply forward at the junction with the cervix
  - With retroflexion, the body is bent slightly back
- Vagina
  - Is the vascularized musculomembranous tube that extends from the external genitals to the uterus; located between the bladder and the rectum
  - Functions as the organ of intercourse, channeling sperm to the cervix so the sperm can meet with the ovum in the fallopian tube
  - Expands with pregnancy to function as a birth canal
  - Acts as a uterine excretory duct for menses and other secretions
  - At the uterine end, there are recesses on all sides of the cervix
    - Anterior fornix — lies at the front of the cervix

Key facts about the vagina

- Vascularized musculomembranous tube that extends from the external genitals to the uterus
- Located between the bladder and the rectum
- Channels sperm to the cervix so they can meet with the ovum in the fallopian tube
- Expands during pregnancy to function as a birth canal
- Acts as a uterine excretory duct for menses and other secretions

Key facts about the fallopian tubes

- Two tubes, each about 12 cm long
- Consist of four layers — peritoneal, subserous, muscular, mucous
- Divided into four portions — interstitial, isthmus, ampulla, fimbria
- Transport ovum from ovary to uterus
- Serve as the site of fertilization
- Provide nourishing environment for zygote

Key facts about the ovaries

- Two almond-shaped glandular structures
- Located on either side of the uterus, below and behind the fallopian tubes
- Produce, mature, and discharge ova
- Ovulation is necessary for maturation of ova and maintenance of secondary sex characteristics

- Posterior fornix — lies behind the cervix; serves as a pool for semen after intercourse to allow a large number of sperm to stay close to the cervix; encourages sperm migration into the cervix
  - Lateral fornices — located at the sides
- Its wall is lined with folds and rugae, which make the vagina very elastic and able to expand during pregnancy to allow a full-term neonate to pass through without tearing
- Blood is supplied by the vaginal artery, which is a branch of the internal iliac artery
- Fallopian tubes
  - Each is about 12 cm long
  - Consist of four layers — peritoneal, subserous, muscular, and mucous
    - Muscular layer produces peristaltic motions that conduct the ova the length of the tube;
    - Ciliated and mucous lining act as lubricant to aid in ova travel and may also act as nourishment for the fertilized egg because the mucus contains protein, water, and salt
  - Divided into four portions — interstitial, isthmus, ampulla, and fimbria
  - Transport the ovum from the ovary to the uterus
  - Serve as the site of fertilization
  - Provide a nourishing environment for zygotes
  - Open at the distal end
    - Provides a direct pathway to the internal organs
    - Makes conception possible but also creates an area where infections of the peritoneum (peritonitis) can occur
    - Creates the need for sterile vaginal examinations during labor and birth and sterile pelvic examinations on nonpregnant women
- Ovaries
  - Two almond-shaped glandular structures on either side of the uterus, below and behind the fallopian tubes
  - Their function is to produce, mature, and discharge ova
    - Ova produce estrogen and progesterone and initiate and regulate the menstrual cycles
      - Estrogen further prevents osteoporosis
      - Because cholesterol is incorporated in estrogen, the production of estrogen is thought to keep cholesterol levels reduced
    - Ovulation is necessary for maturation of ova and maintenance of secondary sex characteristics

Anatomy of the breast

The structure and shape of the breast change with pregnancy and lactation.

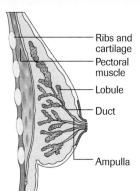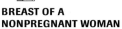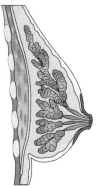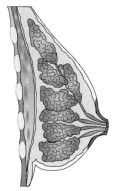

Ribs and cartilage
Pectoral muscle
Lobule
Duct
Ampulla

BREAST OF A NONPREGNANT WOMAN

BREAST OF A PREGNANT WOMAN

BREAST DURING LACTATION

RELATED STRUCTURES

- **Female accessory glands: Breasts**
  - Consist of glandular, fibrous, and adipose tissue
  - Grow and develop from stimulation of secretions from the hypothalamus, anterior pituitary, and ovaries
  - Provide nourishment to the infant and transfer maternal antibodies during breast-feeding
  - Enhance sexual pleasure

(See also *Anatomy of the breast.*)

- **Female pelvis**
  - Supports and protects the reproductive organs
  - Bony ring formed by four united bones
    - Two innominate (flaring hip) bones form the anterior and lateral aspect, each divided into three parts—the ilium, the ischium, and the pubis
      - Ilium—forms the upper and lateral portion; the flaring superior border forms the prominence of the hip
      - Ischium—forms the inferior portion
        - The ischial tuberosities are two projections at the lowest portion
          - ·· Point of fusion between the ischium and the symphysis pubis
          - ·· Important markers when determining lower pelvic width
        - The ischial spines are small projections that mark the midpoint of the pelvis

Key facts about the breasts

- Consist of glandular, fibrous, and adipose tissue
- Grow and develop from stimulation of secretions from the hypothalamus, anterior pituitary, and ovaries
- Provide nourishment to infant and transfer maternal antibodies during breast-feeding
- Enhance sexual pleasure

True and false pelvis

The area below the linea terminalis is the true pelvis; the area above it, the false pelvis. The arrow designates the stovepipe curve that the fetus must travel before it's delivered.

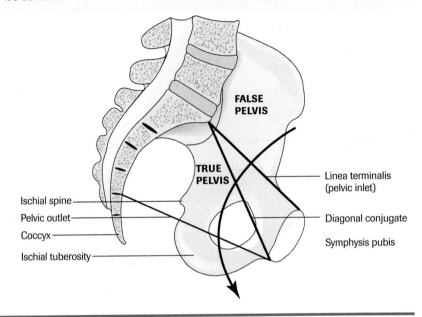

Key facts about the pelvis

- Bony ring formed by four united bones
- Supports and protects the reproductive organs
- Ilium — forms the upper and lateral portion
- Ischium — forms the inferior portion
- Pubis — forms the anterior portion
- The sacrum and coccyx (just below the sacrum) form the posterior aspect
- Further divided into false pelvis and true pelvis (used for obstetric purposes)
- Inlet is the entrance to the true pelvis
- Pelvic cavity is the space between the inlet and the outlet; it's curved so that the passage of the fetus through the cavity is slowed and controlled
- Outlet is the inferior portion of the pelvis; to be delivered vaginally, a fetus must be able to pass through the ring of the pelvic bone and the opening

- Pubis — forms the anterior portion of the innominate bone, the symphysis pubis being the junction of the innominate bones at the front of the pelvis
  – The sacrum and coccyx form the posterior aspect
    - The sacrum forms the upper posterior portion of the pelvic ring
      - Sacral prominence is a marked anterior projection
      - Must be identified when securing pelvic measurements
    - The coccyx is just below the sacrum
      - Made up of five very small bones fused together
      - Can be pressed backward at the sacrococcygeal joint, allowing more room for the fetal head as it passes through the bony pelvic ring at birth
- The pelvis is further divided into the false pelvis and the true pelvis (see *True and false pelvis*)
  – This determination is used only for obstetric purposes
  – The pelves are separated by a false line — the linea terminalis — that is drawn from the sacral prominence at the back to the superior aspect of the symphysis pubis at the front
  – The false pelvis lies above the line

The female pelvis

The female pelvis protects and supports the reproductive and other pelvic organs.

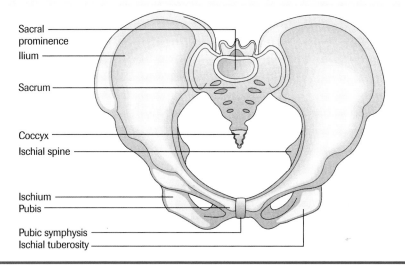

Sacral prominence
Ilium
Sacrum
Coccyx
Ischial spine
Ischium
Pubis
Pubic symphysis
Ischial tuberosity

- Supports the uterus during the late months of pregnancy
- Directs the fetus into the true pelvis for birth
  - The true pelvis lies below the line
- The inlet, the pelvic cavity, and the outlet
  - Inlet—entrance to the true pelvis
    - The upper ring of the bone through which the fetus must pass to be born vaginally
    - The passage appears heart-shaped if you look down the inlet
  - Pelvic cavity—space between the inlet and the outlet
    - Curved so that the passage of the fetus through the cavity is slowed and controlled, to prevent and reduce sudden pressure changes on the fetal head, which could rupture cerebral arteries
    - The snugness of the cavity compresses the fetal chest, helping to push fluid and mucus from the lungs and preparing the lungs for better aeration at birth
  - Outlet—inferior portion of the pelvis
- For a fetus to be delivered vaginally, it must be able to pass through the ring of the pelvic bone and the opening must be sufficient; otherwise the fetus may have to be delivered via cesarean birth

(See also *The female pelvis*.)

Key facts about the reproductive cycle and menstruation

- Purpose is to mature ovum and renew the uterine tissue bed
- Menarche usually occurs between ages 9 and 17
- Average length of menstrual cycle is 28 days
- Average length of menses is 2 to 7 days
- Menses are initiated by release of LHRH
- Under the influence of LHRH, the anterior lobe of the pituitary produces FSH and LH, which further influence the menstrual cycle

Phases of the menstrual cycle

- Menstrual phase (days 1 to 5) —estrogen and progesterone levels decrease, FSH levels rise, estrogen is secreted, and menstrual flow begins
- Proliferative phase (days 6 to 13) — estrogen production increases, leading to proliferation of endometrium and myometrium in preparation for implantation of a fertilized ovum, and FSH production decreases before ovulation
- Secretory phase (days 14 to 25) —the corpus luteum forms, estrogen and progesterone production increase, and the endometrium is prepared for implantation
- Ischemic phase (days 26 to 28) —the corpus luteum degenerates and estrogen and progesterone levels decline if conception doesn't occur

FEMALE REPRODUCTIVE CYCLE

● **Purpose**
- To bring an ovum to maturity and renew the uterine tissue bed that will be responsive to its growth once it's fertilized

● **Menarche (first menstruation)**
- May occur as early as age 9 or as late as age 17

● **The menstrual cycle**
- Varies from woman to woman
  - Average length of the cycle is 28 days, from the beginning of one menstrual flow to the beginning of the next
  - Average length of the menses is 2 to 7 days
- Initiated by the release of luteinizing hormone–releasing hormone (LHRH), also known as gonadotropin-releasing hormone (GnRH), from the hypothalamus
  - Under the influence of LHRH, the anterior lobe of the pituitary produces two hormones that act on the ovaries to further influence the menstrual cycle
    · Follicle-stimulating hormone (FSH)
    · Luteinizing hormone (LH)
- The menstrual cycle has various phases
  - Menstrual phase (days 1 through 5)
    · Estrogen and progesterone levels decrease
    · FSH levels rise, and steady levels of LH influence the ovary to secrete estrogen
    · Menstrual flow begins
  - Proliferative (follicular) phase (days 6 through 13)
    · Estrogen production increases, leading to proliferation of endometrium and myometrium in preparation for possible implantation of a fertilized ovum
    · Follicle secretes estradiol
    · FSH stimulates graafian follicle
    · FSH production decreases before ovulation (around day 14)
  - Secretory (luteal) phase (days 14 through 25)
    · The corpus luteum forms under the influence of LH
    · Estrogen and progesterone production increase
    · The endometrium is prepared for implantation of fertilized ovum
  - Ischemic phase (days 26 through 28)
    · The corpus luteum degenerates if conception doesn't occur
    · Estrogen and progesterone levels decline if conception doesn't occur

MALE REPRODUCTIVE SYSTEM

● **External genitalia**
- Penis
  - Has three layers of erectile tissue — two corpora cavernosa and one corpus spongiosum
  - Consists of the body (shaft) and glans
    - Glans is at the distal end of the penis
    - A retractable casing of skin, or prepuce, protects the glans at birth
    - If an infant undergoes a circumcision, the prepuce is removed shortly after birth
  - Deposits spermatozoa in the female reproductive tract
  - Contains sensory nerve endings that provide sexual pleasure
  - Serves as an outlet for the urinary tract
  - Penile artery supplies blood to the penis
- Scrotum
  - Is a pouch-like structure made up of skin, fascial connective tissue, and smooth-muscle fibers
  - Contains two lateral compartments that house the testes, epididymis, and the lower portion of the spermatic cord
  - Protects the testes and spermatozoa from high body temperature
- Testes
  - Are two oval-shaped glandular organs inside the scrotum
  - Seminiferous tubules produce spermatozoa
  - Leydig's cells produce testosterone, the primary male sex hormone, and other androgens
  - Hypothalamus releases GnRH, which then influences the anterior pituitary to release FSH and LH
  - FSH then is responsible for releasing androgen-producing hormone (APH) and LH for releasing testosterone
  - Sperm can't survive at body temperature; the testes are suspended outside the body where the temperature is approximately 1° F lower than body temperature

● **Internal genitalia**
- Epididymis
  - Although tightly curled, the length totals about 6 m
  - Responsible for conducting sperm from the testis to the vas deferens or storing it
    - Sperm are immobile as they pass through or are stored here
    - Takes at least 12 to 20 days for the sperm to travel the length of the epididymis and a total of 64 days for them to reach maturity

---

Quick guide to male genitalia

- **Bulbourethral glands** — secrete a thick alkaline fluid that neutralizes acidic secretions in the female reproductive tract, thus prolonging spermatozoa survival
- **Epididymis** — stores sperm or conducts them from the testis to the vas deferens
- **Penis** — deposits spermatozoa in female reproductive tract and serves as outlet for urinary tract
- **Prostate gland** — secretes an alkaline fluid that enhances spermatozoa motility and lubricates the urethra during sexual activity
- **Scrotum** — protects testes and spermatozoa from high body temperature
- **Seminal vesicles** — secrete a viscous portion of the semen that aids spermatozoa motility and metabolism
- **Testes** — oval-shaped glandular organs inside scrotum that produce testosterone and other androgens
- **Urethra** — excretory duct for urine and semen
- **Vas deferens** — carries sperm from the epididymis through the inguinal canal into the abdominal cavity where it ends at the seminal vesicles

Male reproductive system and related structures

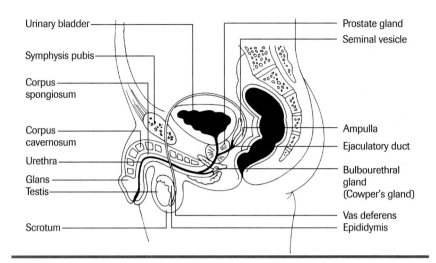

TOP 4

Facts to know about sperm

1. The penis deposits it in the female reproductive tract.
2. The scrotum protects it from high body temperature.
3. The testes keep it 1° F lower than body temperature.
4. The seminal vesicles and the prostate gland secrete alkaline fluid, making it more motile.

- Long length of time for maturity makes response to treatment for aspermia or oligospermia not evident for at least 2 months
- Vas deferens
  - Also called the *ductus deferens*
  - Connects the epididymal lumen and the prostatic urethra
  - Carries sperm from the epididymis through the inguinal canal into the abdominal cavity where it ends at the seminal vesicles into the ejaculatory ducts
  - Sperm mature as they pass through the vas deferens and are immobile at this point
  - Blood vessels and the vas deferens together are referred to as the spermatic cord
- Ejaculatory ducts
  - Located between the seminal vesicles and the urethra
- Urethra
  - Extends from the bladder through the penis to the external urethral opening
  - Serves as the excretory duct for urine and semen
  - Lined with mucous membrane
- Seminal vesicles
  - Are two pouch-like structures between the bladder and the rectum
  - Empty into the urethra by way of the ejaculatory ducts
  - Secrete a viscous portion of the semen that aids in spermatozoa motility and metabolism because the fluid is alkaline and sperm are more motile in an alkaline fluid

- Prostate gland
  - Consists of glandular and muscular tissue
  - Is located just below the bladder
  - Urethra passes through it
  - Is considered homologous to Skene's glands in females
  - Secretes an alkaline fluid that enhances spermatozoa motility and lubricates the urethra during sexual activity
- Bulbourethral glands (Cowper's glands)
  - Are two pea-sized glands that lie beside the prostate and empty into the urethra
  - Secrete a thick alkaline fluid that neutralizes acidic secretions in the female reproductive tract, thus prolonging spermatozoa survival

(See also *Male reproductive system and related structures.*)

NCLEX CHECKS

It's never too soon to begin your NCLEX preparation. Now that you've reviewed this chapter, carefully read each of the following questions and choose the best answer. Then compare your responses to the correct answers.

1. Which structure is the tissue that extends from the clitoris to the posterior fourchette?

- ☐ **A.** Mons pubis
- ☑ **B.** Vaginal vestibule
- ☐ **C.** Clitoris
- ☐ **D.** Labia majora

2. Which three ligaments provide the uterus with support?

- ☐ **A.** Ovarian, broad, and uterosacral ligaments
- ☑ **B.** Broad, round, and uterosacral ligaments
- ☐ **C.** Ovarian, round, and uterosacral ligaments
- ☐ **D.** Broad, ovarian, and round ligaments

3. Which of the following phases are part of the female reproductive cycle?

- ☑ **A.** Menstrual
- ☑ **B.** Proliferative
- ☐ **C.** Premenstrual
- ☑ **D.** Secretory
- ☐ **E.** Premenopausal
- ☑ **F.** Ischemic   *Pg 28*

TOP 8

Items to study for your next test on the reproductive organs

1. The five key external structures of the female genitalia and their functions
2. The four key internal structures of the female genitalia and their functions
3. The four types of uterine deviations with regard to position
4. The role of the female accessory glands in reproduction
5. The components of the female pelvis and their functions
6. The four phases of the female reproductive cycle
7. The three key external structures of the male genitalia and their functions
8. The seven key internal structures of the male genitalia and their functions

4. What are the three layers of the corpus, or body, of the uterus?
- ☐ **A.** Ectoderm, myometrium, mesoderm
- ☐ **B.** Perimetrium, ectoderm, mesoderm
- ☐ **C.** Ectoderm, endoderm, mesoderm
- ☒ **D.** Perimetrium, the myometrium, endometrium

5. Which structure connects the epididymal lumen and the prostatic urethra in the male?
- ☐ **A.** Ejaculatory duct
- ☐ **B.** Cowper's gland
- ☒ **C.** Vas deferens
- ☐ **D.** Skene's gland

ANSWERS AND RATIONALES

1. CORRECT ANSWER: B
The vaginal vestibule is the tissue extending from the clitoris to the posterior fourchette. The mons pubis provides an adipose cushion over the anterior symphysis pubis. The clitoris is located in the anterior portion of the vulva, just above the urethral opening. Labia majora consist of two folds of tissue that converge at the mons pubis and extend down to the posterior commissure.

2. CORRECT ANSWER: B
The uterus receives support from broad, round, and uterosacral ligaments. The ovarian ligament supports the ovary.

3. CORRECT ANSWERS: A, B, D, AND F
The female reproductive cycle has four phases: the menstrual, proliferative, secretory, and ischemic phases. The premenstrual and premenopausal phases aren't part of the female reproductive cycle.

4. CORRECT ANSWER: D
The perimetrium, the myometrium, and the endometrium are the three layers of the corpus, or body, of the uterus. The ectoderm, endoderm, and mesoderm are embryonic germ layers.

5. CORRECT ANSWER: C
The vas deferens connects the epididymal lumen and the prostatic urethra. The ejaculatory ducts are located between the seminal vesicles and the urethra. Cowper's glands are two pea-sized glands opening into the posterior portion of the urethra. Skene's glands are located in the female reproductive tract.

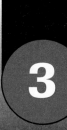

3

Fetal growth and development

LEARNING OBJECTIVES

After studying this chapter, you should be able to:

- Identify the steps involved with gametogenesis.
- Describe the structure and function of the placenta.
- Identify the composition and functions of amniotic fluid and the umbilical cord.
- List the stages of embryonic and fetal development.
- Describe fetal-placental circulation.

CHAPTER OVERVIEW

Intrauterine development begins with gametogenesis and progresses to the term fetus. Fetal growth and development occur over 40 weeks, with the development of specialized structures and events along the way. Certain structures—including fetal membranes, umbilical cord, placenta, and amniotic fluid—are unique to the fetus. Additional specialized structures develop that differentiate fetal circulation from extrauterine circulation.

TOP 6

Things to know about chromosomes

1. They're found in cell nuclei.
2. They reveal genetic makeup.
3. They're made up of DNA.
4. They exist in pairs, except in the germ cells.
5. Normal human cells contain 23 pairs.
6. The first 22 are homologous; the 23rd determines sex.

GENETIC COMPONENTS

● **Chromosomes**
- Structures within the cell nuclei that contain an individual's genetic makeup
- Made up of deoxyribonucleic acid (DNA) and protein, appearing as a network of chromatin granules in the nondividing cell
- Exist in pairs, except in the germ cells (gametes)
    - Here, one chromosome comes from the male germ cell
    - The other, from the female germ cell
- Normal human cells contain 23 pairs
    - 22 pairs are homologous chromosomes
        · Identical in shape, size, and gene location
        · Each chromosome contains genetic information that controls the same characteristics or functions
    - The 23rd pair contains the sex chromosomes, X and Y
        · One chromosome comes from the female germ cell (ovum) and the other from the male germ cell (spermatozoon)
        · The combination of these chromosomes determines sex
          - XX produces a genetic female
          - XY produces a genetic male
        · In the female, the genetic activity of both X chromosomes is essential only during the first few weeks after conception
          - Later development requires just one functional X chromosome
          - The other chromosome is inactive and appears as a dense chromatin mass called a *Barr body* attached to the nuclear membrane in the cells of the normal female

● **Genes**
- Individual carriers of heredity information
- Each is arranged in a linear fashion on a double-stranded chain of DNA
- Occur in pairs on homologous chromosomes
- The location of a specific gene on a chromosome is called the *gene locus*
    - Alleles are alternate forms of a gene that can occupy a gene locus
    - Only one allele can occupy a specific locus
    - When alleles are identical at the corresponding loci, the person is homozygous for the trait
    - When alleles differ at corresponding loci, the person is heterozygous for the trait
- Not all genes have an equal probability of expression

– When different genes occur at corresponding loci on homologous chromosomes, these genes must compete for expression
  · The gene expressed is dominant
  · The gene not expressed is recessive
– Dominant genes can be expressed and transmitted to offspring, even if only one parent possesses the gene
– When two recessive genes occur at corresponding loci, the recessive trait is expressed
– Recessive genes are expressed only when both parents transmit them to the offspring
– In some cases — for example the genes that direct specific types of hemoglobin synthesis in red blood cells — genes are codominant allowing expression of both alleles
• Some are sex-linked
  – They're carried on the sex chromosome
  – Most appear on the X chromosome and are recessive
  – In the male, sex-linked genes act like dominant genes because no second X chromosome exists

Genetic expression

• A person with two like genes for a trait is homozygous for that trait
  – If the trait is dominant, the person is homozygous dominant
  – If the trait is recessive, the person is homozygous recessive
• A person with two different genes for a trait is heterozygous for that trait; therefore, the dominant gene would be expressed
• Genotype refers to a person's genetic makeup, which is determined at fertilization
• Phenotype refers to a person's outward appearance based on the expression of the person's genes
  – The offspring of parents who are both homozygous dominant or both homozygous recessive would demonstrate a phenotype and genotype similar to that of the parents
  – The offspring of a parent who is homozygous dominant for a trait and a parent who is homozygous recessive for a trait would demonstrate a phenotype for the dominant trait; the genotype would be heterozygous (a gene for the dominant trait and a gene for the recessive trait)
  – The offspring of a parent who is homozygous dominant and a parent who is heterozygous would exhibit a phenotype for the dominant trait; the child would have a 50% chance of being homozygous dominant or 50% chance of being heterozygous
  – The offspring of parents who are both heterozygous for a trait would exhibit a phenotype for the dominant trait 3 out of 4 times (75%) and a phenotype for the recessive trait 1 out of 4 times

(25%); the child would have a 25% chance of being homozygous recessive, a 50% chance of being heterozygous, and a 25 % chance of being homozygous dominant
- Karyotype refers to a visual presentation (photograph) of the person's actual chromosomal pattern

CELL REPRODUCTION

● Mitosis
- Refers to the equal division of nuclear material followed by division of the cell body
  - Division of the nuclear material is called *karyokinesis*
  - Division of the cell body is called *cytokinesis*
- All cells of the body (except the germ cells, or gametes) undergo mitosis
- Occurs in five phases
  - Interphase—inactive phase when many normal cellular functions occur
  - Prophase—active phase when chromatin shorten and thicken, centrioles separate, and the nuclear membrane begins to break down
  - Metaphase—active phase when the nuclear membrane completely dissolves and chromosomes line up in the center of the cell
  - Anaphase—active phase when chromatids move to opposite poles of the cell
  - Telophase—active phase that results in the formation of two identical daughter cells
- Results in the two daughter cells, each of which contains 23 pairs of chromosomes, or 46 individual chromosomes (the diploid number)

(See also *Five phases of mitosis.*)

● Meiosis
- Refers to the division of the germ cells, or gametes
  - *Gametogenesis* is the production of specialized sex cells, called *gametes*
  - As gametes mature, the number of chromosomes they contain is halved (through meiosis) from 46 to 23
- Intermixes genetic material between homologous chromosomes, producing four daughter cells
- Has two divisions separated by a resting phase
  - The first division has six phases
    · It begins with a parent cell
    · It ends with two daughter cells

Key facts about mitosis

- Equal division of nuclear material (karyokinesis) followed by division of the cell body (cytokinesis)
- Most body cells undergo mitosis
- Occurs in five phases
- Results in two daughter cells that each contains 23 pairs of chromosomes, or 46 individual chromosomes

Key facts about meiosis

- Division of the germ cells, or gametes (sex cells)
- As gametes mature, the number of chromosomes they contain is halved (through meiosis) from 46 to 23
- Intermixes genetic material between homologous chromosomes, producing four daughter cells
- Has two divisions separated by a resting phase
- The first division has six phases
- The second division, which resembles mitosis, has four phases

Five phases of mitosis

Through the process of mitosis, the nuclear content of all body cells (except gametes) reproduces and divides. The result is the formation of two new daughter cells, each containing the diploid (46) number of chromosomes.

INTERPHASE

During *interphase*, the nucleus and nuclear membrane are well defined, and the nucleolus is visible. As chromosomes replicate, each forms a double strand that remains attached at the center by a centromere.

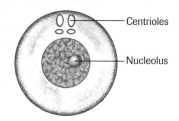

Centrioles

Nucleolus

PROPHASE

In *prophase*, the nucleolus disappears and the chromosomes become distinct. *Chromatids*, halves of each duplicated chromosome, remain attached by the centromere. Centrioles move to opposite sides of the cell and radiate spindle fibers.

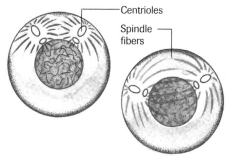

Centrioles

Spindle fibers

METAPHASE

Metaphase occurs when chromosomes line up randomly in the center of the cell between the spindles, along the *metaphase plate*. The centromere of each chromosome then replicates.

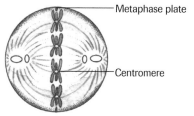

Metaphase plate

Centromere

ANAPHASE

Anaphase is characterized by centromeres moving apart, pulling the separate chromatids (now called *chromosomes*) to opposite ends of the cell. The number of chromosomes at each end of the cell equals the original number.

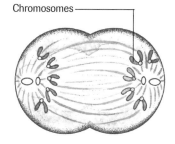

Chromosomes

TELOPHASE

During telophase, the final stage of mitosis, a nuclear membrane forms around each end of the cell and spindle fibers disappear. The cytoplasm compresses and divides the cell in half. Each new cell contains the diploid (46) number of chromosomes.

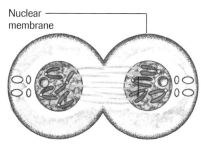

Nuclear membrane

Phases of mitosis

- Interphase – inactive phase when normal cellular functions occur
- Prophase – active phase when chromatin shorten and thicken, centrioles separate, and nuclear membrane begins to break down
- Metaphase – active phase when the nuclear membrane dissolves and chromosomes line up in the center of the cell
- Anaphase – active phase when chromatids move to opposite poles of the cell
- Telophase – active phase that results in the formation of two identical daughter cells

Meiosis: Step-by-step

Meiosis has two divisions separated by a resting phase. By the end of the first division, there are two daughter cells that each contain the haploid (23) number of chromosomes. When the second division ends, each of the two daughter cells from the first division divides, resulting in four daughter cells, each containing the haploid number of chromosomes.

FIRST DIVISION

First division has six phases. Here is what happens during each one.

Interphase
1. Chromosomes replicate, forming a double strand attached at the center by a centromere.
2. Chromosomes appear as an indistinguishable matrix within the nucleus.
3. Centrioles appear outside the nucleus.

Prophase I
1. Nucleolus and nuclear membrane disappear.
2. Chromosomes are distinct, with chromatids attached by the centromere.
3. Homologous chromosomes move close together and intertwine; exchange of genetic information (genetic recombination) may occur.
4. Centrioles separate and spindle fibers appear.

Metaphase I
1. Pairs of synaptic chromosomes line up randomly along the metaphase plate.
2. Spindle fibers attach to each chromosome pair.

Anaphase I
1. Synaptic pairs separate.
2. Spindle fibers pull homologous, double-stranded chromosomes to opposite ends of the cell.
3. Chromatids remain attached.

Telophase I
1. Nuclear membrane forms.
2. Spindle fibers and chromosomes disappear.
3. Cytoplasm compresses and divides the cell in half.
4. Each new cell contains the haploid (23) number of chromosomes.

Interkinesis
1. Nucleus and nuclear membrane are well defined.
2. Nucleolus is prominent, and each chromosome has two chromatids that don't replicate.

SECOND DIVISION

Second division closely resembles mitosis and is characterized by these four phases.

Prophase II
1. Nuclear membrane disappears.
2. Spindle fibers form.
3. Double-stranded chromosomes appear as thin threads.

Metaphase II
1. Chromosomes line up along the metaphase plate.
2. Centromeres replicate.

Anaphase II
1. Chromatids separate (now a single-stranded chromosome).
2. Chromosomes move away from each other to the opposite ends of the cell.

Telophase II
1. Nuclear membrane forms.
2. Chromosomes and spindle fibers disappear.
3. Cytoplasm compresses, dividing the cell in half.
4. Four daughter cells are created, each of which contains the haploid (23) number of chromosomes.

- Each daughter cell contains the haploid number of chromosomes
  - The second division, which resembles mitosis, has four phases
    - It begins with the two daughter cells
    - It ends with four new haploid cells
    - In each cell, the two chromatids of each chromosome separate to form new daughter cells
    - Each cell entering the second division has only 23 chromosomes; therefore each daughter cell formed has only 23 chromosomes

(See also *Meiosis: Step-by-step.*)

GAMETOGENESIS

● Spermatogenesis

- When the male sex hormones are stimulated, mature sperm cells are formed continuously within the seminiferous tubules
- Begins when a male reaches puberty and normally continues throughout life
- The process involves several steps
  - Primary germinal epithelial cells, spermatogonia, grow and develop into primary spermatocytes
    - Spermatogonia and spermatocytes contain 46 chromosomes
    - Of the 46 chromosomes, 44 are autosomes and 2 are sex chromosomes (X and Y)
  - Primary spermatocytes divide to form secondary spermatocytes
    - No new chromosomes are formed
    - Each secondary spermatocyte contains one-half the number of autosomes (22)
    - One secondary spermatocyte contains an X chromosome and the other a Y chromosome
  - Each secondary spermatocyte divides again to form spermatids
  - Spermatids undergo a series of structural changes that transform them into mature spermatozoa (sperm)
    - Each spermatozoa is made up of a head, neck, body, and tail
    - The head contains the nucleus
    - The tail contains a large amount of adenosine triphosphate, which provides energy for sperm motility
  - Newly mature sperm pass from the seminiferous tubules through the vasa recta into the epididymis where they mature
    - Only a few sperm can be stored in the epididymis
    - Most sperm move into the vas deferens, where they're stored until sexual stimulation triggers emission

Key facts about spermatogenesis

- When male sex hormones are stimulated, mature sperm cells are formed continuously within the seminiferous tubules
- Begins at puberty and normally continues throughout life
- It takes about 75 days for a mature sperm to develop from a germinal cell
- The process:
- Spermatogonia grow and develop into primary spermatocytes (contain 46 chromosomes, 44 of which are autosomes and 2 of which are sex chromosomes [X and Y])
- Primary spermatocytes divide to form secondary spermatocytes (each with one-half the number of autosomes [22]; one with an X chromosome and one with a Y)
- Each secondary spermatocyte divides again to form spermatids
- Spermatids undergo structural changes that transform them into mature spermatozoa (made up of a head, neck, body, and tail)
- Newly mature sperm pass from the seminiferous tubules into the epididymis
- Most sperm then move into the vas deferens, where they're stored until sexual stimulation triggers emission

Steps to oocyte maturation

1. They develop in the fetus.
2. They begin meiosis in the fetus but then stop.
3. Until puberty, they're immature and inactive.
4. Hormones stimulate them.
5. They begin to grow again

Key facts about fertilization

- Fusion of a sperm and an ovum
- Fertilized egg is called a *zygote*
- The diploid number of chromosomes (44 autosomes and 2 sex chromosomes) is restored when the zygote is formed
- Male zygote forms with fertilization by a sperm carrying a Y chromosome
- Female zygote forms with fertilization by a sperm carrying an X chromosome
- Cellular multiplication occurs when the zygote undergoes mitosis
- The morula forms and enters the uterus
- After the morula enters the uterus, a cavity forms within the dividing cells, thus changing the morula into a blastocyst
- Blastocyst cells differentiate into trophoblasts or the inner cell mass, a discrete cell cluster enclosed within the trophoblast that later forms the embryo

- It takes about 75 days for a mature sperm to develop from a germinal cell

● **Oogenesis**
- At birth, an ovary contains about 2 million immature primary oocytes
  - These primary oocytes develop from oogonia in the fetus
  - Oogonia undergo mitosis in the fetal ovaries before birth forming primary oocytes, each with 46 chromosomes
  - Primary follicles are formed when a single layer of cells surround the oocytes
  - The oocytes begin meiosis during fetal development but stop dividing, remaining inactive until puberty
- Under stimulation of follicle-stimulating hormone (FSH) and luteinizing hormone (LH) at puberty, primary follicles become activated and begin to grow
  - The cellular layer around the follicle increases
  - The zona pellucida forms on the surface of the oocyte
  - Fluid accumulates in the cellular layer forming a central-filled cavity, leading to the formation of the graafian follicle (mature follicle)
- At ovulation, the oocyte is released and travels to the fallopian tube where it is propelled via cilia and peristaltic contractions
  - Normally, only one follicle matures and is ovulated
  - The oocyte completes the first meiotic division resulting in the formation of a secondary oocyte and a first polar body
  - The secondary oocyte is a haploid cell that contains 23 chromosomes and the majority of cytoplasm
  - The first polar body contains the remaining 23 chromosomes and no cytoplasm
- The secondary oocyte begins the second meiotic division
  - Completion of this division occurs with fertilization, resulting in a mature ovum and a second polar body
  - Regardless of whether fertilization occurs with the secondary oocyte, the first polar body immediately undergoes a second meiotic division resulting in two additional polar bodies; these polar bodies degenerate
  - Overall, one oocyte and three polar bodies are formed

CONCEPTION

● **Fertilization**
- Occurs with the fusion of a spermatozoon and an ovum (oocyte) in the ampulla of the fallopian tube
(See *How fertilization occurs.*)
- The fertilized egg is called a *zygote*

How fertilization occurs

Fertilization begins when the spermatozoon is activated upon contact with the ovum.

The spermatozoon has a covering called the *acrosome* that develops small perforations through which it releases enzymes necessary for the sperm to penetrate the protective layers of the ovum before fertilization.

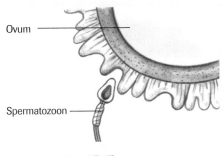

Ovum

Spermatozoon

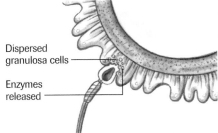

Dispersed granulosa cells

Enzymes released

The spermatozoon then penetrates the zona pellucida (the inner membrane of the ovum). This triggers the ovum's second meiotic division (following meiosis), making the zona pellucida impenetrable to other spermatozoa.

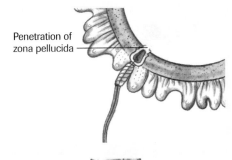

Penetration of zona pellucida

After the spermatozoon penetrates the ovum, its nucleus is released into the ovum, its tail degenerates, and its head enlarges and fuses with the nucleus of the ovum. This fusion provides the fertilized ovum, called a *zygote*, with 46 chromosomes.

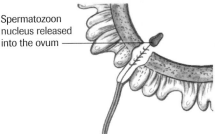

Spermatozoon nucleus released into the ovum

Quick guide to fertilization

- Fertilization begins when the sperm reaches the ovum.
- The acrosome releases enzymes that help to penetrate the ovum.
- The sperm penetrates the zona pellucida.
- The ovum becomes impenetrable to other sperm.
- The sperm releases its nucleus into the ovum.
- The sperm tail disintegrates.
- The sperm head fuses with the nucleus of the ovum, and zygote is formed.

- The diploid number of chromosomes (44 autosomes and 2 sex chromosomes) is restored when the zygote is formed
    - A male zygote is formed if the ovum is fertilized by a spermatozoon carrying a Y chromosome

– A female zygote is formed if the ovum is fertilized by a spermatozoon carrying an X chromosome
- Cellular multiplication occurs when the zygote undergoes *mitosis,* dividing into two cells, four cells, and so on
    – These cells, called *blastomeres,* eventually form the *morula,* a solid ball of cells
    – After the morula enters the uterus, a cavity forms within the dividing cells, thus changing the morula into a blastocyst
    – The blastocyst cells differentiate into one of two forms — trophoblast, which develop into fetal membranes and contribute to placenta formation, or the inner cell mass, a discrete cell cluster enclosed within the trophoblast, which will form the embryo (late blastocyst)

● Implantation
- *Implantation* occurs when the cellular wall of the blastocyst (the trophoblast) implants itself in the endometrium of the anterior or posterior fundal region, 7 to 9 days after fertilization after the zona pellucida degenerates
- Primary villi appear within weeks after implantation
- The trophoblast, in contact with the endometrial lining, proliferates and invades the underlying endometrium by separating and dissolving endometrial cells
- The invading blastocyst sinks below the surface of the endometrium
- Continuity of the surface is restored as the site of penetration heals (See *Tracing implantation.*)
- After implantation, the endometrium is called the *decidua*

● Placentation
- In *placentation,* the chorionic villi invade the decidua
- This becomes the fetal portion of the future placenta

STAGES OF FETAL DEVELOPMENT

● Pre-embryonic period
- Begins with fertilization and lasts about 3 weeks
- As the zygote passes through the fallopian tube, it undergoes a series of mitotic divisions, or cleavage
- Once formed, the zygote develops into the morula and then blastocyst, eventually becoming attached to the endometrium

● Embryonic period
- Begins with the fourth week of gestation and ends with the seventh week
- During this period, the zygote begins to take on a human shape
- The zygote is now called an *embryo*

Key facts about implantation

- Cellular wall of the blastocyst implants itself in the endometrium after the zona pellucida degenerates (7 to 9 days after fertilization)
- Primary villi appear within weeks after implantation
- The trophoblast proliferates and invades the underlying endometrium by separating and dissolving endometrial cells
- Invading blastocyst sinks below the surface of the endometrium
- Continuity of the surface is restored as the site of penetration heals
- After implantation, the endometrium is called the *decidua*

Tracing implantation

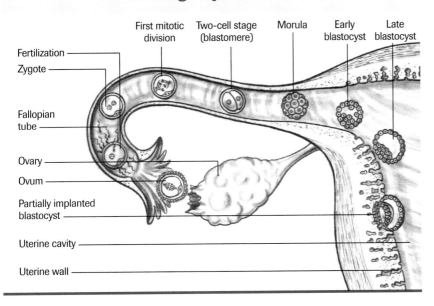

Labels on diagram:
- First mitotic division
- Two-cell stage (blastomere)
- Morula
- Early blastocyst
- Late blastocyst
- Fertilization
- Zygote
- Fallopian tube
- Ovary
- Ovum
- Partially implanted blastocyst
- Uterine cavity
- Uterine wall

- Germ layers develop, giving rise to organ systems
- The embryo is highly vulnerable to injury from maternal drug use, certain maternal infections, and other factors

● **Fetal period**
- Begins with the 8th week of gestation and continues until birth
- During this period, the embryo, now called a *fetus,* matures, enlarges, and grows heavier
  - The head of the fetus is disproportionately larger when compared to its body
  - The fetus also lacks subcutaneous fat

EMBRYONIC AND FETAL STRUCTURES

● **Decidua**
- Refers to the endometrial lining during pregnancy
- Provides a nesting place for the developing ovum
- Has some endocrine functions
  - Secretes prolactin to promote lactation
  - Secretes relaxin, which relaxes the connective tissue of the symphysis pubis and pelvic ligaments; also promotes cervical dilation
  - Secretes prostaglandin, a potent hormone like fatty acid, important for mediating several physiologic functions
- Is divided into three separate layers
  - Decidua basalis—lies directly under the embryo; it's where the trophoblasts connect to the maternal blood vessels

Stages of fetal development

1. Pre-embryonic period — fertilization to 3 weeks
2. Embryonic period — 4th to 7th week of gestation
3. Fetal period — 8th week of gestation to birth

Endocrine functions of the decidua

- Secretes prolactin
- Secretes relaxin
- Secretes prostaglandin

Layers of the decidua

- Decidua basalis – directly under the embryo; where trophoblasts connect to maternal blood vessels
- Decidua capsularis – stetches over the trophoblast and enlarges as embryo grows
- Decidua vera – remaining area of the endometrial lining

Key facts about fetal membranes

- Chorion is closest to the uterine wall.
- Chorion becomes the placenta and forms the outer wall of the blastocyst.
- Amnion is the inner fetal membrane.
- Amnion lines the amniotic sac.

Embryonic germ layers

- Layers developed during the embryonic period that later become specific organs and tissues
- Ectoderm – outermost layer
- Endoderm – innermost layer
- Mesoderm – middle layer

– Decidua capsularis—stretches over or forms a capsule over the trophoblast; enlarges as the embryo grows, eventually coming into contact and fusing with the opposite side of the uterine wall
– Decidua vera—is the remaining area of the endometrial lining

● **Fetal membranes**
- The chorion is the fetal membrane closest to the uterine wall
  – It gives rise to the placenta
  – It forms the outer wall of the blastocyst
  – Vascular projections, called *chorionic villi,* arise from its periphery
  – As the chorionic vesicle enlarges, villi arising from the superficial portion of the chorion (the chorion laeve) atrophy, leaving the surface smooth
  – Villi arising from the deeper part of the chorion (the chorion fondosum) proliferate, projecting into the large blood vessels within the decidua basalis, through which the maternal blood flows
  – Blood vessels form within the villi as they grow, becoming connected with blood vessels formed in the chorion and in the body of the embryo
  – Blood flows through this developing network of vessels as soon as the embryo's heart begins to beat
- The amnion is the thin, tough inner fetal membrane that lines the amniotic sac

● **Embryonic germ layers**
- Three germ layers develop during the embryonic period, each giving rise to specific organ and tissues
  – Ectoderm
    · The outermost layer
    · Generates the epidermis, nervous system, pituitary gland, salivary glands, optic lens, lining of the lower portion of the anal canal, hair, and tooth enamel
  – Endoderm
    · The innermost layer
    · Generates the epithelial lining of the larynx, trachea, bladder, urethra, prostate gland, auditory canal, liver, pancreas, and alimentary canal
  – Mesoderm
    · The middle layer
    · Generates the connective and sclerous tissues; blood and the vascular system; musculature; teeth (except enamel); mesothelial lining of the pericardial, pleural, and peritoneal cavities; kidneys and ureters

Yolk sac

- Forms next to the endoderm of the germ disk
- A portion is incorporated into the developing embryo and forms the GI tract
- Another portion develops into primitive germ cells, which travel to the developing gonads and eventually form the oocytes or spermatocytes after sex has been determined
- Also forms blood cells during the early embryonic period
- Eventually undergoes atrophy and disintegrates

Amniotic sac

- Is enclosed within the chorion
- Gradually increases in size and surrounds the embryo
- Expands into the chorionic cavity as it enlarges
- Fuses with the chorion by the 8th week of gestation
- Contains fluid, known as *amniotic fluid*
  - With the sac, helps provide the fetus with a buoyant, temperature-controlled environment
  - Serves as a fluid wedge that helps to open the cervix during birth
  - Early in pregnancy, comes from three sources
    - Fluid is filtered into the amniotic sac from maternal blood as it passes through the uterus (most)
    - Fluid is filtered into the sac from fetal blood passing through the placenta
    - Fluid diffuses into the sac from the fetal skin and respiratory tract
  - Later in pregnancy, when the fetal kidneys begin to function, the fetus urinates into the amniotic fluid; fetal urine then becomes the major source of amniotic fluid
  - Replaced every 3 hours
    - Production of amniotic fluid from maternal and fetal sources balances amniotic fluid lost through the fetal GI tract
    - Normally, the fetus swallows up to several hundred milliliters of amniotic fluid per day
    - This fluid is absorbed into the fetal circulation from the fetal GI tract
    - Some is transferred from the fetal circulation to the maternal circulation and excreted in maternal urine
  - Contains albumin, lanugo, urea, creatinine, bilirubin, fat, fructose, protein, enzymes, lecithin, sphingomyelin, and leukocytes
  - Prevents heat loss, preserves constant fetal body temperatures, cushions the fetus, facilitates symmetrical fetal growth and devel-

Key facts about the yolk sac

- A portion is incorporated into the embryo and becomes the GI tract.
- Another part becomes the oocytes or spermatocytes.
- It forms blood cells.
- It eventually atrophies and disintegrates.

Functions of amniotic fluid

- Provides buoyancy and temperature control
- Prevents heat loss
- Preserves constant fetal body temperatures
- Cushions the fetus
- Facilitates symmetrical fetal growth and development
- Provides a source of oral fluid
- Provides a repository for fetal waste
- Helps open the cervix during birth

opment, provides a source of oral fluid, and serves as a repository for fetal waste
– At term, the uterus contains 800 to 1,200 ml of amniotic fluid, which is clear and yellowish and has a specific gravity of 1.007 to 1.025 and a pH of 7.0 to 7.25

● Umbilical cord

Key facts about the umbilical cord

- Lifeline for the embryo
- Has two arteries and one vein
- Blood flows at 400 ml/minute
- Wharton's jelly helps prevent kinking

- Serves as the lifeline from the embryo to the placenta
- Measures from 30.5 to 90 cm in length and 2 cm in diameter at full-term
- Contains two arteries and one vein
    - The umbilical arteries transport blood from the fetus to the placenta
    - The umbilical vein returns blood to the fetus from the placenta
- Contains Wharton's jelly, a gelatinous substance that helps prevent kinking of the cord in utero
- Blood flows through the cord at about 400 ml/minute

● Placenta

Functions of the placenta

- Receives maternal oxygen via diffusion
- Produces hormones
- Supplies the fetus with carbohydrates, water, fats, protein, minerals, and inorganic salts
- Carries end products of fetal metabolism to maternal circulation for excretion
- Transfers passive immunity via maternal antibodies

- A flat disk-shaped structure formed from the chorion, chorionic villi, and adjacent decidua basalis
- Contains 15 to 20 subdivisions called *cotyledons*
- Weighs 450 to 600 g, measures from 15 to 25.5 cm in diameter, and is 2.5 to 3 cm thick at full-term
- Has a rough texture; appears red on the maternal surface and shiny and gray on the fetal surface
- Functions as a transport mechanism between the mother and the fetus, from the 3rd month of pregnancy until birth
    - The placenta's life span and function depend on oxygen consumption and maternal circulation; circulation to the fetus and placenta improves when the mother lies on her left side
    - The placenta receives maternal oxygen via diffusion
    - It produces hormones, including human chorionic gonadotropin, human placental lactogen, gonadotropin-releasing hormone, thyrotropin-releasing factor, corticotropin, estrogen, and progesterone
    - It supplies the fetus with carbohydrates, water, fats, protein, minerals, and inorganic salts
    - It carries end products of fetal metabolism to the maternal circulation for excretion
    - It transfers passive immunity via maternal antibodies

Hormones produced in the placenta

- Human chorionic gonadotropin
- Human placental lactogen
- Gonadotropin-releasing hormone
- Thyrotropin-releasing factor
- Corticotropin
- Estrogen
- Progesterone

● Fetal circulation structures

(See *Fetal blood circulation.*)

- *Umbilical vein* carries oxygenated blood to the fetus from the placenta

GO WITH THE FLOW

Fetal blood circulation

The three flowcharts below illustrate fetal blood circulation. The first chart shows the flow of blood from the placenta to the inferior vena cava. After the blood reaches the inferior vena cava, most of the blood flows back to the placenta, as shown in the second chart. However, a small amount of blood flows differently, taking the path shown in the third chart.

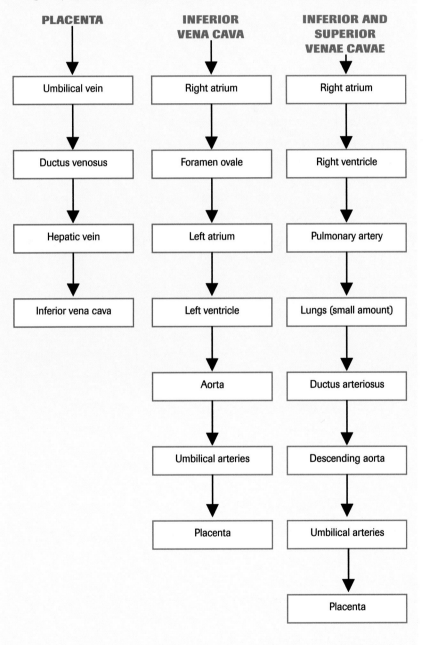

PLACENTA	INFERIOR VENA CAVA	INFERIOR AND SUPERIOR VENAE CAVAE
Umbilical vein	Right atrium	Right atrium
Ductus venosus	Foramen ovale	Right ventricle
Hepatic vein	Left atrium	Pulmonary artery
Inferior vena cava	Left ventricle	Lungs (small amount)
	Aorta	Ductus arteriosus
	Umbilical arteries	Descending aorta
	Placenta	Umbilical arteries
		Placenta

Developmental milestones: 4 weeks

- Head accounts for one-third of embryo.
- Embryo appears C-shaped.
- Heart appears in rudimentary form (bulge on anterior surface).
- Eyes, ears, and nose appear.
- Extremities appear as buds.
- Nervous system begins to form.

Developmental milestones: 8 weeks

- Organ formation is complete.
- Head accounts for one-half of total mass.
- Heart beats and has a septum and valves.
- Arms and legs are developed.
- Abdomen is large with evidence of fetal intestines.
- Facial features are readily visible.
- Gestational sac is visible on ultrasound.

Developmental milestones: 12 weeks

- Nail beds begin to form on extremities.
- Arms appear in normal proportions.
- Heartbeat can be heard using a Doppler ultrasound stethoscope.
- Kidney function begins.
- Tooth buds are present.
- Placenta formation is complete (fetal circulation established).
- Sex is distinguishable with external genitalia's outward appearance.

- *Umbilical arteries* carry deoxygenated blood from the fetus to the placenta
- *Foramen ovale* serves as the septal opening between the atria of the fetal heart
- *Ductus arteriosus* connects the pulmonary artery to the aorta, allowing blood to shunt around the fetal lungs
- *Ductus venosus* carries oxygenated blood from the umbilical vein to the inferior vena cava, bypassing the liver

EMBRYONIC AND FETAL DEVELOPMENT

● Characteristics
- As the embryo grows, different patterns and structures develop
- By the 4th week of gestation, a normal fetus begins to show noticeable signs of growth in all areas assessed
(See *Fetal development by gestational age.*)
- The fetus typically achieves specific developmental milestones by the end of certain gestational weeks
- Failure to feel fetal movement after the 20th week of gestation must be investigated by a health care provider

● 4 weeks' gestation
- Head becomes prominent, accounting for about one-third of the entire embryo
- Head is bent to such a degree that it appears as if it is touching the tail; embryo appears in a **C** shape
- Heart appears in a rudimentary form as a bulge on the anterior surface
- Eyes, ears, and nose appear in a rudimentary form
- Nervous system begins to form
- Extremities appear as buds

● 8 weeks' gestation
- Organ formation is complete
- Head accounts for about one-half of the total mass
- Heart is beating and has a septum and valves
- Arms and legs are developed
- Abdomen is large with evidence of fetal intestines
- Facial features readily visible; eye folds are developed
- Gestational sac visible on ultrasound

● 12 weeks' gestation
- Nail beds are beginning to form on extremities; arms appear in normal proportions
- Heartbeat can be heard using a Doppler ultrasound stethoscope

(Text continues on page 52.)

Fetal development by gestational age

This chart highlights significant areas of fetal growth and development by body system, along with changes in appearance and weight and crown-to-rump measurements. Weeks are approximate.

BODY SYSTEM	GESTATIONAL AGE (WEEKS)	DEVELOPMENT
Respiratory	4 to 7	Primary lung, tracheal, and bronchi buds appear. Nasal pits form. Abdominal and thoracic cavities are separated by the diaphragm.
	8 to 12	Bronchioles branch. Pleural and pericardial cavities appear. Lungs assume definitive shape.
	13 to 20	Terminal and respiratory bronchioles appear.
	21 to 28	Nostrils open. Surfactant production begins. Respiratory movements are possible. Alveolar ducts and sacs appear.
	38 to 40	Pulmonary branching is two-thirds complete. Lecithin-sphingomyelin ratio is 2:1.
Genitourinary	4 to 7	Rudimentary ureteral buds are present.
	8 to 12	Bladder and urethra separate from rectum; bladder expands as a sac. Kidneys secrete urine.
	13 to 20	Kidneys are in proper position with definitive shape.
	36	Nephron formation ceases.
Nervous	4	Midbrain flexure is well-marked.
	8	Cerebral cortex, meninges, ventricular foramens, and cerebrospinal fluid circulation are differentiated.
	12 to 16	Brain structural configuration is roughly completed. Cerebral lobes are delineated. Cerebellum assumes prominence.
	20 to 24	Brain is grossly formed. Myelination of spinal cord begins. Spinal cord ends at S1.
	28 to 36	Cerebral fissures and convolutions appear. Spinal cord ends at L3.
	40	Myelination of brain begins.
Gastrointestinal	4	Oral cavity and primitive jaw are present. Stomach, ducts of pancreas, and liver form. Esophagus and trachea division begins.
	8 to 11	Intestinal villi form. Small intestines coil in umbilical cord.

(continued)

Fetal development by gestational age *(continued)*

BODY SYSTEM	GESTATIONAL AGE (WEEKS)	DEVELOPMENT
Gastrointestinal *(continued)*	12 to 16	Bile is secreted. Intestines withdraw from umbilical cord to normal position. Meconium is present in bowel. Anus opens.
	20	Enamel and dentin are deposited. Ascending colon appears. Fetus can suck and swallow. Peristaltic movements begin.
Hepatic	4	Liver function begins.
	6	Liver hematopoiesis begins.
Endocrine	2 to 3	Thyroid tissue appears.
	4	Thyroid can synthesize thyroxine.
	10	Islets of Langerhans differentiated.
	12	Thyroid secretes hormones. Insulin present in pancreas.
Reproductive	2 to 3	Sex is determined.
	6 to 8	Sex glands appear and begin differentiation into ovaries or testes. External genitalia appear similar.
	12 to 24	Testes descend into the inguinal canal. External genitalia are distinguishable.
Musculoskeletal	4	Limb buds appear.
	8	Ossification (mandible, humerus, occiput) is identifiable.
	12	Some bones are well outlined. Ossification continues.
	16	Joint cavities are present. Muscular movements are detectable.
	20	Ossification of sternum is identifiable. Mother can detect fetal movements (quickening).
	28 to 32	Ossification continues. Fetus can turn head to side.
	36	Muscle tone is developed; fetus can turn and elevate head.
Cardiovascular	2 to 4	Heart formation begins. Blood circulation begins. Primitive red blood cells circulate. Fetus has tubular heartbeat by 24 days.
	5 to 7	Atria divide. Heart chambers are present. Fetal heartbeat is detectable. Blood cell groups are identifiable.

Fetal development by gestational age *(continued)*

BODY SYSTEM	GESTATIONAL AGE (WEEKS)	DEVELOPMENT
Cardiovascular *(continued)*	8	Heart development is complete. Fetal circulation follows two intra-embryonic and four extra-embryonic circuits.
	12 to 20	Fetal heart tones are audible with Doppler (12 weeks) and fetoscope (16 to 20 weeks).
External appearance	4	Body is C-shaped; eyes pigmented; auditory pit enclosed.
	8	Eyes, ears, nose, and mouth recognizable; flat nose; eyes far apart; digits well formed.
	12	Nails appear; skin is pink and delicate; lacrimal ducts developing.
	16	Head is dominant; scalp hair present; sweat glands developing.
	20	Vernix, lanugo, and sebaceous glands appear; legs considerably lengthened.
	24	Skin red and wrinkled; eyes structurally complete.
	28	Eyelids open.
	32	Subcutaneous fat increases; skin pink and smooth.
	36	Lanugo disappearing; earlobes soft with little cartilage.
	40	Vernix is copious; hair is moderate to profuse; lanugo on shoulders and upper body; ear lobes stiffer with cartilage.

GESTATIONAL AGE (WEEKS)	WEIGHT (g)	CROWN-TO-RUMP LENGTH (cm)
4	0.4	0.4 to 0.5
8	2	2.5 to 3.0
12	19	6.0 to 9.0
16	100	11.5 to 13.5
20	300	16.0 to 18.5
24	600	23
28	1,100	27
32	1,800 to 2,100	31
36	2,200 to 2,900	35
40	3,200+	40

Developmental milestones: 16 to 24 weeks

- Fetal heart sounds are audible.
- Fetal urine is present in amniotic fluid.
- Mother feels spontaneous movement of fetus.
- Hair begins to form.
- Fetus demonstrates sleep-awake patterns.
- Lower extremities are fully formed.
- Lungs produce surfactant.
- Passive antibody transfer from the mother begins.

Developmental milestones: 24 to 32 weeks

- Surfactant appears in amniotic fluid.
- Alveoli in the lungs begin to mature.
- Skin appears red.
- Fetus begins to appear more rounded as more subcutaneous fat is deposited.
- Moro reflex is active.
- Vernix caseosa becomes thick.

Developmental milestones: 32 to 40 weeks

- Subcutaneous fat continues to be deposited.
- Lanugo decreases in amount.
- Skin on face and body smooths.
- Fetus begins to kick actively and forcefully.
- Vernix caseosa is fully formed.
- Soles have creases.
- Conversion of fetal hemoglobin to adult hemoglobin begins.

- Kidney function is beginning; fetal urine may be present in amniotic fluid
- Tooth buds are present
- Placenta formation is complete with establishment of fetal circulation
- Sex is distinguishable with external genitalia's outward appearance

● 16 weeks' gestation

- Fetal heart sounds are audible with stethoscope
- Lanugo present and well formed
- Fetus demonstrates active swallowing of amniotic fluid
- Fetal urine is present in amniotic fluid
- Skeleton begins ossification
- Intestines assume normal position in the abdomen

● 20 weeks' gestation

- Mother is able to feel spontaneous movements by the fetus
- Hair begins to form, including that of the eyebrows and scalp hair
- Fetus demonstrates definite sleep and awake patterns
- Brown fat begins to form
- Sebum is produced by the sebaceous glands
- Meconium is evident in the upper portion of the intestines
- Lower extremities are fully formed
- Vernix caseosa covers the skin

● 24 weeks' gestation

- Well-defined eyelashes and eyebrows are visible
- Eyelids are open and pupils can react to light
- Meconium may be present in the rectum
- Hearing is developing with the fetus being able to respond to a sudden sound
- Lungs are producing surfactant
- Passive antibody transfer from the mother begins (possibly as early as 20 weeks' gestation)

● 28 weeks' gestation

- Surfactant appears in amniotic fluid
- Alveoli in the lungs begin to mature
- In the male, the testes start to move from the lower abdomen into the scrotal sac
- The eyelids can open and close
- Skin appears red

● 32 weeks' gestation

- Fetus begins to appear more rounded as more subcutaneous fat is deposited
- Moro reflex is active
- Fetus may assume a vertex or breech position in preparation for birth

- Iron stores are beginning to develop
- Fingernails increase in length, reaching the tips of the fingers
- Vernix caseosa becomes thick

36 weeks' gestation
- Subcutaneous fat continues to be deposited
- Soles of feet have one or two creases
- Lanugo begins to decrease in amount
- The fetus is storing additional glycogen, iron, carbohydrate, and calcium
- Skin on the face and body begins to smooth

40 weeks' gestation
- Fetus begins to kick actively and forcefully, causing maternal discomfort
- Vernix caseosa is fully formed
- Soles of feet demonstrate creases covering at least two-thirds of the surface
- Conversion of fetal hemoglobin to adult hemoglobin begins
- Testes descend fully into the scrotal sac

NCLEX CHECKS

It's never too soon to begin your NCLEX preparation. Now that you've reviewed this chapter, carefully read each of the following questions and choose the best answer. Then compare your responses to the correct answers.

1. Where is the female gamete produced?
- ☐ **A.** Fallopian tube
- ☐ **B.** Seminiferous tubules
- ☐ **C.** Endometrium
- ☑ **D.** Graafian follicle

2. What is the endometrium called after implantation of the blastocyst?
- ☐ **A.** Blastocyte
- ☑ **B.** Decidua
- ☐ **C.** Blastomere
- ☐ **D.** Morula

3. What are the two fetal membranes?
- ☑ **A.** Chorion and amnion
- ☐ **B.** Ectoderm and mesoderm
- ☐ **C.** Chorion and endoderm
- ☐ **D.** Amnion and mesoderm

TOP 9

Items to study for your next test on fetal development

1. The chromosomal makeup of a normal human cell
2. The meaning of homozygous and heterozygous
3. The five phases of mitosis and what occurs in each
4. The steps involved with spermatogenesis and oogenesis
5. The three stages of embryonic and fetal development and the duration of each
6. The structure and function of the placenta
7. The composition and function of amniotic fluid and the umbilical cord
8. The five structures involved in fetal-placental circulation and the roles they play
9. The major developmental milestones and when they occur

4. Which structure is responsible for supplying the fetus with nutrients and removing wastes?

- ☐ **A.** Yolk sac
- ☒ **B.** Placenta
- ☐ **C.** Amniotic fluid
- ☐ **D.** Ductus arteriosus

5. Which factors affect placental function?

- ☒ **A.** Oxygen consumption and maternal circulation
- ☐ **B.** Oxygen consumption and fetal circulation
- ☐ **C.** Amount of amniotic fluid
- ☐ **D.** Position of fetus

6. Which structure carries deoxygenated blood from the fetus to the placenta?

- ☐ **A.** Foramen ovale *septal opening*
- ☐ **B.** Umbilical veins *oxygenated*
- ☒ **C.** Umbilical arteries
- ☐ **D.** Ductus venosus *inferior vena cava*

7. At 12 weeks' gestation, what fetal development would you expect to find? Select all that apply.

- ☒ **A.** Thyroid secretes hormones.
- ☐ **B.** Eyelids are open. *28 wks*
- ☒ **C.** Insulin is present in the pancreas.
- ☒ **D.** Nails appear.
- ☐ **E.** Vernix caseosa is copious. *40 wks*
- ☒ **F.** Skin is pink and delicate.

ANSWERS AND RATIONALES

1. CORRECT ANSWER: D

The female gamete is produced in the graafian follicle of the ovary. Fertilization occurs in the fallopian tubes. The male gamete is produced in the seminiferous tubules of the testes. The endometrium is where implantation of the blastocyte occurs.

2. CORRECT ANSWER: B

After implantation, the endometrium is called the *decidua*. After the morula enters the uterus, a cavity forms within the dividing cells, thus changing the morula into a blastocyst. Blastomeres are cells that result after cellular multiplication occurs and eventually form the morula. The morula is a solid ball of cells.

3. CORRECT ANSWER: A

The chorion and the amnion are the two fetal membranes. The ectoderm and the mesoderm are embryonic germ layers. The ectoderm generates the epidermis, nervous system, pituitary gland, salivary glands, optic lens, lining of the lower portion of the anal canal, hair, and tooth enamel. The mesoderm generates the connective and sclerous tissues; blood and the vascular system; musculature; teeth (except enamel); mesothelial lining of the pericardial, pleural, and peritoneal cavities; kidneys and ureters.

4. CORRECT ANSWER: B

The placenta is a flat disk-shaped structure that uses the umbilical cord to provide nutrients to and remove wastes from the fetus from the third month of pregnancy until birth. The yolk sac forms next to the endoderm of the germ disk; a portion of it is incorporated into the developing embryo and forms the GI tract, whereas another portion develops into primitive germ cells, which travel to the developing gonads and eventually form the oocytes or spermatocytes after sex has been determined. The amniotic fluid provides the fetus with a buoyant, temperature-controlled environment and serves a fluid wedge that helps to open the cervix during birth. The ductus arteriosus, a fetal heart structure, connects the pulmonary artery to the aorta, allowing blood to shunt around the fetal lungs.

5. CORRECT ANSWER: A

Oxygen consumption and maternal circulation affect placental function. Fetal circulation, the amount of amniotic fluid, and the position of the fetus don't affect placental function.

6. CORRECT ANSWER: C

The umbilical arteries carry deoxygenated blood from the fetus to the placenta. The foramen ovale serves as the septal opening between the atria of the fetal heart. The umbilical veins carry oxygenated blood to the fetus from the placenta. The ductus venosus carries oxygenated blood from the umbilical vein to the inferior vena cava, bypassing the liver.

7. CORRECT ANSWERS: A, C, D, AND F

At 12 weeks' gestation, the thyroid gland secretes hormones, the pancreas secretes insulin, the nails appear, and the skin is pink and delicate. The eyelids don't open until 28 weeks' gestation. Vernix caseosa is copious at 40 weeks' gestation.

4

The normal prenatal period

The normal
prenatal period

LEARNING OBJECTIVES

After studying this chapter, you should be able to:

● Describe the physiologic and psychological adaptations to pregnancy.
● Explain causes of and interventions for common discomforts of pregnancy.
● Describe common methods for assessing fetal status.
● Identify major points to include when counseling a pregnant patient.
● Describe the nutritional needs of the pregnant patient.

CHAPTER OVERVIEW

A woman who's pregnant experiences presumptive, probable, and positive signs and symptoms of pregnancy. Pregnancy causes normal physiologic changes in each body system and psychosocial adaptations. Many discomforts of pregnancy are related to these physiologic changes. Nursing care during the normal prenatal period involves obtaining a thorough maternal history and physical examination, and educating the patient about health promotion activities, nutrition, and danger signs to be reported.

SIGNS AND SYMPTOMS OF PREGNANCY

● **Presumptive**
- Amenorrhea (in about 80% of patients) or slight, painless spotting of unknown cause in early gestation (in about 20% of patients)
- Nausea and vomiting
- Urinary frequency and urgency
- Breast enlargement and tenderness
- Fatigue
- Quickening
- Thinning and softening of fingernails
- Intensified skin pigmentation

● **Probable**
- Uterine enlargement
- Goodell's sign (softening of the cervix)
- Chadwick's sign (bluish mucous membranes of the vagina, cervix, and vulva)
- Hegar's sign (softening of the lower uterine segment)
- Braxton Hicks contractions (painless uterine contractions that recur throughout pregnancy)
- Ballottement (passive fetal movement in response to tapping of the lower portion of the uterus or cervix)
- Laboratory test results indicating pregnancy
- Sonogram results showing the characteristic ring of the gestational sac (visible as early as 4 to 6 weeks' gestation)
- Palpable fetal outline

● **Positive**
- Fetal heartbeat detected by 17 to 20 weeks' gestation
- Ultrasonography results as early as 6 weeks' gestation
- Fetal movements felt by examiner after 16 weeks' gestation
- Visualization of fetus and fetal outline

OVERVIEW OF THE TRIMESTERS OF PREGNANCY

● **First trimester**
- Lasts from weeks 1 through 12 and is a critical time in the pregnancy
- Rapid cell differentiation makes the developing embryo or fetus highly susceptible to the teratogenic effects of viruses, alcohol, cigarettes, caffeine, and other drugs
- The woman usually experiences physical changes, such as amenorrhea, urinary frequency, nausea and vomiting (more severe in the morning or when the stomach is empty), breast swelling and tenderness, fatigue, increased vaginal secretions, and constipation

TOP 6
Pregnancy indicators
1. Amenorrhea or spotting
2. Uterine enlargement
3. Cervical softening (Goodell's sign)
4. Bluish mucous membranes (Chadwick's sign)
5. Softening of lower uterine segment (Hegar's sign)
6. Fetal heartbeat

Positive pregnancy signs
- Fetal heartbeat (by 17 to 20 weeks)
- Ultrasonography results (as early as 6 weeks)
- Fetal movements felt by examiner (after 16 weeks)
- Visualization of fetus and fetal outline

First trimester facts

- Weeks 1 through 12 (critical time)
- Rapid fetal cell differentiation occurs
- Maternal physical changes occur (amenorrhea, urinary frequency, nausea and vomiting, breast swelling and tenderness, fatigue, increased vaginal secretions, constipation)
- 10 days after conception, a serum pregnancy test can usually detect hCG
- Uterine enlargement, Chadwick's sign, and Hegar's sign present at 9 weeks

Second trimester facts

- Weeks 13 through 27
- Uterine and fetal size increase substantially
- By week 20, the patient feels quickening

Third trimester facts

- Weeks 28 through 40
- The patient experiences Braxton Hicks contractions
- Increasing uterine size may displace pelvic and intestinal structures, causing indigestion, protrusion of the umbilicus, shortness of breath, and insomnia
- The patient's center of gravity changes (may cause backaches)

- 7 to 10 days after conception, a serum pregnancy test can usually detect the presence of human chorionic gonadotropin (hCG)
- A pelvic examination, performed 6 to 8 weeks later, shows uterine enlargement, Chadwick's sign, and Hegar's sign

Second trimester
- Lasts from weeks 13 through 27
- Uterine and fetal size increase substantially
  - The woman gains weight, the waistline thickens, and the abdomen enlarges
  - Reddish streaks (striations) may become apparent as abdominal skin stretches
  - Pigment changes may cause skin alterations, such as linea nigra, melasma (or mask of pregnancy) and a darkening of the areolae of the nipples
  - Other physical changes include diaphoresis, increased salivation, indigestion, continuing constipation, hemorrhoids, nosebleeds, and some dependent edema
  - The breasts become larger and heavier, and about 19 weeks after the last menses they may secrete colostrum
- By week 20, the fetus is large enough for the mother to feel its movements (quickening)

Third trimester
- Lasts from weeks 28 through 40
- The woman experiences Braxton Hicks contractions—sporadic episodes of painless uterine tightening—which help strengthen uterine muscles in preparation for labor
- Increasing uterine size may displace pelvic and intestinal structures, causing indigestion, protrusion of the umbilicus, shortness of breath, and insomnia
- The woman's center of gravity changes; she may experience backaches because she walks with a swaybacked posture to counteract her frontal weight

PHYSIOLOGIC ADAPTATIONS TO PREGNANCY

Cardiovascular system
- Cardiac hypertrophy from increased blood volume and cardiac output
- Displacement of the heart upward and to the left from pressure on the diaphragm
- Progressive increase in blood volume, peaking in the third trimester at 30% to 50% of prepregnancy levels
- Increased heart rate

- Gradual increase during the second trimester, possibly reaching 10 to 15 beats/minute above the prepregnancy rate
- During the third trimester, rate may increase 15 to 20 beats/minute above the prepregnancy rate
• Smooth-muscle relaxation and arteriole dilation, resulting in vasodilation
  - Due to increased progesterone levels in early pregnancy
  - Systolic and diastolic pressures may decrease 5 to 10 mm Hg
    · Reach their lowest levels during the second half of the second trimester
    · Gradually return to first trimester levels during the third trimester
• Increased cardiac output
    · Up to a 50% increase by the 32nd week of pregnancy
    · Results from an increased tissue demand for oxygen and increased stroke volume
    · Highest when the patient is lying on her side (side-lying position reduces pressure on the great vessels, which increases venous return to the heart)
    · Lowest when she's lying on her back
• Pulmonic systolic and apical systolic murmurs, resulting from decreased blood viscosity and increased blood flow
• S_1 tends to exhibit a pronounced splitting, and each component tends to be louder; an occasional S_3 sound may occur after 20 weeks of pregnancy
• Supine hypotension
  - Results from obstructed blood flow from the lower extremities due to the weight of the growing uterus pressing the vena cava against the vertebrae when the patient lies in a supine position
  - Causes a decrease in blood return to the heart and, consequently, immediate decreased cardiac output and hypotension
• Increased femoral venous pressure caused by impaired circulation from the lower extremities, which results from the pressure of the enlarged uterus on the pelvic veins and inferior vena cava
• Edema in the legs and, possibly, varicosities in the legs, rectum, and vulva
• Enlargement of vessels surrounding the spinal cord's dura mater, which decreases cerebrospinal fluid space
• Increased fibrinogen levels (up to 50% at term) from hormonal influences
• Increased levels of blood coagulation factors VII, IX, and X, leading to a hypercoagulable state

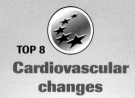

TOP 8
Cardiovascular changes

1. Cardiac hypertrophy
2. Displacement of the heart
3. Increased blood volume
4. Increased heart rate
5. Supine hypotension
6. Increased fibrinogen levels
7. Decreased hematocrit
8. Increased hemoglobin level

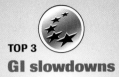

TOP 3

GI slowdowns

1. Delayed intestinal motility
2. Delayed gallbladder and gastric emptying time
3. Constipation

• Increase of about 33% in total red blood cell volume, despite hemodilution and decreased erythrocyte count
• Hematocrit decrease of about 7%
• Hemoglobin level increase of 12% to 15%, which is less than the overall plasma volume increase, thus reducing hemoglobin levels and leading to physiologic anemia of pregnancy
• Leukocyte production equal to or slightly greater than blood volume increase
  – Average leukocyte count is 10,000 to 11,000/µl
  – Count peaks at 25,000/µl during labor, possibly through an estrogen-related mechanism

● **Gastrointestinal system**
• Gum swelling from increased estrogen levels; gums may be spongy and hyperemic
• Lateral and posterior displacement of the intestines
• Superior and lateral displacement of the stomach
• Delayed intestinal motility and gastric and gallbladder emptying time from smooth-muscle relaxation caused by high levels of placental progesterone
• Hemorrhoids in late pregnancy from venous pressure
• Constipation from increased progesterone levels, resulting in increased water absorption from the colon
• Displacement of the appendix from McBurney's point (making diagnosis of appendicitis difficult)
• Increased tendency of gallstone formation caused by the gallbladder's inability to empty as a result of pressure from the increasing size of the uterus (especially if patient had previous stone formation)

● **Endocrine system**
• Increased basal metabolic rate (up 25% at term)
  – Caused by demands of the fetus and uterus
  – Also caused by increased oxygen consumption
• Increased iodine metabolism from slight hyperplasia of the thyroid, caused by estrogen levels
• Slight parathyroidism from increased requirement for calcium and vitamin D
• Elevated plasma parathyroid hormone levels, peaking between 15 and 35 weeks of gestation
• Slightly enlarged pituitary gland
• Increased production of prolactin by the pituitary gland
• Increased estrogen levels and hypertrophy of the adrenal cortex
• Increased cortisol levels to regulate protein and carbohydrate metabolism

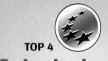

TOP 4

Endocrine increases

1. Increased basal metabolic rate
2. Increased production of prolactin
3. Increased estrogen levels
4. Increased cortisol levels

- Decreased maternal blood glucose levels
- Decreased insulin production in early pregnancy
- Increased production of estrogen, progesterone, and human chorionic somatomammotropin by the placenta
- Increased levels of maternal cortisol, which reduce the mother's ability to use insulin, thus ensuring an adequate glucose supply for the fetus and placenta

● **Respiratory system**
- Increased vascularization of the respiratory tract caused by increased estrogen levels
- Shortening of the lungs caused by the enlarging uterus
- Upward displacement of the diaphragm by the uterus
- Increased tidal volume, causing slight hyperventilation
- Increased chest circumference (by about $2\frac{3}{8}$″ [6 cm])
- Altered breathing, with abdominal breathing replacing thoracic breathing as pregnancy progresses
- Slight increase (2 breaths/minute) in respiratory rate
- Increased pH from a lowered threshold for carbon dioxide from increased estrogen and progesterone levels
  - Leads to mild respiratory alkalosis
  - A decreased bicarbonate level partially or completely compensates for this tendency

● **Metabolic system**
- Increased water retention
  - Caused by higher levels of steroidal sex hormones
  - Leads to edema-dependent carpal tunnel syndrome
- Decreased serum protein levels
- Increased intracapillary pressure and permeability
- Increased levels of serum lipids, lipoproteins, and cholesterol
- Increased iron requirements caused by fetal demands
- Increased carbohydrate needs
- Increased protein retention from hyperplasia and hypertrophy of maternal tissues
- Weight gain of 25 to 30 lb (11.3 to 13.6 kg)
  - Commonly estimated at 3-, 12-, and 12-lb (1.4-, 5.4-, and 5.4-kg) gains for first, second, and third trimesters, respectively
  - Caused by fetus (7.5 lb [3.4 kg]), placenta and membranes (1.5 lb [0.7 kg]), amniotic fluid (2 lb [0.9 kg]), uterus (2.5 lb [1.1 kg]), breasts (3 lb [1.4 kg]), blood volume (2 to 4 lb [0.9 to 1.8 kg]), and extravascular fluid and fat reserves (4 to 9 lb [1.8 to 4.1 kg])

● **Integumentary system**
- Hyperactive sweat and sebaceous glands

TOP 3

Respiratory changes

1. Upward displacement of diaphragm
2. Increased tidal volume
3. Slight hyperventilation

Reasons for water retention during pregnancy

- Higher levels of steroidal sex hormones
- Decreased serum protein levels
- Increased intracapillary pressure and permeability

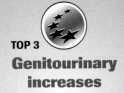

- Hyperpigmentation
  - From the increase of melanocyte-stimulating hormone caused by increased estrogen and progesterone levels
  - Nipples, areola, cervix, vagina, and vulva darken
  - Nose, cheeks, and forehead show pigmentary changes known as *facial chloasma*
  - Striae gravidarum (red or pinkish streaks on the sides of the abdominal wall and sometimes on the thighs) and linea nigra (a dark line extending from the umbilicus or above to the mons pubis)
- Breast changes such as leaking of colostrum
- Palmar erythema and increased angiomas
- Hair and nails grow faster but become thinner and softer

● **Genitourinary system**
- Dilated ureters and renal pelvis caused by progesterone and pressure from the enlarging uterus
- Increased glomerular filtration rate (GFR) and renal plasma flow (RPF) early in pregnancy
  - GFR is elevated until delivery
  - RPF returns to a near-normal level by term
- Increased clearance of urea and creatinine from increased renal function
- Decreased blood urea and nonprotein nitrogen values from increased renal function
- Glycosuria from increased glomerular filtration without an increase in tubular reabsorptive capacity
- Decreased bladder tone
- Increased sodium retention from hormonal influences
- Increases uterine dimension
  - From 6.5 to 32 cm ($2\frac{1}{2}$″ to $12\frac{1}{2}$″) in length
  - From 4 to 24 cm ($1\frac{1}{2}$″ to $9\frac{1}{2}$″) in width
  - From 22 to 25 cm ($8\frac{5}{8}$″ to 10″) in depth
  - From 56.5 to 1,191 g (2 to 42 oz) in weight
  - From 4 ml to 5,028 ml ($\frac{1}{8}$ to 170 oz) in volume
- Hypertrophied uterine muscle cells (5 to 10 times normal size)
- Increased vascularity, edema, hypertrophy, and hyperplasia of the cervical glands
- Increased vaginal secretions with a pH of 3.5 to 6
- Discontinued ovulation and maturation of new follicles
- Thickening of vaginal mucosa, loosening of vaginal connective tissue, and hypertrophy of small-muscle cells
- Changes in sexual desire

- Typically decreased during the first trimester, secondary to nausea, fatigue, and breast tenderness
- Markedly increased during the second trimester due to increased pelvic blood flow
- Possibly increased during the third trimester or possibly decreased due to difficulty finding a comfortable position secondary to the increased size of the abdomen

● **Musculoskeletal system**
  • Lumbosacral curve increases accompanied by a compensatory curvature in the cervicodorsal region
  • Increasing sex hormones (and possibly the hormone relaxin) relax the sacroiliac, sacrococcygeal, and pelvic joints causing the gait to change
  • Enlarged breasts pull the shoulders forward, producing a stoop-shouldered stance
  • The rectus abdominis muscles separate in the third trimester, allowing the abdominal contents to protrude at the midline

PSYCHOLOGICAL RESPONSES TO PREGNANCY

● **General characteristics**
  • Varied psychological responses due to hormonal changes, altered body image, anticipation of role changes, emotional makeup, sociocultural background, and reactions of family and friends
  • Common responses include ambivalence, grief, narcissism, introversion or extroversion, stress, and emotional lability
  • Patient experiences mixed feelings (even if the pregnancy was planned) due to unresolved emotional conflicts between the patient and her mother, fear of pending role changes or of labor and delivery, and the need to alter career plans
  • Growing acceptance of the pregnancy as the patient sees her physical appearance change, experiences quickening, and hears fetal heart tones
  • Focusing of woman's attention toward self to prepare for the birth
    – Normal response
    – May strain the relationship if her partner misinterprets introversion as rejection
  • Wide mood swings can strain marital or familial relationships, possibly causing the partner or family members to withdraw, leaving the patient feeling rejected
● **Ambivalence**
  • Normal response in both the woman and her partner

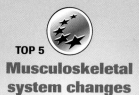

TOP 5
Musculoskeletal system changes

1. Lumbosacral curve increases
2. Compensatory curvature in the cervicodorsal region develops
3. Sacroiliac, sacrococcygeal, and pelvic joints relax
4. Shoulders pull forward
5. Rectus abdominis muscles separate

General psychological responses to pregnancy

● Psychological responses vary
● Feelings are mixed due to unresolved emotional conflicts between the patient and her mother, fear of role changes or of labor and delivery, and the need to alter career plans
● Acceptance of the pregnancy grows with physical appearance changes, quickening, and presence of fetal heart tones
● Patient focuses on self
● Mood swings can strain relationships

Common maternal responses to pregnancy

- Ambivalence – normal response; discomforts of pregnancy cause mixed feelings; fear
- Grief – role adjustment
- Narcissism – woman focuses on self and changing body
- Introversion or extroversion – woman focuses on self or becomes more outgoing
- Stress – pregnancy interferes with ability to perform daily tasks such as caring for other family members; support systems can alleviate some stress and aid adaptation to pregnancy
- Emotional lability – mood changes; influenced by hormones; avoiding fatigue and reducing stress can help

- Changes occurring as a result of pregnancy may lead to discomforts and alterations that can leave the woman feeling less than positive about the experience
- The woman, although desiring to be pregnant, may not enjoy the experience
- Her partner may feel ambivalent because of anxieties or fears related to the pregnancy
    - May feel reluctant to voice concerns about the pregnancy for fear of increasing his partner's anxiety
    - May have an underlying fear that he should already know what to do or how to act
- Lack of knowledge of or preparation for parenthood and children may also contribute to ambivalence

Grief
- Commonly occurs as a result of changes in the woman's role
- With pregnancy, the woman must alter her current roles
    - No longer assumes the role of just being someone's wife or daughter
    - Must integrate her new role as mother with those of her current roles
- Her partner also experiences a similar reaction in role adjustment

Narcissism
- Narcissism occurs as the woman becomes focused on herself and the changes occurring in her body
- Common response during early pregnancy
- May be reflected by the increased time that the woman spends on dressing or self-care activities, changes in activities, or additional measures used to avoid injury
- Signifies an effort by the woman to protect her body and the fetus
- Her partner also may experience narcissism by decreasing participation in risky behaviors and activities so that he'll be available for his child

Introversion or extroversion
- Some pregnant women become introverted during pregnancy, focusing entirely on their bodies and themselves
- Other women become extroverted
    - May increase their participation in activities and appear more outgoing
    - May view their expanding abdomen with a sense of fulfillment

Stress reaction
- For some women pregnancy can be a time of stress

- The woman or her partner may view the pregnancy as interfering with his or her ability to accomplish daily tasks
- Others, for example, children or older parents, dependent on the woman or her partner may to contribute to this feeling of stress
- Family members, such as siblings, need to be prepared for changes in the family that may occur during the pregnancy and also after the baby is born
- Adequate support systems can help to alleviate some of this stress and aid in adapting to the pregnancy

● **Emotional lability**
- Mood changes occur frequently
- May be the result of the woman's introversion and narcissism
- Additionally, hormonal changes, specifically increased estrogen and progesterone, contribute to this lability
- Avoiding fatigue and reducing the stress level are helpful in reducing the incidence of mood swings

● **Couvade syndrome**
- Response in which the partner identifies with the woman's pregnancy
- Partner may experience discomforts such as nausea, vomiting, fatigue, or weight gain, similar to or possibly more intense than those that the pregnant woman experiences
- These discomforts are normal and temporary and become problematic only if the partner becomes delusional or emotionally disruptive

DEVELOPMENTAL TASKS OF PREGNANCY

● **General characteristics**
- Depending on the woman's age, tasks may include acceptance and comfort with body image, development of a personal value system, adjustment to an adult identity, and internalization of sexual role and identity
- Other tasks include acceptance of the pregnancy's termination at the time of delivery and the maternal role, and resolution of fears about childbirth and bonding
- The woman's partner also achieves these same developmental tasks

● **First trimester: Acceptance of the pregnancy**
- Pregnancy confirmation may leave some couples with disbelief, shock, or amazement
- The woman and her partner must learn to accept the reality of the pregnancy
- Most couples experience some degree of ambivalence

Factors affecting emotional lability

- Introversion
- Narcissism
- Hormonal changes
- Fatigue
- Stress

Facts about couvade syndrome

- Paternal response to pregnancy
- Partner identifies with woman's pregnancy
- May experience such discomforts as nausea, vomiting, fatigue, or weight gain
- Temporary and rarely problematic

Pregnancy "to do" list

- Accept the pregnancy—first trimester
- Accept the baby—second trimester
- Prepare for parenthood—third trimester

- Feeling the fetus move or seeing the fetus on an ultrasound can help the couple achieve acceptance
- In accepting the pregnancy, the partner also accepts the woman as she undergoes the changes associated with pregnancy

● **Second trimester: Acceptance of the baby**
- The woman and her partner work to accept the baby
- Acceptance of the baby refers to acknowledgment that the fetus is a distinct individual, separate from the mother
- Feeling the fetus move or hearing its heart beat demonstrates that the fetus is an active being
- Anticipatory role playing, for example with the woman or partner imagining what type of parent she or he will be, may occur
- The woman and her partner begin active preparations for the baby
- The partner may feel left out with all the information being focused on the woman and fetus; time is needed to ensure that the partner is given the information and support required

● **Third trimester: Preparation for parenthood**
- The couple work on preparing to become parents
- The couple begin to demonstrate "nesting" behaviors, such as preparing the baby's room, shopping for necessary baby items, and discussing names
- The couple may attend childbirth education classes
- The couple may review relationships with their own parents and engage in role-playing and fantasizing about being a parent

COMMON DISCOMFORTS DURING THE FIRST TRIMESTER

● **Nausea and vomiting**
- Called "morning sickness," but it may occur anytime during the day
- Causes
  - Hormonal changes
  - Fatigue
  - Emotional factors
  - Changes in carbohydrate metabolism
- Patient teaching
  - Instruct patient to avoid greasy, highly seasoned food
  - Encourage her to eat small, frequent meals
  - Advise her to eat dry toast or crackers before getting out of bed in the morning
  - Suggest intake of complex carbohydrates with the onset of nausea

TOP 4
Ways to beat nausea and vomiting

1. Avoid greasy, highly seasoned foods.
2. Eat small, frequent meals.
3. Eat dry toast or crackers before getting out of bed.
4. Eat complex carbohydrates when nausea sets in.

Nasal stuffiness, discharge, or obstruction
- Cause
  - Edema of the nasal mucosa from elevated estrogen levels
- Patient teaching
  - Encourage the use of a cool-moist humidifier
  - Suggest the use of normal saline nose drops or nasal spray
  - Advise patient to apply cool compresses to the nasal area

Breast enlargement and tenderness
- Cause
  - Increased estrogen and progesterone levels
- Patient teaching
  - Encourage the use of a well-fitting bra with wide shoulder straps for support
  - Reinforce the need for maintaining good posture
  - Advise the patient to wash her breast and nipple area with water only

Urinary frequency and urgency
- Cause
  - Pressure of the enlarging uterus on the bladder
  - Around the 12th week the uterus rises into the abdominal cavity, causing symptoms to disappear
  - Symptoms recur in the third trimester as the uterus again presses on the bladder
- Patient teaching
  - Suggest to the patient that she decrease fluid intake in the evening to minimize nocturia
  - Encourage her to limit intake of caffeinated beverages
  - Reinforce the need to promptly respond to the urge to void in order to prevent bladder distention and urine stasis
  - Teach her how to perform Kegel exercises
  - Teach her the signs and symptoms of urinary tract infection and instruct her to promptly report any she experiences

Increased leukorrhea
- Causes
  - Hyperplasia of vaginal mucosa
  - Increased mucus production by the endocervical glands
- Patient teaching
  - Encourage the woman to bathe daily and avoid using soap on the vulvar area
  - Reinforce the need to wipe from front to back
  - Urge her to wear loose, absorbent cotton underwear and to avoid tight pants and pantyhose

TOP 3

Ways to beat nasal discomforts

1. Use a cool-mist humidifier.
2. Use normal saline nose drops or nasal spray.
3. Apply cool compresses to the nasal area.

TOP 3

Ways to cope with breast changes

1. Wear a well-fitting bra with wide shoulder straps.
2. Maintain good posture.
3. Wash breast and nipple area with water only.

TOP 4

Ways to beat urinary frequency and urgency

1. Decrease fluid intake in the evening.
2. Limit intake of caffeinated beverages.
3. Promptly respond to the urge to void.
4. Perform Kegel exercises.

Ways to fight fatigue

1. Have frequent rest periods.
2. Obtain rest during the day.
3. Eat a balanced diet and take iron supplements.
4. Engage in moderate regular exercise.

Ways to avoid heartburn

1. Eat small, frequent meals.
2. Avoid fatty and fried foods.
3. Remain upright for 1 hour after meals.

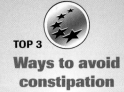

Ways to avoid constipation

1. Exercise.
2. Drink plenty of fluids.
3. Increase daily intake of fiber.

– Suggest the use of panty liners or perineal pads and frequent changing if discharge is bothersome
– Caution her to avoid douching
– Instruct the woman to notify her health care provider immediately if the discharge changes in color or odor

● **Increased fatigue**
- Causes
  – The increased effort of the body to manufacture the placenta
  – The need to adjust to the many other physical and emotional demands of pregnancy
- Patient teaching
  – Encourage frequent rest periods as much as possible
  – Offer suggestions to obtain rest during the day at home or at work
  – Encourage intake of a balanced diet with iron supplementation
  – Suggest the use of warm milk or warm shower or bath before going to bed at night to aid in relaxation
  – Advise engaging in moderate regular exercise

COMMON DISCOMFORTS DURING THE SECOND AND THIRD TRIMESTERS

● **Heartburn**
- Causes
  – Relaxation of the cardiac sphincter
  – Decreased GI motility
  – Increased production of progesterone
  – Gastric displacement
- Patient teaching
  – Encourage the woman to eat small, frequent meals spaced throughout the day
  – Caution her to avoid fatty and fried foods and caffeine products
  – Suggest that she remain upright for at least 1 hour after eating
  – Encourage her to check with her health care provider before using a over-the-counter antacid

● **Constipation**
- Causes
  – Oral iron supplements
  – Displacement of the intestines by the fetus
  – Bowel sluggishness caused by increased progesterone and steroid metabolism
- Patient teaching
  – Encourage the woman to engage in moderate daily exercise
  – Advise the increased intake of fluids and foods high in fiber

– Urge the woman to maintain regular elimination patterns and avoid ignoring the urge to defecate

– Caution the woman to avoid the use of mineral oil, which can deplete her level of fat-soluble vitamins

Hemorrhoids

- Cause
    – Pressure on the pelvic veins by the enlarging uterus, which interferes with venous circulation
    – Increased pressure secondary to constipation
- Patient teaching
    – Describe ways to avoid constipation
    – Caution the woman against prolonged standing and wearing constrictive clothing
    – Suggest the use of a topical ointment or anesthetic if allowed
    – Encourage the use of witch hazel compresses
    – Teach the woman how to perform sitz baths or apply warm soaks
    – Encourage the woman to lie on her left side with her feet slightly elevated

Backache

- Cause
    – Postural adjustments of pregnancy secondary to curvature of the lumbosacral vertebrae that increases with uterine enlargement
- Patient teaching
    – Teach the woman how to use proper body mechanics
    – Encourage the woman to maintain good posture
    – Suggest that she wear low- to mid-heel shoes
    – Recommend that the woman walk with her pelvis tilted forward
    – Advise the woman to apply local heat to the back if necessary
    – Suggest sleeping on a firmer mattress or using a board under the current mattress to add firmness
    – Teach the woman how to do pelvic rocking or tilting exercises

Leg cramps

- Causes
    – Pressure from the enlarging uterus
    – Poor circulation
    – Fatigue
    – Balance in the calcium-phosphorus ratio
- Patient teaching
    – If necessary, assist woman with measures to alter calcium and phosphorus intake
    – Encourage frequent rest periods with the legs slightly elevated
    – Encourage her to wear warm clothing

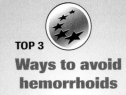

TOP 3

Ways to avoid hemorrhoids

1. Avoid prolonged standing.
2. Lie on left side with feet slightly elevated.
3. Avoid constrictive clothing.

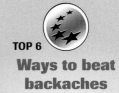

TOP 6

Ways to beat backaches

1. Use proper body mechanics.
2. Maintain good posture.
3. Wear low- to mid-heel shoes.
4. Walk with pelvis tilted forward.
5. Use a board under the current mattress to add firmness.
6. Perform pelvic rocking or tilting exercises.

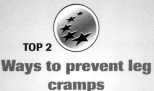

TOP 2

Ways to prevent leg cramps

1. Rest with legs slightly elevated.
2. Wear warm clothing.

Ways to avoid ankle edema

- Lie on the left side in bed to enhance glomerular filtration rate of the kidneys.
- Avoid wearing tight, constrictive clothing.
- Elevate legs during rest periods.
- Dorsiflex the feet when standing or sitting for prolonged periods.
- Get up and move about every 1 to 2 hours when sitting for long periods.

Calculating estimated date of delivery using Nägele's rule

- Determine the first day of the woman's last menses.
- Subtract 3 months.
- Add 7 days.

– Teach her what to do during a leg cramp: pull the toes up toward the leg while pressing down on the knee

● **Shortness of breath**
- Caused by pressure of the uterus on the diaphragm
- Patient teaching
    – Encourage the woman to maintain proper posture, especially when standing
    – Suggest that the woman use semi-Fowler's position when sleeping and use additional pillows for support
    – Encourage a balance of activity and rest

● **Ankle edema**
- Causes
    – Poor venous return from the lower extremities; aggravated by prolonged sitting or standing and by warm weather
    – Fluid retention
- Patient teaching
    – Recommend that the woman lie on her left side in bed to enhance glomerular filtration rate of the kidneys
    – Encourage the woman to avoid wearing tight, constrictive clothing
    – Advise her to elevate her legs during rest periods
    – Urge her to dorsiflex her feet when standing or sitting for prolonged periods
    – Suggest that she get up and move about every 1 to 2 hours when sitting for long periods

ESTIMATED DATE OF DELIVERY

● **Nägele's rule**
- Nägele's rule determines the estimated date of delivery and is considered the standard method
- The procedure is as follows:
    – Ask the woman to state the first day of her last menses
    – Subtract 3 months from this first day of the last menses
    – Add 7 days (for example, October 5 − 3 months = July 5 + 7 days = July 12)

● **Other methods**
- Gestational age wheels
    – Similar to a circular slide rule
    – The circular device consists of the days of the month for a year and arrows to identify the day of the last menses
    – After placing the arrow on the proper date, the user can quickly locate the arrow for the 40th week of gestation to determine the estimated date of delivery

- Calculators that actually determine the estimated birth date
- Computer software programs
  - Determines the estimated date of delivery based on the woman's last menses and information obtained from ultrasound
  - Can be used to determine estimated fetal weight

GESTATIONAL AGE ASSESSMENTS

Fetal movement
- Also called *quickening;* described as a light fluttering
- Is usually felt first between 16 and 22 weeks of gestation
- Typically follows a consistent pattern, usually on the average of at least 10 times per day

Fetal heart sounds (rate)
- Can be detected at 12 weeks of gestation with a Doppler ultrasound
- Can be auscultated at 16 to 20 weeks with a fetoscope (see *Assessing fetal heart rate,* page 72)
- Normal fetal heart rate (FHR) ranges from 120 to 160 beats/minute

Fetal crown-to-rump measurements
- Determined by ultrasonography
- Can be used to assess the fetus's age until the head can be defined

Biparietal diameter
- The widest transverse diameter of the fetal head; a side-to-side measurement obtained using ultrasound
- Measurements can be made by 12 to 13 weeks' gestation
- Typically, if the biparietal diameter is 8.5 cm or more, the fetus will weigh more than 5.5 lb (2,500 g)

Fundal height
- Difficult to interpret
- The measurement can be affected by the patient's weight, polyhydramnios, more than one fetus (multiple gestation), and the fetus's size
- Measuring the height of the uterus above the symphysis pubis reflects the progress of fetal growth and provides a gross estimate about the duration of pregnancy (see *Measuring fundal height,* page 73)
  - The uterus is usually palpable just over the symphysis pubis at 12 to 14 weeks' gestation; at the umbilicus at 20 to 22 weeks' gestation; at the xiphoid process at 36 weeks' gestation
  - The fundus reaches its highest point at about 36 weeks' gestation and then drops about 4 cm by 40 weeks' gestation, when lightening occurs
- McDonald's rule
  - Uses fundal height to determine the duration of a pregnancy in either lunar months or weeks

TOP 3

Ways to assess gestational age

1. Measure the fetus from crown to rump.
2. Measure biparietal diameter.
3. Use McDonald's rule.

Factors affecting fundal height measurements

- Patient's weight
- Polyhydramnios
- Multiple gestation
- Fetus's size

Quick guide to fetal monitoring techniques

- **Amniocentesis** – Transabdominal aspiration of amniotic fluid for analysis
- **CVS** – Removal and analysis of tissue specimen from fetal portion of placenta
- **Ultrasonography** – Noninvasive use of sound waves to determine fetal presence, size, position, and presentation and to detect abnormalities
- **NST** – Noninvasive detection of fetal heart accelerations in response to fetal movement
- **Stress test (OCT)** – Evaluation of fetal ability to withstand decreased oxygen supply and physiologic stress of contractions (simulating labor)
- **Nipple stimulation test** – Noninvasive stress test in which nipple stimulation is used to initiate contractions
- **Vibroacoustic stimulation** – Noninvasive use of vibration and sound to detect fetal reactivity
- **Biophysical profile** – Assessment of fetal breathing, body movements, and muscle tone; amniotic fluid volume; FHR reactivity; and placental grade
- **Fetal blood flow studies** – Use of umbilical or uterine Doppler velocimetry to measure speed of red blood cells
- **PUBS** – Sampling of fetal blood obtained by insertion of needle into uterine wall
- **MSAFP** – Evaluation of maternal blood sample to determine alpha fetoprotein level
- **Triple screen** – Blood sampling to measure maternal serum alpha fetoprotein, unconjugated estriol, and hCG

Assessing fetal heart rate

Fetal heart rate provides important information about fetal well-being. It can be assessed by auscultating the mother's abdomen with a Doppler ultrasound stethoscope or a fetoscope.

After assisting the woman to the supine position and providing privacy, apply water-soluble lubricant to her abdomen or to the monitoring device.

DOPPLER ULTRASOUND STETHOSCOPE
1. Place the earpieces in your ears (if there are no earpieces, turn on the device and adjust the volume).
2. Press the bell or transducer gently on the woman's abdomen.
3. Begin to listen at the midline, midway between the umbilicus and symphysis pubis.

FETOSCOPE
1. Place the earpieces in your ears.
2. Position the fetoscope centrally on your forehead.
3. Gently press the bell about ½″ (1 cm) into the woman's abdomen.
4. Move the instrument slightly from side to side to locate the loudest heart tones.
5. Simultaneously assess the mother's pulse rate for at least 15 seconds.
6. If the maternal pulse rate and fetal heart rate are the same, reposition the device slightly and listen again.
7. If you encounter difficulty, try to locate the fetal thorax by using Leopold's maneuvers.

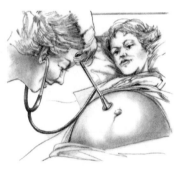

- Fundal height in cm $\times \frac{2}{7}$ = duration of pregnancy in lunar months
- Fundal height in cm $\times \frac{8}{7}$ = duration of pregnancy in weeks
  – Becomes inaccurate during the third trimester because the fetal weight is increasing more than fetal height

MONITORING FETAL STATUS

● **Amniocentesis**
- Refers to a needle insertion into the uterus transabdominally to aspirate amniotic fluid for analysis
- Performed between the 14th and 20th weeks of gestation, when amniotic fluid is sufficient and the uterus has moved into the abdominal cavity

Measuring fundal height

To measure fundal height, use a pliable but nonstretchable tape measure or pelvimeter and follow these steps:
- Help the woman into a supine position and drape her appropriately to provide privacy; expose her abdomen.
- Position one end of the tape measure at the notch of the symphysis pubis.
- Pull the tape measure up and over the woman's abdomen to the top of the fundus, being careful not to tip the corpus of the fundus back.
- Measure the distance in centimeters.

Typically, between the 20th and 32nd weeks of gestation, the fundal height in centimeters corresponds to the week of gestation. Fundal heights greater than or less than the gestational week may suggest a complication. For example, if the fundal height is significantly greater than what is expected, the woman may have a multiple pregnancy, polyhydramnios, or a large-for-gestational-age fetus, or her estimated date of delivery may have been miscalculated. If the measurement is less than what is expected, a small-for-gestational-age fetus, intrauterine growth retardation, or an anomaly may be suspected.

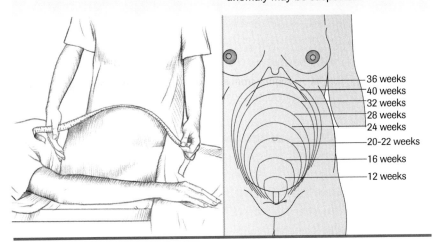

- 36 weeks
- 40 weeks
- 32 weeks
- 28 weeks
- 24 weeks
- 20-22 weeks
- 16 weeks
- 12 weeks

- Is indicated for women age 35 and older and women with family history of chromosomal or neural tube defects or inborn errors of metabolism
- Used for assessment, diagnosis, and evaluation
  - Gestational age assessment via a lecithin-sphingomyelin ratio, presence of phosphatidyl glycerol, creatinine levels, or the delta optical density of bilirubinoid pigments
  - Prenatal diagnosis of genetic disorders, such as chromosomal aberrations, sex-linked disorders, inborn errors of metabolism, and neural tube defects
  - Diagnosis and evaluation of isoimmune disease, including Rh sensitization and ABO incompatibility; Rh negative mothers must receive RhoGAM after amniocentesis
- Contraindicated when the anterior uterine wall is completely covered by the placenta or when amniotic fluid is insufficient

Why use amniocentesis?

- To assess gestational age
- To diagnose genetic disorders
- To diagnose and evaluate isoimmune disease

Maternal complications of amniocentesis

- Amniotic fluid embolism
- Hemorrhage
- Infection
- Abruptio placentae
- Placenta or umbilical cord trauma
- Premature labor
- Bladder or intestinal puncture
- Rh isoimmunization

Rare fetal complications of amniocentesis

- Intrauterine fetal death
- Amnionitis
- Injury from needle puncture
- Amniotic fluid leakage
- Bleeding
- Spontaneous abortion
- Premature birth

Benefits of chorionic villi sampling

- Provides early diagnosis of fetal abnormalities
- Provides complete results within a few days
- Produces less social and psychological stress

- An ultrasound is performed before the amniocentesis to locate the fetus, placenta, and fluid
  - If the woman is under 20 weeks' gestation, ultrasound using a full bladder may be necessary to hold the uterus steady
  - If the woman is over 20 weeks' gestation, typically an empty bladder is necessary for the ultrasound to reduce the risk of bladder puncture
- Amniotic fluid should be clear but may contain white flecks of vernix caseosa when the fetus is near term (see *Amniotic fluid analysis findings*)
- After the procedure, the FHR and uterine activity is monitored frequently for at least 30 minutes using an external fetal monitor
- Maternal complications include amniotic fluid embolism, hemorrhage, infection, abruptio placentae, placenta or umbilical cord trauma, premature labor, bladder or intestinal puncture, and Rh isoimmunization
- Fetal complications, although rare, include intrauterine fetal death, amnionitis, injury from needle puncture, amniotic fluid leakage, bleeding, spontaneous abortion, and premature birth

● **Chorionic villi sampling (CVS)**
- Involves the removal and analysis of a small tissue specimen from the fetal portion of the placenta to determine the genetic makeup of the fetus
  - Chorionic villi are fingerlike projections that surround the embryonic membrane and eventually give rise to the placenta
  - Cells obtained from the sample are fetal (not maternal) allowing analysis for fetal abnormalities (see *Understanding CVS*, page 76)
- Provides an earlier diagnosis because it's best performed between 8 and 10 weeks' gestation), allows an earlier and safer abortion if chosen, and produces less social and psychological stress than amniocentesis because results are received earlier in gestation
  - Preliminary results may be available within hours with complete results in a few days
  - Results of amniocentesis aren't available for at least 2 weeks
- Complications are similar to those for amniocentesis
  - Carries the risk of spontaneous abortion, infection, hematoma, and intrauterine death
  - Research has reported limb malformations in neonates of mothers who have undergone CVS
- Rh-negative mother must receive RhoGAM following CVS

● **Ultrasonography**
- Uses sound waves reflected by tissues of different densities; signals are amplified and displayed on an oscilloscope or screen

Amniotic fluid analysis findings

Amniotic fluid analysis can provide information about the condition of the mother, fetus, and placenta. This table shows normal findings and abnormal findings and their implications.

TEST COMPONENT	NORMAL FINDINGS	FETAL IMPLICATIONS OF ABNORMAL FINDINGS
Color	Clear, with white flecks of vernix caseosa in a mature fetus	Blood of maternal origin is usually harmless. "Port wine" fluid may indicate abruptio placentae. Fetal blood may indicate damage to the fetal, placental, or umbilical cord vessels.
Bilirubin	Absent at term	High levels indicate hemolytic disease of the newborn.
Meconium	Absent	Presence indicates fetal hypotension or distress.
Creatinine	More than 2 mg/dl (SI, 177 µmol/L, in a mature fetus	Decrease may indicate fetus less than 37 weeks.
Lecithin-sphingomyelin ratio	More than 2	Less than 2 indicates pulmonary immaturity.
Phosphatidyl glycerol	Present	Absence indicates pulmonary immaturity.
Glucose	Less than 45 mg/dl (SI, 2.3 mmol/L)	Excessive increases at term or near term indicate hypertrophied fetal pancreas.
Alpha-fetoprotein	Variable, depending on gestational age and laboratory technique	Inappropriate increases indicate neural tube defects, such as spina bifida or anencephaly, impending fetal death, congenital nephrosis, or contamination of fetal blood.
Bacteria	Absent	Presence indicates chorioamnionitis.
Chromosome	Normal karyotype	Abnormal karyotype indicates fetal chromosome disorders.
Acetylecholinesterase	Absent	Presence may indicate neural tube defects, exomphalos, or other serious malformations.

- Noninvasive and painless, obtained abdominally or transvaginally
- Provides immediate results without potential harm to the fetus or the mother
  - Information about fetal presence, size, position, and presentation, placental location, and amniotic fluid
  - Gestational maturity via biparietal measurements
  - Evidence of normal fetal growth or possible defects or malformations

Benefits of ultrasonography

- Noninvasive and painless
- Provides immediate results without potential harm to fetus or mother
- Provides information about fetal presence, size, position, and presentation; placental location; amniotic fluid; and gestational maturity
- Can detect fetal death, malpresentation, placental abnormalities, multiple gestation, and hydramnios or oligohydramnios

Understanding CVS

To collect a chorionic villi sample, place the patient in the lithotomy position. The physician checks the placement of the uterus bimanually, inserts a Graves' speculum, and swabs the cervix with an antiseptic solution. If necessary, he may use a tenaculum to straighten an acutely flexed uterus, permitting cannula insertion. Guided by ultrasound and possibly endoscopy, he directs the catheter through the cannula to the villi. He applies suction to the catheter to remove about 30 mg of tissue from the villi. Next, he withdraws the sample, places it in a Petri dish, and examines it with a microsope. Part of the sample is then cultured for further testing.

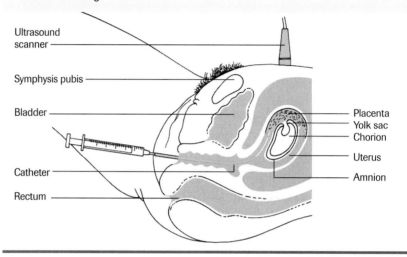

Ultrasound scanner
Symphysis pubis
Bladder
Catheter
Rectum
Placenta
Yolk sac
Chorion
Uterus
Amnion

     – Fetal sex (if a penis is observed)
- Can detect fetal death, malpresentations, placental abnormalities, multiple gestation, and hydramnios or oligohydramnios
- For an abdominal ultrasound, the woman needs to have a full bladder to ensure that the uterus is held steady and that the best sound wave transmission is obtained; for a transvaginal ultrasound, a full bladder is unnecessary

● **Fetal movement**
- Can be identified by the patient 90% of the time
- Is an indicator of fetal well-being
  - An actively moving fetus indicates well-being
  - Changes in the pattern of fetal movement, such as a decrease in frequency or intensity or stoppage, may indicate fetal compromise
- Can be determined using any one of various methods
  - The woman is instructed to count movements while in a comfortable side-lying position, usually after a meal
  - Generally the fetus is expected to move at least 10 times in 1 hour

- Is affected by drugs, cigarette use, sound, time of day, sleep patterns, and blood glucose levels
    - Nicotine has been found to decrease fetal movements
    - Maternal food intake has been found to increase fetal movements

Nonstress test (NST)

- Noninvasive; used to detect fetal heart accelerations either spontaneously or in response to fetal movement
- Provides immediate results simply and inexpensively without contraindications or complications with the use of indirect electronic fetal monitoring
    - Fetal movement typically results in an increase in FHR of about 15 beats/minute
    - This increase should be sustained for about 15 seconds and return to baseline or average when the fetus quiets down
    - Absence of an increase in FHR with movement is highly suggestive of fetal hypoperfusion
- Indicated for suspected fetal distress or uteroplacental insufficiency
- Usually ordered during the third trimester
- Provides information about the possibility of fetal hypoxia, fetal sleep cycle, or the effects of drugs (see *Interpreting NST and OCT results*, page 79)
- Usually performed over 20 to 40 minutes
    - If fetus doesn't move within this time span, possibly because of sleeping, mother may be given a carbohydrate snack to raise her glucose levels, thus stimulating fetal movement
    - Sound may be applied to awaken the fetus or stimulate fetal movement

Stress test (oxytocin challenge test [OCT])

- Method of evaluating fetal ability to withstand decreased oxygen supply and the physiologic stress of an oxytocin-induced contraction before true labor begins
    - I.V. oxytocin is administered, usually starting at 0.5 mU/minute and increasing by 0.5 mU/minute at 15- to 20-minute intervals until three high-quality uterine contractions are obtained within 10 minutes
    - FHR is assessed to evaluate the placenta's ability to provide sufficient oxygen to the fetus
    - FHR pattern is evaluated for early, late, and variable decelerations
- Can be used at 32 to 34 weeks' gestation
- Used for a patient at risk for placental insufficiency or fetal compromise from diabetes, heart disease, hypertension, history of previous stillbirth, renal disease, or a nonreactive NST

Indications for a nonstress test

- Suspected fetal distress
- Suspected uteroplacental insufficiency

Uses for a nonstress test

- Detects fetal heart accelerations
- Checks for fetal hypoxia
- Obtains information about the fetal sleep cycle
- Obtains information about the effects of drugs

What a stress test tells you

- Fetal ability to withstand decreased oxygen supply and physiologic stress of oxytocin-induced contraction
- Late FHR decelerations during two or more contractions or late decelerations that are inconsistent indicate the risk of fetal hypoxia

Stress test results indicating risk of fetal hypoxia

- Late fetal heart rate decelerations during two or more contractions
- Inconsistent late decelerations

Actions in a nipple stimulation stress test

- Sensory receptors in the areola are activated.
- Oxytocin is released.
- Contractions are induced.

Key facts about vibroacoustic stimulation

- Noninvasive
- Quick results
- Artificial larynx or fetal acoustic stimulator applied to abdomen

- Doesn't apply to those with previous classical cesarean delivery or third-trimester bleeding or those at high risk for preterm labor
- Involves the use of an external fetal monitoring system (fetal monitor applied to the mother's abdomen to assess FHR and patter; a tokodynamometer applied to the mother's lower abdomen to monitor contractions)
  - A baseline recording is made, then FHR is monitored and recorded continuously for 20 minutes
  - Oxytocin is administered I.V. as ordered
  - FHR and contractions are monitored and recorded
  - Oxytocin infusion is discontinued to determine the FHR response to the contractions; FHR monitoring is continued for 30 minutes as uterine movements return to normal
- A normal stress test results when FHR is within the normal range of 120 to 160 beats/minute, indicating that the fetus can tolerate the stress of labor (see *Interpreting NST and OCT results*)
  - Maternal hypotension can produce false-positive results
  - A full bladder can displace the uterus and interfere with monitoring
- Late FHR decelerations during two or more contractions or late decelerations that are inconsistent indicate the risk of fetal hypoxia
- Use of oxytocin may precipitate the onset of labor

● **Nipple stimulation stress test (breast self-stimulation test)**
- Noninvasive, less expensive, and less time-consuming than the OCT but carries the risk of hyperstimulation or embarrassment because it can't be controlled if there's hyperstimulation
- May require nipple rolling or application of warm washcloths to one nipple
- Induces contractions by activating sensory receptors in the areola, triggering the release of oxytocin by the posterior pituitary gland
- Exhibits the same reactive pattern as the reactive NST result and the same positive pattern as the abnormal OCT result

● **Vibroacoustic stimulation**
- Noninvasive and convenient; offers quick results
- Uses vibration and sound to induce fetal reactivity during an NST
- Sound is produced using an artificial larynx or fetal acoustic stimulator to apply stimulation for 1 to 5 seconds to the mother's abdomen over the fetus's head

● **Biophysical profile**
- Noninvasive and relatively quick to perform; considered a more accurate assessment than the nonstress test or oxytocin challenge test alone

Interpreting NST and OCT results

This chart lists the possible interpretations of results from a nonstress test (NST) and an oxytocin challenge test (OCT), commonly called a stress test. Appropriate actions are also included.

	INTERPRETATION	ACTION
NST result		
Reactive	Two or more fetal heart rate (FHR) accelerations of 15 beats/minute lasting 15 seconds or more within 20 minutes; related to fetal movement	Repeat NST biweekly or weekly, depending on rationale for testing.
Nonreactive	Tracing without FHR accelerations or with accelerations of fewer than 15 beats/minute lasting less than 15 seconds throughout fetal movement	Repeat in 24 hours or perform a biophysical profile immediately.
Unsatisfactory	Quality of FHR recording inadequate for interpretation	Repeat in 24 hours or perform a biophysical profile immediately.
OCT result		
Negative	No late decelerations; three contractions every 10 minutes; fetus would probably survive labor if it occurred within 1 week	No further action needed now.
Positive	Persistent and consistent late decelerations with more than half of contractions	Induce labor; fetus is at risk for perinatal morbidity and mortality.
Suspicious	Late decelerations with less than half of contractions after an adequate contraction pattern has been established	Repeat test in 24 hours.
Hyperstimulation	Late decelerations with excessive uterine activity (occurring more often than every 2 minutes or lasting longer than 90 seconds)	Repeat test in 24 hours.
Unsatisfactory	Poor monitor tracing or uterine contraction pattern	Repeat test in 24 hours.

- Assesses several variables
  - A total of 4 to 6 variables may be used
  - These variables include fetal breathing movements, fetal body movements, fetal muscle tone, amniotic fluid volume, FHR reactivity, and placental grade
- Each variable is scored as 0 or 2, with 0 indicating an abnormal finding and 2 indicating a normal finding; some institutions use a scoring system of 0, 1, and 2
- The total score is then calculated

Variables assessed in a biophysical profile

- Fetal breathing movements
- Fetal body movements
- Fetal muscle tone
- Amniotic fluid volume
- Fetal heart rate reactivity
- Placental grade

- If 4 variables are measured, then a total score of 8 is considered perfect
- If 5 or 6 variables are measured, then a total score of 10 to 12, respectively, is considered perfect; commonly 5 variables are evaluated
- When using 5 variables, a fetal score of 8 or more indicates a healthy fetus; a score of 6 or less indicates fetal compromise
- This profile is commonly referred to as the fetal Apgar score because scoring is similar to that of the neonatal Apgar score
- Can detect central nervous system depression

● **Fetal blood flow studies**
- Measures the speed at which red blood cells flow through the uterine and fetal blood vessels, using umbilical or uterine Doppler velocimetry
- Aid in evaluating fetal status, especially in patients with hypertension, diabetes, isoimmunization, or lupus
  - Increased vascular resistance may result in placental insufficiency
  - Decreased velocity suggests fetal compromise and is related to a poor outcome
- Indications for testing include the fetus with suspected congenital anomalies or cardiac arrhythmias

● **Percutaneous umbilical blood sampling (PUBS)**
- An invasive procedure during which a needle is inserted through the mother's abdomen and uterine wall into a vessel in the umbilical cord, under direct ultrasound guidance
- Provides direct access to the fetal circulation to obtain fetal blood samples or to transfuse the fetus in utero
  - Fetal karyotyping can be done rapidly
  - Access to the fetal circulation allows for direct drug administration to the fetus
- Used when the fetus is at risk for congenital and chromosomal abnormalities, congenital infection, or anemia
- Also used to assess acid-base balance of fetuses with intrauterine growth retardation
- Can be done anytime after 16 weeks' gestation
- Rh-negative mothers must receive RhoGAM following PUBS

● **Maternal serum alpha fetoprotein (MSAFP) screen**
- Requires a blood sample obtained via venipuncture to evaluate the level of alpha fetoprotein in the mother's serum
  - The fetal liver produces alpha fetoprotein
  - This protein crosses the placenta and appears in the mother's serum
- Elevated MSAFP levels suggest a neural tube defect or other neural tube anomaly

Purposes of PUBS
- To obtain fetal blood sample
- To transfuse blood to the fetus in utero
- To perform fetal karyotyping
- To administer drugs to fetus
- To assess acid-base balance of fetus with intrauterine growth retardation

Fetal complications associated with high MSAFP levels
- Intrauterine death
- Anencephaly
- Spina bifida
- Duodenal atresia
- Omphalocele
- Tetralogy of Fallot
- Turner's syndrome

– Alpha fetoprotein levels rise sharply in 90% of fetuses with anencephaly and in 50% of those with spina bifida

– High MSAFP levels may indicate intrauterine death or anomalies such as duodenal atresia, omphalocele, tetralogy of Fallot, or Turner's syndrome

- Decreased MSAFP levels are associated with Down syndrome
- Definitive diagnosis requires ultrasonography and amniocentesis

● **Triple screen**

- Involves a blood sample that tests three parameters: maternal serum for alpha fetoprotein, unconjugated estriol, and hCG
- May be done in lieu of MSAFP to obtain more accurate and reliable results, usually between 15 to 22 weeks' gestation
- Estimates the likelihood of occurrence of birth anomalies, such as neural tube defects, Down syndrome, or other chromosomal defects such as trisomy 18 and 21
- Decreased levels of all three parameters is considered an abnormal test result

MATERNAL ASSESSMENT

● **Maternal physical examination**

- Breasts
  - Inspection
  - Palpation
- Abdomen
  - Inspection
  - Auscultation
  - Percussion
  - Palpation
- External genitalia
  - Inspection of pubic hair, skin, labia, clitoris, urethral orifice, perineum, and anus
  - Palpation of the mons pubis, inguinal lymphatics, labia, and Skene's and Bartholin's glands
- Speculum examination
  - Cervix
  - Papanicolaou smear
  - Vaginal mucosa
  - Vaginal and rectal culture for group B streptococcus
- Bimanual abdominovaginal palpation
  - Cervix
  - Uterus
  - Cul-de-sac

Triple screen facts

- Tests three parameters: maternal serum alpha fetoprotein, unconjugated estriol, and hCG
- More accurate than MSAFP in measuring maternal serum alpha fetoprotein
- Estimates likelihood of birth anomalies, such as neural tube defects, Down syndrome, or other chromosomal defects (trisomy 18 and 21)
- Decreased levels of all three parameters are considered abnormal

---

Elements of a maternal physical examination

- Breasts
- Abdomen
- External genitalia
- Speculum examination
- Bimanual abdominovaginal palpation
- Rectovaginal palpation
- Smears for cytology

TOP 9

Maternal assessment points

1. Medical problems (past and current)
2. Personal or family history of multiple births, congenital diseases, or deformities
3. Use of prescription and non-prescription drugs
4. First day of last menses
5. History of infections
6. Rubella titer
7. Screen for blood type, Rh, and abnormal antibodies
8. Hepatitis B screen
9. Vaginal and rectal culture for group B streptococcus

Taking the obstetric history

When taking the pregnant patient's obstetric history, ask her about:
- genital tract anomalies
- medications used during pregnancy
- history of hepatitis, pelvic inflammatory disease, acquired immunodeficiency syndrome, blood transfusions, herpes, or sexually transmitted diseases in the patient or her partner
- previous abortions
- history of infertility
- full-term or preterm pregnancies
- duration of labor
- type of delivery
- complications during previous pregnancies and labors
- birthplace, condition, and weight of fetus
- rhesus factor of previous babies
- postpartum problems she experienced after previous pregnancies
- problems with previous infants during first several days after birth.

   – Adnexal area
- Rectovaginal palpation
   – Uterus
   – Adnexal area
   – Cul-de-sac
- Smears for cytology
   – Cervical
   – Endocervical
   – Vaginal

● **Maternal medical and obstetric history**
- Medical history
   – Childhood diseases
   – Surgical procedures
   – Medical problems (such as hypertension, renal, or cardiac disease)
- Family medical history
   – History of multiple births, congenital diseases, or deformities
   – Significant medical problems
- Present medical status
   – Use of prescription and nonprescription drugs
   – Use of alcohol, tobacco, or illegal drugs
   – Conditions that could negatively affect pregnancy (for example, viral infection)
   – Presence of disease, such as diabetes or cardiac disease
- Obstetric history (see *Taking the obstetric history*)
   – Number of pregnancies, abortions (spontaneous and induced), and living children; list total number of pregnancies, number of premature deliveries, number of abortions and miscarriages, number of living children (see *Summarizing pregnancy information*)

Summarizing pregnancy information

Typically, an abbreviation system is used to summarize a woman's pregnancy information. Although many variations exist, a common abbreviation system consists of five digits — GTPAL.

Gravida = the number of pregnancies, including the present one.
Term = the total number of infants born at term or 37 or more weeks.
Preterm = the total number of infants born before 37 weeks.
Abortions = the total number of spontaneous or induced abortions.
Living = the total number of children currently living.

For example, if a woman pregnant once with twins delivers at 35 weeks' gestation and the neonates survive, the abbreviation that represents this information is "10202." During her next pregnancy, the abbreviation would be "20202."

An abbreviated but less informative version reflects only the **G**ravida (the number of times the woman has been pregnant, including the current pregnancy) and **P**ara (the number of pregnancies that reached the age of viability — generally accepted to be 24 weeks regardless of whether the babies were born alive or not). In some cases, the number of abortions may also be included. For example, "G3, P2, Ab1" represents a woman who has been pregnant three times, has had two deliveries after 24 weeks' gestation, and has had one abortion. "G2, P1" represents a woman who has been pregnant 2 times and has delivered once after 24 weeks' gestation.

- History of previous pregnancies (antepartum, intrapartum, and postpartum)
    - Perinatal status of previous neonates
- Current pregnancy
    - First day of last menses
    - Abnormal symptoms (cramping, vaginal bleeding)
    - Attitude toward pregnancy
- Gynecologic history
    - History of infections (cervical, vaginal, or sexually transmitted)
    - Age at menarche; typical menstrual-cycle characteristics
    - Contraceptive use
- Partner's history
    - Age
    - Genetic or medical disorders
    - Alcohol or drug use
- Personal information
    - Age, religion, economic status, and educational level
    - History of emotional or psychiatric disorders
    - Diet practices

● Routine maternal laboratory testing
- Rubella titer to assess immunity to rubella
- Complete blood count to detect anemia or infection

Questions to ask about the current pregnancy

- When was the first day of your last menses?
- Have you been experiencing cramping or bleeding?
- How are you feeling about your pregnancy?

- Blood type, Rh, and abnormal antibodies to identify the fetus at risk for erythroblastosis fetalis or hyperbilirubinemia
- Rapid plasma reagin to detect untreated syphilis
- Serum glucose level to detect gestational diabetes
- Urinalysis and urine culture to test for glucose, protein, blood, acetone, and asymptomatic bacteriuria
- Hepatitis B to screen for hepatitis B surface antigen
- Gonorrhea and chlamydia smears to detect sexually transmitted diseases
- Triple screen between 15 and 20 weeks to identify fetus at increased risk for Down syndrome and neural tube defects
- Vaginal and rectal culture for group B streptococcus

PATIENT COUNSELING

Patient counseling topics

- Prenatal care and birth planning
- Fetal growth and development
- Nutrition
- Available birth settings and alternative methods of birth
- Process and events of labor and delivery
- Perineal and abdominal exercises
- Breathing exercises
- Comfort measures
- Breast-feeding
- Postpartum care

● **Childbirth and parenthood education**
- Classes address the learning needs of the parents-to-be
- Topics include prenatal care and birth planning; fetal growth and development; nutrition; available birth settings and alternative methods of birth; process and events of labor and delivery; perineal and abdominal exercises; breathing exercises; comfort measures, such as anesthesia and analgesia; breast-feeding; and postpartum care
- Various methods are used, including individual teaching and counseling, group discussions and classes, and facility tours presenting available options and services
- Pain management is a key area of childbirth education programs (see *Highlighting childbirth education methods*)
- Classes are also available for siblings and grandparents

● **Danger signs to report immediately**
- Severe vomiting
- Frequent, severe headaches
- Epigastric pain
- Fluid discharge from vagina
- Fetal movement changes or cessation after quickening
- Swelling of the fingers or face
- Vision disturbances
- Signs of vaginal or urinary tract infection
- Unusual or severe abdominal pain
- Seizures or muscular irritability
- Preterm signs of labor such as rhythmic contractions

● **Dental care**
- A dental checkup early in pregnancy and routine examinations and cleaning are encouraged

Highlighting childbirth education methods

Regardless of the childbirth education method used, all methods incorporate the need for a well-informed woman entering labor who is knowledgeable about breathing exercises, able to relax her abdomen, and alter her pain perception by using appropriate techniques. Some of the more common methods are highlighted below.

- Dick-Read method – emphasizes the use of abdominal breathing with contractions to relax the body and reduce pain.
- Bradley method – focuses on muscle-toning exercises during pregnancy combined with the limitation or elimination of foods containing preservatives, animal fat, or large amounts of salt; emphasizes the partner's role in all aspects of the pregnancy and neonatal period; incorporates abdominal breathing and ambulating during labor.
- Kitzinger method – encourages the woman to go with the contractions of labor and delivery rather than fight against them by incorporating progressive relaxation and breathing.
- Lamaze method – incorporates the stimulus response theory for pain control; emphasizes the use of controlled breathing techniques, such as conscious relaxation, cleansing breath, and consciously controlled and second-stage breathing with effleurage (light abdominal stroking), imagery, and focusing to reduce pain.

- Nausea and vomiting, heartburn, and hyperemia of gums may lead to poor oral hygiene and dental caries
- The fetus receives calcium and phosphorus from the pregnant patient's diet, not from her teeth; the belief that a patient loses a tooth for every pregnancy is a fallacy
- Nutritious snacks, such as fresh fruits and vegetables, are recommended to avoid excessive contact of sugar with the teeth

● **Immunizations**
- Immunizations with attenuated live viruses (including mumps and rubella vaccines) shouldn't be given during pregnancy because of their teratogenic effect on the developing embryo
- Vaccinations with killed viruses (including varicella, hepatitis, influenza, tetanus, and diphtheria vaccines) may be given during pregnancy

● **Clothing**
- Clothes should be nonconstrictive
- Low- to mid-heeled shoes are recommended to prevent backache and poor balance
- Comfort is the key

● **Substance abuse**
- Increases the risk of gross structural fetal defects
- Risk is greatest in the first trimester, during organogenesis

TOP 11

Danger signs during pregnancy

1. Severe vomiting
2. Frequent, severe headaches
3. Epigastric pain
4. Fluid discharge from vagina
5. Fetal movement changes or cessation after quickening
6. Swelling of the fingers or face
7. Vision disturbances
8. Signs of vaginal or urinary tract infection
9. Unusual or severe abdominal pain
10. Seizures or muscular irritability
11. Preterm signs of labor such as rhythmic contractions

Vaccinations allowed during pregnancy

- Varicella
- Hepatitis
- Influenza
- Tetanus
- Diphtheria

- Nicotine in cigarettes
  - Causes vasoconstriction
  - Alters maternal and fetal heart rate
  - Alters blood pressure and cardiac output
  - Increases the incidence of low-birth-weight infants
- Alcohol and illicit or recreational drugs
  - Abuse of alcohol can lead to fetal alcohol syndrome
  - Use of illicit or recreational drugs can lead to a wide range of effects in the neonate; it can also increase the mother's risk for infection with hepatitis B or human immunodeficiency virus
  - Cocaine is associated with spontaneous abortion, preterm labor, and intrauterine growth retardation; children may experience learning difficulties

Medications

- A pregnant patient should consult her health care provider before taking any medication
- Prescription medications are categorized as A, B, C, D, and X by the risk to the pregnant woman
  - Category D drugs are those that have clear health risks for the fetus and include alcohol, lithium (used to treat manic depression), and phenytoin (Dilantin), which is used to treat seizure disorders
  - Category X drugs are those that have been shown to cause birth defects and should never be taken during pregnancy
    - Isotretinoin (Accutane) is used to treat skin conditions
    - Diethylstilbestrol (DES), which is used to treat miscarriages
- Over-the-counter medications may also pose a risk to the fetus
  - Aspirin and other drugs containing salicylates aren't recommended during pregnancy
  - Herbal remedies aren't recommended because their effects on pregnancy and the fetus are unknown

Sexuality

- Sexual behavior (coital and noncoital) is usually unrestricted in complication-free pregnancies
- Sexual desire may decrease during the first trimester from discomforts and fatigue
- Sexual desire may increase in the second trimester, when discomforts commonly wane; the woman may have greater sexual satisfaction than before pregnancy because of vascular congestion of the pelvis
- Sexual desire may decrease in the third trimester from increasing fatigue and abdominal size; changes in position and use of water-soluble lubricant may be necessary

---

Nicotine's effects on pregnancy

- Causes vasoconstriction
- Alters maternal and fetal heart rate
- Alters blood pressure and cardiac output
- Increases the incidence of low-birth-weight infants

Medication categories contraindicated in pregnant women

- Category D — these medications create a health risk to the fetus
- Category X — these medications have been shown to cause birth defects

Sexual desire by trimester

- First trimester — may decrease due to discomfort and fatigue
- Second trimester — may increase as discomforts wane
- Third trimester — may decrease due to increasing fatigue and abdominal size

TIME-OUT FOR TEACHING

Teaching about the prenatal period

Be sure to include these topics in your teaching plan for the pregnant patient during the prenatal period:
- physiologic changes and psycho-social adaptations
- possible diagnostic procedures
- common discomforts
- danger signs
- self-care and health promotion activities
- avoidance of medication use
- nutritional requirements and appropriate food choices.

Physical activities
- Exercise promotes circulation and a feeling of well being
- Prenatal exercises increase muscle strength in preparation for delivery and promote restoration of muscle tone after delivery
- Kegel exercises strengthen the pubococcygeal muscle and increase its elasticity
- Walking is considered the best exercise for the pregnant woman
- Swimming is allowed as long as membranes haven't ruptured

Precautions
- The work site should be checked for potential environmental hazards, such as pesticides, anesthetic gas, and such heavy metals as lead and mercury
- Development of obstetric complications may interfere with employment during pregnancy
- Work duties may have to be altered to avoid excessive physical strain; rest periods need to be scheduled to avoid fatigue
- When riding in a car, seat belts should be worn low, under the abdomen
- If a long trip is planned, the woman should get out of the car every hour to walk around
- Airplane travel is permissible in planes with well-pressurized cabins; some airlines have restrictions for women over 7 months pregnant

Breast care
- Proper breast support promotes comfort, retains breast shape, and prevents back strain
- Washing the breasts with clear water and no soap daily is recommended
- Gauze or breast pads may be needed if the woman's secretion of colostrum is significant; these should be changed frequently to avoid excoriation (for additional teaching tips, see *Teaching about the prenatal period*)

Recommended exercises for pregnant patients
- Kegel exercises – strengthen pubococcygeal muscle and increase its elasticity
- Walking – considered best exercise
- Swimming – permitted if membranes haven't ruptured

Precautions for a pregnant patient
- Check the work site for potential environmental hazards, such as pesticides, anesthetic gas, and such heavy metals as lead and mercury.
- Alter work duties to avoid excessive physical strain. Schedule rest periods to avoid fatigue.
- When riding in a car, wear seat belts low, under the abdomen.
- On a long car trip, get out of the car every hour to walk around.
- Travel by air in airplanes with well-pressurized cabins. Note that some airlines have restrictions for women over 7 months pregnant.

TOP 6

Ways to stay nutritionally fit during pregnancy

1. Increase caloric intake to 2,400 kcal/day.
2. Increase protein intake to 60 g/day.
3. Incorporate sources of linoleic acid into the diet.
4. Get plenty of folic acid (800 mg/day).
5. Drink fluoridated water or take a fluoride supplement.
6. Increase sodium intake to 2,469 mg/day.

Good sources of folic acid

- Green, leafy vegetables
- Eggs
- Milk
- Whole-grain breads

NUTRITION DURING PREGNANCY

- **Calories**
  - Requirement exceeds prepregnancy needs by 300 calories/day (from 2,100 kcal/day to 2,400 kcal/day)
    - To support maternal-fetal tissue synthesis
    - To meet increased basal metabolic needs
    - To provide optimal use of protein and tissue growth (see *The Food Guide Pyramid for the pregnant female*)

- **Protein**
  - Requirement exceeds prepregnancy needs by 14 to 16 g/day (from 44 to 46 g/day to 60 g/day)
    - For expansion of blood volume
    - For tissue growth
    - For adequate amino acid intake for fetal development

- **Fats**
  - 20% to 35% of woman's daily calorie intake
  - Linoleic acid
    - Essential for new cell growth
    - Must be supplied by the diet
    - Found in vegetable oils, such as corn, olive, peanut, and safflower oils

- **Vitamins**
  - Intake of all vitamins should be increased
    - Necessary for tissue synthesis and energy production
    - Requirements for fat- and water-soluble vitamins increase
  - Intake of a varied, healthy diet usually supplies the requirements for all of the vitamins except folic acid
  - Folic acid is particularly important
    - Promotes fetal growth and prevents anemia
    - Intake should be increased from 400 to 800 mg/day
    - Sources include green, leafy vegetables; eggs; milk; and whole-grain breads

- **Minerals**
  - Intake of all minerals should be increased, including iodine, calcium, phosphorus, and zinc
  - Drinking fluoridated water is important to aid in tooth formation; if fluoridated water is unavailable, a fluoride supplement should be prescribed

The Food Guide Pyramid for the pregnant female

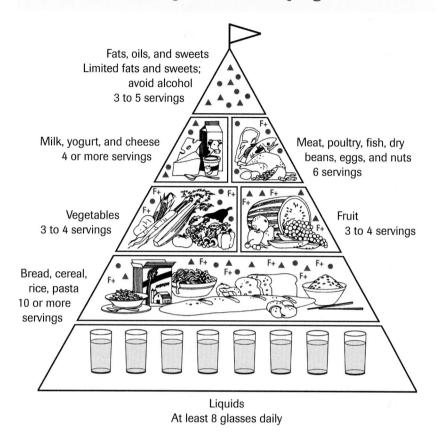

Fats, oils, and sweets
Limited fats and sweets;
avoid alcohol
3 to 5 servings

Milk, yogurt, and cheese
4 or more servings

Meat, poultry, fish, dry
beans, eggs, and nuts
6 servings

Vegetables
3 to 4 servings

Fruit
3 to 4 servings

Bread, cereal,
rice, pasta
10 or more
servings

Liquids
At least 8 glasses daily

Key:
● Fat (naturally occurring and added)
▲ Sugars (added)
F+ Fiber (should be present)

- The average American diet doesn't provide enough iron to prevent iron deficiency anemia; recommended supplemental iron intake is 30 to 60 mg per day
- Sodium restriction is no longer advocated because it has been associated with hormonal and biochemical changes
  - The National Research Council recommends an increase in daily sodium intake of 69 mg over the normal dietary requirement of 2,400 mg
  - Excessive sodium may lead to hypertension by altering fluid and electrolyte balance

The sodium balancing act

- Too little sodium can cause hormonal and biochemical changes.
- Too much sodium may lead to hypertension.

NCLEX CHECKS

It's never too soon to begin your NCLEX preparation. Now that you've reviewed this chapter, carefully read each of the following questions and choose the best answer. Then compare your responses to the correct answers.

1. Which signs are considered presumptive signs of pregnancy? Select all that apply.

- ☐ **A.** Goodell's sign
- ☐ **B.** Uterine enlargement
- ☐ **C.** Ballottement
- ☑ **D.** Nausea with vomiting
- ☑ **E.** Quickening
- ☑ **F.** Linea nigra

2. During pregnancy, what happens to the heart from displacement of the diaphragm? It moves:

- ☐ **A.** upward and to the left.
- ☐ **B.** upward and to the right.
- ☐ **C.** downward and to the left.
- ☐ **D.** downward and to the right.

3. What is a common endocrine system response to pregnancy?

- ☐ **A.** Decreased cortisol levels
- ☐ **B.** Decreased production of prolactin
- ☐ **C.** Increased plasma parathyroid hormone levels
- ☐ **D.** Increased maternal blood glucose levels

4. Which is a common discomfort of the second and third trimesters?

- ☐ **A.** Urinary frequency
- ☑ **B.** Backache
- ☐ **C.** Nasal stuffiness
- ☐ **D.** Nausea and vomiting

5. Which method of estimating date of delivery and gestational age assessments uses measurement of the widest transverse diameter of the fetal head?

- ☑ **A.** Biparietal diameter
- ☐ **B.** Nägele's rule
- ☐ **C.** McDonald's rule
- ☐ **D.** Crown-to-rump measurements

6. What must be done before an amniocentesis?

- ☑ **A.** Ultrasound
- ☐ **B.** Nonstress test
- ☐ **C.** Fundal height measurement
- ☐ **D.** Biparietal diameter

TOP 6

Items to study for your next test on the normal prenatal period

1. Key features of the first, second, and third trimesters of pregnancy
2. Body system responses to pregnancy
3. Ways to cope with the common discomforts associated with pregnancy
4. Way to determine an estimated date of delivery
5. Maternal complications associated with amniocentesis
6. Food sources of folic acid

7. What should the pregnant woman immediately report to her health care provider?

☐ **A.** Heartburn
☒ **B.** Rhythmic regular contractions
☐ **C.** Ankle swelling
☐ **D.** Leg cramps

8. Which test would be used to evaluate the pregnant woman for gestational diabetes?

☐ **A.** Triple screen
☐ **B.** Rapid plasma reagin
☐ **C.** Rubella titer
☒ **D.** Serum glucose level

ANSWERS AND RATIONALES

1. CORRECT ANSWERS: D, E, AND F
Nausea, vomiting, quickening, and linea nigra are presumptive signs of pregnancy. Goodell's sign, uterine enlargement, and ballottement are all probable signs of pregnancy.

2. CORRECT ANSWER: A
During pregnancy, the heart is displaced upward and to the left from pressure of the pregnant uterus on the diaphragm. The heart isn't displaced to the right nor does it move downward.

3. CORRECT ANSWER: C
During pregnancy, plasma parathyroid hormone levels increase, peaking between 15 and 35 weeks of gestation. Cortisol levels and prolactin production increase and the maternal blood glucose level decreases during pregnancy.

4. CORRECT ANSWER: B
A backache is a common discomfort during the second and third trimesters because curvature of the lumbosacral vertebrae increases affecting maternal posture. Urinary frequency and urgency, nasal stuffiness, and nausea and vomiting are common discomforts of the first trimester.

5. CORRECT ANSWER: A
The biparietal diameter uses measurement of the widest transverse diameter of the fetal head. Nägele's rule uses the first day of the patient's last menses, subtracts 3 months and adds 7 days to get the estimated date of delivery. McDonald's rule uses fundal height to determine the duration of a pregnancy. Crown-to-rump measurements are done by ultrasonography and are used to assess the fetal age until the head can be defined.

6. CORRECT ANSWER: A

Before an amniocentesis is performed, an ultrasound must be done to locate the fetus, placenta, and amniotic fluid. A nonstress test is used to assess fetal heart rate accelerations in response to fetal movement. Fundal height measurement is used to roughly assess gestational growth and development. Biparietal diameter is performed during an ultrasound.

7. CORRECT ANSWER: B

Rhythmic regular contractions are considered a danger sign of pregnancy, suggesting the onset of preterm labor. Heartburn, ankle swelling, and leg cramps are common discomforts associated with pregnancy.

8. CORRECT ANSWER: D

Routinely, serum glucose levels are used to screen pregnant women for gestational diabetes. A triple screen is used to identify a fetus at risk for Down syndrome or neural tube defects. Rapid plasma reagin is used to detect untreated syphilis. Rubella titer is used to assess the woman's immunity to rubella.

5

Complications and high-risk conditions of the prenatal period

LEARNING OBJECTIVES

After studying this chapter, you should be able to:

- Describe potential complications of pregnancy.
- Identify the role of the nurse when caring for a patient whose pregnancy is complicated.
- Describe the impact of preexisting conditions on pregnancy.

CHAPTER OVERVIEW

Many women experience complications or are placed at high risk during pregnancy as the result of either a preexisting condition or from the pregnancy itself. These problems may place both the mother and fetus at risk. Nursing care focuses on minimizing the risk to the mother and fetus and ensuring the best possible outcome.

FACTORS CONTRIBUTING TO COMPLICATIONS AND HIGH-RISK STATUS

- **Overview**
  - Most women progress through pregnancy without problems, entering the pregnancy in good health and giving birth to a healthy neonate

Common high-risk conditions in pregnant adolescents younger than age 15

- Pregnancy-induced hypertension
- Anemia
- Labor dysfunction
- Cephalopelvic disproportion
- Low-birth-weight and preterm neonates

Factors that can complicate a pregnancy

- Maternal age
- No recent pregnancies (8 years or more)
- More than five pregnancies of at least 20 weeks' duration
- Pregnancy occurring within 3 months of last delivery
- Presence of a chronic or acute medical condition (especially sickle cell anemia or Tay-Sachs disease)
- Inadequate nutrition
- Exposure to toxic substances
- Cigarette smoking
- Substance abuse

- In some cases problems develop, placing the woman and her fetus in jeopardy
  - These problems may result from a chronic illness that the mother has, a complication that develops during the pregnancy, or some external factor that impacts the health and well-being of the mother or the fetus
  - The cause of the problem may be known or unknown
  - The condition may be the direct result of the pregnancy
  - A preexisting condition may affect the course of the pregnancy and the fetus

● **Factors that place the woman at high risk**
  - Age
    - Adolescents younger than age 15
      - Increased incidence of low-birth-weight and preterm neonates
      - Increased risk of pregnancy-induced hypertension (PIH), anemia, labor dysfunction, and cephalopelvic disproportion
    - Nulliparas who are age 35 and older and multiparas who are age 40 and older
      - Increased risk of placenta previa, hydatidiform mole, and vascular, neoplastic, and degenerative diseases
      - Increased risk of having fraternal twins or infants with genetic abnormalities, especially Down syndrome (trisomy 21)
  - Maternal parity with at least one of the following
    - 8 years or more since last pregnancy
    - Five or more pregnancies of at least 20 weeks' duration
    - Pregnancy occurring within 3 months of last delivery
  - Presence of chronic or acute medical condition
  - Maternal obstetric and gynecologic history with any of the following
    - Two or more premature deliveries or spontaneous abortions
    - One or more still births at term
    - One or more neonates born with gross anomalies
    - Pelvic inadequacy or abnormal shaping
    - Uterine incompetency, position, or structure
    - History of multiple gestations, placental anomalies, amniotic fluid abnormalities, or poor weight gain
    - History of gestational diabetes, PIH, or infection
    - History of delivery of preterm or postterm neonate
    - History of dystocia, precipitous delivery, cervical or vaginal lacerations due to labor and delivery, cephalopelvic disproportion, hemorrhage during labor and delivery, or retained placenta
    - Lack of previous prenatal care or preparation for labor or birth
    - Poor self-care practices

– Pregnancy occurring within 3 years of menarche (increased risk of mortality and morbidity; such a pregnancy also places the patient at risk for delivering a neonate who is small for his gestational age)

- Maternal medical history
  – Exacerbation of a current medical problem
    - Peptic ulcer disease
      - Gastric reflux due to stomach displacement by the gravid uterus
      - Cardiac sphincter relaxation and decreased GI motility caused due to increased progesterone
    - Heart disease
      - Overtaxing cardiac workload due to increase in blood volume and increased cardiac output
      - Potential adverse effect on placental perfusion and subsequently fetal nutrition for a woman with severe heart disease, subsequently leading to the birth of a low-birth-weight neonate
    - Maternal hypertension leading to an increased risk of abruptio placentae
    - Diabetes mellitus
      - Development of insulin resistance, which may require increased amounts of insulin
      - Fetus typically large due to increased insulin production necessary to counteract the overload of maternal glucose, which acts as a stimulator for growth
      - Possibly cephalopelvic disproportion and dystocia for the mother
    - Abdominal trauma possibly leading to premature rupture of membranes or abruptio placentae
- Maternal lifestyle and habits
  – Inadequate nutrition possibly leading to deficiency of iron (associated with low fetal birth weight and preterm birth), folic acid (associated with neural tube defects), or protein (associated with poor fetal development and growth restriction)
  – Exposure to toxic substances such as lead, organic solvents, certain gases (for example, carbon monoxide), and radiation possibly resulting in fetal malformations
  – Ingestion of over-the-counter and prescription drugs detrimental to the fetus
  – Cigarette smoking associated with intrauterine growth retardation and low-birth-weight neonates

Family influences on pregnancy

- Cultural background (sickle cell anemia, Tay-Sachs disease)
- Religious practices (no dairy, immunizations)
- Family history of multiple births, congenital diseases or deformities, and mental disability
- Paternal exposure to environmental hazards
- Environment (history of abuse, lack of support or finances)

– Substance abuse with illicit drugs and alcohol possibly leading to fetal anomalies; when born, neonatal drug withdrawal possible
– Involvement with substance abuse via injection posing an increased the risk of infection with hepatitis B and human immunodeficiency virus
- Family culture and ethnicity
  – Sickle cell anemia occurring primarily in people of African and Mediterranean descent
  – Tay-Sachs disease affecting people of Eastern European Jewish (Ashkenazi) ancestry about 100 times more common than in the general population
  – Religious practices, such as exclusion of dairy products (Seventh-Day Adventists) or no immunizations for communicable diseases such as rubella (Amish) possibly leading to problems with fetal bone growth or development of congenital anomalies (if exposed), respectively
- Family history
  – Some conditions and disorders, such as family history of multiple births, congenital diseases or deformities, and mental disability are considered familial
  – Father's family medical history important because some fetal congenital anomalies are traceable to the father's exposure to environmental hazards
  – Family environment, such as a history of battery or abuse, lack of support, inadequate housing, or lack of adequate finances may increase pregnancy risks

HYPEREMESIS GRAVIDARUM

Definition
- Severe and unremitting nausea and vomiting that persists after the first trimester
- Usually occurs with the first pregnancy and commonly affects pregnant women with conditions that produce high levels of human chorionic gonadotropin (hCG), such as gestational trophoblastic disease or multiple gestations

Pathophysiology
- Exact cause is unknown, but it's linked to trophoblastic activity, gonadotropin production, and psychological factors
- Various possible causes
  – Pancreatitis (elevated serum amylase levels are common)
  – Biliary tract disease
  – Decreased secretion of free hydrochloric acid in the stomach

Key facts about hyperemesis gravidarum

- Severe, unremitting nausea and vomiting after first trimester
- Usually occurs with the first pregnancy
- Exact cause is unknown
- Possible causes include pancreatitis, biliary tract disease, decreased secretion of free hydrochloric acid in the stomach, decreased gastric motility, vitamin deficiency, and psychological factors

– Decreased gastric motility
– Drug toxicity
– Inflammatory obstructive bowel disease
– Vitamin deficiency (especially of B_6)
– Psychological factors (in some cases)
– Transient hyperthyroidism

Assessment findings
- Unremitting nausea and vomiting (cardinal sign), with the vomitus usually containing undigested food, mucus, and small amounts of bile initially, progressing to containing only bile and mucus and, finally, blood and material resembling coffee grounds
- Reports of report substantial weight loss and eventual emaciation
- Thirst
- Hiccups
- Oliguria
- Vertigo
- Headache
- Electrolyte imbalance
- Dehydration
- Metabolic acidosis
- Jaundice

Diagnostic test findings
- Decreased serum protein, chloride, sodium, and potassium levels
- Increased blood urea nitrogen levels
- Elevated hemoglobin levels
- Elevated white blood cell count
- Ketonuria and slight proteinuria

Management
- Restoration of fluid and electrolyte balance with I.V. fluid therapy
- Control of vomiting with an antiemetic
- Maintenance of adequate nutrition and rest
- Progression of diet to oral feedings as tolerated (clear liquid diet, then a full liquid diet and, finally, small, frequent meals of high-protein solid foods); if necessary, total parenteral nutrition

Nursing interventions
- Administer I.V. fluids as ordered until the patient can tolerate oral feedings
- Monitor fluid intake and output, vital signs, skin turgor, daily weight, serum electrolyte levels, and urine ketone levels; anticipate the need for electrolyte replacement therapy
- Provide frequent mouth care

Key interventions for hyperemesis gravidarum

- Administer I.V. fluids as ordered.
- Monitor fluid intake and output, vital signs, skin turgor, daily weight, serum electrolyte levels, and urine ketone levels.
- Suggest decreased liquid intake at mealtime.
- Instruct the patient to remain upright for 45 minutes after eating.
- Suggest that the patient eat two or three dry crackers on awakening.
- Provide reassurance and a calm, restful atmosphere.
- Encourage the patient to discuss her feelings.
- Help the patient develop effective coping strategies.
- Teach the patient measures to conserve energy.

Key facts about gestational trophoblastic disease

- Anomaly of the placenta that converts the chorionic villi into a mass of clear vesicles
- Also called *molar pregnancy*
- Two types: complete (neither embryo nor amniotic sac) or partial (embryo with abnormalities and amniotic sac)
- Major cause of second trimester bleeding
- Associated with choriocarcinoma
- Exact cause unknown

- Consult a dietitian to provide a diet high in dry, complex carbohydrates
- Suggest company, diversionary conversation, and decreased liquid intake at mealtime
- Instruct the patient to remain upright for 45 minutes after eating to decrease reflux
- Suggest that the patient eat two or three dry crackers on awakening in the morning, before getting out of bed, to alleviate nausea
- Provide reassurance and a calm, restful atmosphere
- Encourage the patient to discuss her feelings about her pregnancy and the disorder
- Help the patient develop effective coping strategies
  - Refer her to a mental health professional for additional counseling, if necessary
  - Refer her to the social service department for help in caring for other children at home, if appropriate
- Teach the patient protective measures to conserve energy and promote rest, including relaxation techniques; the importance of fresh air and moderate exercise, if tolerated; and activities to prevent fatigue

● Possible complications

- Substantial weight loss
- Starvation, with ketosis and acetonuria
- Dehydration, with subsequent fluid and electrolyte imbalances (hypokalemia)
- Acid-base imbalances (acidosis and alkalosis)
- Retinal, neurologic, and renal damage

GESTATIONAL TROPHOBLASTIC DISEASE

● Definition

- Developmental anomaly of the placenta that converts the chorionic villi into a mass of clear vesicles; also called *molar pregnancy*
- Two types of moles
  - Complete moles—there's neither an embryo nor an amniotic sac
  - Partial mole—there's an embryo (usually with multiple abnormalities) and amniotic sac (see *Comparing complete and partial moles*)
- Gestational trophoblastic disease is a major cause of second trimester bleeding
- Early detection is necessary because it's associated with choriocarcinoma, a fast growing, highly invasive malignancy

● Pathophysiology

- Exact cause is unknown

Comparing complete and partial moles

Gestational trophoblastic disease may be classified as a complete or partial mole based on chromosomal analysis.

A *complete mole* is characterized by swelling and cystic formation of all trophoblastic cells. No fetal blood is present. If an embryo did develop, it was most likely only 1 to 2 mm in size and died early on. A complete mole is highly associated with the development of choriocarcinoma.

A *partial mole* is characterized by edema of a layer of the trophoblastic villi with some of the villi forming normally. Fetal blood may be present in the villi and an embryo up to the size of 9 weeks' gestation may be present. Typically, a partial mole has 69 chromosomes in which there are three chromosomes for every one pair.

- Researchers believe the condition may be associated with poor maternal nutrition, specifically an insufficient intake of protein and folic acid, a defective ovum, chromosomal abnormalities, or hormonal imbalances
  - About 50% of patients with choriocarcinoma have had a preceding molar pregnancy
  - In the remaining 50%, the disease is usually preceded by a spontaneous or induced abortion, ectopic pregnancy, or normal pregnancy
- With this disorder, the trophoblastic villi cells rapidly increase in size and fill with fluid
  - Trophoblast cells are the cells located in the outer ring of the blastocyst (the structure that develops via cell division around the 3rd to 4th day after fertilization)
  - These cells eventually become part of the structure that forms the placenta and fetal membranes
  - As the cells begin to deteriorate they become filled with fluid
  - The cells become edematous, appearing as grapelike clusters of vesicles
  - As a result, the embryo fails to develop past the early primitive stages

● **Assessment findings**
- Disproportionate enlargement of the uterus; possible grapelike clusters noted in vagina on pelvic examination
- Excessive nausea and vomiting
- Intermittent or continuous bright red or brownish vaginal bleeding by the 12th week of gestation
- Passage of tissue resembling grapelike clusters
- Symptoms of PIH before the 20th week of gestation
- No fetal heart tones

TOP 6

Assessment findings for gestational trophoblastic disease

1. Disproportionate enlargement of the uterus; possible grapelike clusters noted in vagina on pelvic examination
2. Excessive nausea and vomiting
3. Intermittent or continuous bright red or brownish vaginal bleeding by the 12th week of gestation
4. Passage of tissue resembling grapelike clusters
5. Symptoms of PIH before the 20th week of gestation
6. Absence of fetal heart tones

TOP 4
Things to know about gestational trophoblastic disease

1. It causes second trimester bleeding.
2. Early detection is critical.
3. It's associated with choriocarcinoma.
4. Tissue clusters are a key assessment finding.

Key interventions for gestational trophoblastic disease

- Assess the patient's vital signs to obtain a baseline.
- Observe the patient for signs of complications (hemorrhage, uterine infection, vaginal passage of vesicles).
- Encourage the patient and her family to express their feelings, and offer support.
- Help the patient and her family develop effective coping strategies.
- Help obtain baseline information (pelvic examination, chest X-ray, serum hCG levels).
- Stress the need for regular monitoring of hCG levels.
- Instruct the patient to promptly report any new signs and symptoms and to use contraceptives to prevent pregnancy for at least 1 year after hCG levels return to normal.

● **Diagnostic test findings**
- Radioimmunoassay of hCG levels extremely elevated for early pregnancy
- Histologic examination of possible vesicles helps confirm diagnosis
- Ultrasonography performed after the 3rd month revealing grapelike clusters rather than a fetus, no fetal skeleton detected by ultrasound, and evidence of a snowflakelike pattern
- Hemoglobin level, hematocrit, red blood cell (RBC) count, prothrombin time, partial thromboplastin time, fibrinogen levels, and hepatic and renal function findings are all abnormal
- White blood cell count and erythrocyte sedimentation rate increased

● **Management**
- Induced abortion if a spontaneous one doesn't occur
- Follow-up care vital because of increased risk of choriocarcinoma
- Weekly monitoring of hCG levels until they remain normal for 3 consecutive weeks
- Periodic follow-up for 1 to 2 years
- Pelvic examinations and chest X-rays at regular intervals
- Emotional support for the couple who are grieving for the lost pregnancy and an unsure obstetric and medical future
- Avoidance of pregnancy until hCG levels are normal (may take up to 1 year)

● **Nursing interventions**
- Assess the patient's vital signs to obtain a baseline for future comparison
- Preoperatively, observe the patient for signs of complications, such as hemorrhage and uterine infection, and vaginal passage of vesicles, saving any expelled tissue for laboratory analysis
- Prepare the patient for surgery
- Postoperatively, monitor vital signs, fluid intake and output, and patient for signs of hemorrhage
- Encourage the patient and her family to express their feelings about the disorder
- Offer emotional support and help them through the grieving process for their lost infant
- Help the patient and her family develop effective coping strategies, referring them to a mental health professional for additional counseling, if needed
- Help obtain baseline information, including pelvic examination, chest X-ray, and serum hCG levels and help with ongoing monitoring

- When evaluating the serum hCG levels in a woman who has had gestational trophoblastic disease, keep in mind that gradually declining levels suggest no further disease; levels that plateau for three times or increase at any one time, on the other hand, may indicate malignancy
- Stress the need for regular monitoring of hCG levels and chest X-rays to detect any malignant changes
- Instruct the patient to promptly report new signs and symptoms (for example, hemoptysis, cough, suspected pregnancy, nausea, vomiting, and vaginal bleeding)
- Explain to the patient that she must use contraceptives to prevent pregnancy for at least 1 year after hCG levels return to normal and her body reestablishes regular ovulation and menstrual cycles

● **Possible complications**
- Choriocarcinoma

PLACENTA PREVIA

● **Definition**
- Occurs when the placenta implants in the lower uterine segment where it encroaches on the internal cervical os
  - Low implantation—the placenta implants in the lower uterine segment
  - Partial placenta previa—the placenta partially occludes the cervical os
  - Total placenta previa—the placenta totally occludes the cervical os
- One of the most common causes of bleeding during the second half of pregnancy

(See also *Placenta previa,* page 102)

● **Pathophysiology**
- Exact cause is unknown; may be linked to uterine fibroid tumors or uterine scars from surgery
- Factors that may affect the site of the placenta's attachment to the uterine wall include:
  - Defective vascularization of the decidua
  - Multiple gestations (the placenta requires a larger surface for attachment)
  - Previous uterine surgery
  - Multiparity
  - Advanced maternal age

Factors affecting placental attachment

- Defective vascularization of the decidua
- Multiple gestations (the placenta requires a larger surface for attachment)
- Previous uterine surgery
- Multiparity
- Advanced maternal age

Key assessment findings for placenta previa

- Painless, bright red vaginal bleeding after the 20th week of gestation that starts without warning and stops spontaneously
- Bleeding increases with each successive incident
- Soft, nontender uterus
- Leopold's maneuver reveals various malpresentations

Placenta previa

These illustrations show the various forms of placenta previa.

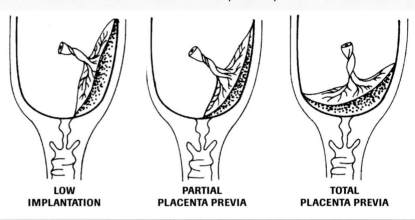

LOW IMPLANTATION   PARTIAL PLACENTA PREVIA   TOTAL PLACENTA PREVIA

- The lower uterine segment of the uterus fails to provide as much nourishment as the fundus
- Placenta tends to spread out, seeking the blood supply it needs, becoming larger and thinner than normal
- Placental villi are torn from the uterine wall as the lower uterine segment contracts and dilates in the third trimester
- As the internal cervical os effaces and dilates, uterine vessels are torn
- Uterine sinuses are exposed at the placental site and bleeding occurs

● Assessment findings

- Painless, bright red vaginal bleeding is most common after the 20th week of gestation, especially during the third trimester
- Initially, scant bleeding is noted, beginning before the onset of labor
  - Typically episodic, starting without warning and stopping spontaneously
  - Bleeding increases with each successive incident
- Palpation may reveal a soft, nontender uterus
- Abdominal examination using Leopold's maneuver reveals various malpresentations due to interference with the descent of the fetal head caused by the placenta's abnormal location
  - Minimal descent of the fetal presenting part may indicate placenta previa
  - The fetus remains active, however, with good heart tones audible on auscultation

● Diagnostic test findings

- Pelvic examination under a double setup (preparations for an emergency cesarean delivery) — because of the likelihood of hemorrhage — to confirm the diagnosis

– Performed only immediately before delivery

– In most cases, only the cervix is visualized

- Laboratory studies may reveal decreased maternal hemoglobin levels (due to blood loss)
- Transvaginal ultrasound scanning is used to determine placental position
- Radiologic tests, such as femoral arteriography, retrograde catheterization, or radioisotope scanning or localization, may be done to locate the placenta

  – These tests have limited value and are risky

  – They're usually performed only when ultrasound is unavailable

Management

- Dependent on when the first episode occurred and the amount of bleeding
- Limitation of maternal activities
- Monitoring of all relevant vital signs
- Emotional support
- Rectal or vaginal examination, which could stimulate uterine activity, shouldn't be performed unless equipment is available for vaginal and cesarean delivery; the placenta can be located via ultrasound
- Vaginal delivery is considered only when the bleeding is minimal and the placenta previa is marginal or when the labor is rapid
- Immediate cesarean delivery performed as soon as the fetus is sufficiently mature or in the case of intervening severe hemorrhage

Nursing interventions

- Teach the patient to immediately identify and report signs and symptoms of placenta previa (bleeding, cramping)
- If the patient with placenta previa shows active bleeding, continuously monitor her blood pressure, pulse rate, respirations, central venous pressure, intake and output, and amount of vaginal bleeding, as well as the fetal heart rate and rhythm
- Anticipate the need for electronic fetal monitoring and assist with application as indicated
- Have oxygen readily available for use should fetal distress occur, evidenced by bradycardia, tachycardia, or late or variable decelerations
- If the patient is Rh-negative, administer $Rh_o(D)$ immune globulin (RhoGAM) after every bleeding episode
- Institute complete bed rest
- Prepare the patient and her family for a possible cesarean delivery and the birth of a preterm neonate, thoroughly explaining postpartum care so the patient and her family know what measures to expect

Managing placenta previa

- Limit activity.
- Monitor vital signs.
- Provide emotional support.
- Refrain from performing rectal and vaginal examinations.

Signs of fetal distress

- Bradycardia
- Tachycardia
- Late or variable decelerations

TOP 3

Life-saving measures for placenta previa

1. Oxygen for fetal distress
2. $Rh_o(D)$ immune globulin for bleeding in Rh-negative patients
3. Betamethasone for fetal lung maturity

Key facts about abruptio placentae

- Premature separation of the placenta from the uterine wall
- Usually occurs after 24 weeks of pregnancy
- Most common in multigravidas
- Fetal prognosis depends on the gestational age and amount of blood lost
- Maternal prognosis is good if hemorrhage can be controlled
- Classified according to the degree of placental separation

- If the fetus isn't mature, expect to administer an initial dose of betamethasone to aid in promoting fetal lung maturity; explain that additional doses may be given again in 24 hours, and possibly in 1 to 2 weeks
- Provide emotional support during labor
  - Because of the neonate's prematurity, the patient may not be given an analgesic and labor pain may be intense
  - Reassure her of her progress throughout labor
  - Keep her informed of the fetus's condition
- Anticipate the need for a referral for home care once the patient's bleeding ceases and she has to return home on bed rest
- During the postpartum period, monitor the patient for signs of hemorrhage and shock caused by the uterus's diminished ability to contract
- Tactfully discuss the possibility of neonatal death
  - Tell the mother that the neonate's survival depends primarily on gestational age, the amount of blood lost, and associated hypertensive disorders
  - Assure her that frequent monitoring and prompt management greatly reduce the risk of death
- Encourage the patient and her family to verbalize their feelings, help them to develop effective coping strategies, and refer them for counseling, if necessary

● Possible complications
- Postpartum hemorrhage
- Infection

ABRUPTIO PLACENTAE

● Definition
- Refers to the premature separation of the normally implanted placenta from the uterine wall
- Usually occurs after 20 to 24 weeks of pregnancy but may occur as late as during first or second stage of labor
- Is most common in multigravidas—usually in women age 35 and older—and is a common cause of bleeding during the second half of pregnancy
- Diagnosis is confirmed when there's heavy maternal bleeding, which generally necessitates termination of the pregnancy
  - Fetal prognosis depends on the gestational age and amount of blood lost
  - Maternal prognosis is good if hemorrhage can be controlled

Degrees of placental separation in abruptio placentae

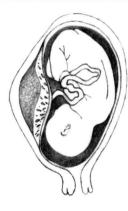 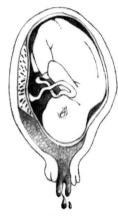 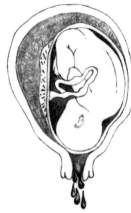

MILD SEPARATION
Mild separation begins with small areas of separation and internal bleeding (concealed hemorrhage) between the placenta and uterine wall.

MODERATE SEPARATION
Moderate separation may develop abruptly or progress from mild to extensive separation with external hemorrhage.

SEVERE SEPARATION
With severe separation, external hemorrhage occurs, along with shock and possible fetal cardiac distress.

- May be classified according to the degree of placental separation and the severity of maternal and fetal symptoms (see *Degrees of placental separation in abruptio placentae*)

● Pathophysiology

- Primary cause is unknown
- Contributing factors include multiple gestations, hydramnios, cocaine use, decreased blood flow to the placenta, and trauma to the abdomen; women with low serum folic acid levels, vascular or renal disease, or PIH are at risk
- Blood vessels at the placental bed rupture spontaneously due to a lack of resiliency or to abnormal changes in uterine vasculature
- An enlarged uterus, which can't contract sufficiently to seal off the torn vessels, and hypertension complicate the situation
- Consequently, bleeding continues unchecked, possibly shearing off the placenta partially or completely
    - Bleeding is external, or marginal (in about 80% of patients), if a peripheral portion of the placenta separates from the uterine wall
    - It's internal, or concealed (in about 20%), if the central portion of the placenta becomes detached and the still-intact peripheral portions trap the blood

Factors contributing to abruptio placentae

- Multiple gestations
- Hydramnios
- Cocaine use
- Decreased blood flow to the placenta
- Trauma to the abdomen
- Low serum folic acid levels
- Vascular or renal disease
- Pregnancy-induced hypertension

Signs and symptoms of abruptio placentae

- **Mild:** gradual onset, mild to moderate bleeding, vague lower abdominal discomfort, mild to moderate abdominal tenderness and uterine irritability, strong and regular fetal heart tones
- **Moderate:** gradual or abrupt onset, moderate, dark red vaginal bleeding, continuous abdominal pain, tender uterus that remains firm between contractions, barely audible or irregular and bradycardic fetal heart tones, possible signs of shock
- **Severe:** abrupt onset of agonizing, unremitting uterine pain; boardlike, tender uterus; moderate vaginal bleeding; rapidly progressive shock; absence of fetal heart tones

Managing abruptio placentae

- Monitoring: maternal vital signs, fetal heart rate, uterine contractions, vaginal bleeding
- Vaginal delivery (depending on the degree and timing of separation) or cesarean delivery (for moderate to severe placental separation)
- Fluid and electrolyte replacement therapy
- Blood transfusion
- Emotional support

- As blood enters the muscle fibers, complete relaxation of the uterus becomes impossible, increasing uterine tone and irritability
- If bleeding into the muscle fibers is profuse, the uterus turns blue or purple and the accumulated blood prevents its normal contractions after delivery (Couvelaire uterus, or uteroplacental apoplexy)

● **Assessment findings**
- Mild abruptio placentae
    - Gradual onset of mild to moderate bleeding
    - Vague lower-abdominal discomfort
    - Mild to moderate abdominal tenderness and uterine irritability
    - Fetal heart tones strong and regular
- Moderate abruptio placentae (about 50% placental separation)
    - Gradual or abrupt onset of moderate, dark red, vaginal bleeding
    - Continuous abdominal pain
    - Tender uterus that remains firm between contractions
    - Barely audible or irregular and bradycardic fetal heart tones
    - Possible signs of shock
    - Onset of labor usually within 2 hours and usually proceeding rapidly
- Severe abruptio placentae (70% placental separation)
    - Abrupt onset of agonizing, unremitting uterine pain (described as tearing or knifelike)
    - Boardlike, tender uterus
    - Moderate vaginal bleeding
    - Rapidly progressive shock
    - Absence of fetal heart tones

● **Diagnostic test findings**
- Pelvic examination under double setup (preparations for an emergency cesarean delivery) and ultrasonography rule out placenta previa
- Decreased hemoglobin levels and platelet counts
- Periodic assays for fibrin split products to monitor progression of abruptio placentae and detect disseminated intravascular coagulation

● **Management**
- Monitoring of maternal vital signs, fetal heart rate (FHR), uterine contractions, and vaginal bleeding
- Likelihood of vaginal delivery depends on the degree and timing of separation in labor
- Cesarean delivery indicated for moderate to severe placental separation
- Evaluation of maternal laboratory values
- Fluid and electrolyte replacement therapy; blood transfusion
- Emotional support

Nursing interventions

- Assess the patient's extent of bleeding and monitor fundal height every 30 minutes for changes
- Draw a line at the level of the fundus, and check it every 30 minutes (if the level of the fundus increases, suspect abruptio placentae)
- Count the number of pads that the patient uses, weighing them as necessary to determine the amount of blood loss
- Monitor maternal blood pressure, pulse rate, respirations, central venous pressure, intake and output, and amount of vaginal bleeding every 10 to 15 minutes
- Begin electronic fetal monitoring to continuously assess FHR
- Have equipment for emergency cesarean delivery readily available
  - Prepare the patient and family members for the possibility of an emergency cesarean delivery, the delivery of a premature neonate, and the changes to expect in the postpartum period
  - Offer emotional support and an honest assessment of the situation
- If vaginal delivery is elected, provide emotional support during labor
  - Because of the neonate's prematurity, the mother may not receive an analgesic during labor and may experience intense pain
  - Reassure the patient of her progress through labor and keep her informed of the fetus's condition
- Tactfully discuss the possibility of neonatal death
  - Tell the mother that the neonate's survival depends primarily on gestational age, the amount of blood lost, and associated hypertensive disorders
  - Assure her that frequent monitoring and prompt management greatly reduce the risk of death
- Encourage the patient and her family to verbalize their feelings
- Help them to develop effective coping strategies, referring them for counseling if necessary

Possible complications

- Maternal mortality is about 6%, dependent on the severity of the bleeding, the presence of coagulation defects, hypofibrinogenemia, and the time lapse between placental separation and delivery
- Postpartum patients at risk for vascular spasm, intravascular clotting or hemorrhage, and renal failure from shock
- Perinatal mortality dependent on the degree of placental separation and fetal level of maturity
- Most serious neonatal complications stem from hypoxia, prematurity, and anemia

---

Key interventions for abruptio placentae

- Assess extent of bleeding and monitor fundal height every 30 minutes for changes.
- Determine the amount of blood loss.
- Monitor maternal blood pressure, pulse rate, respirations, central venous pressure, intake and output, and amount of vaginal bleeding every 10 to 15 minutes.
- Begin electronic fetal monitoring.
- Have equipment for emergency cesarean delivery readily available.
- Reassure the patient of her progress through labor and keep her informed of the fetus's condition.
- Tactfully discuss the possibility of neonatal death.
- Encourage the patient and her family to verbalize their feelings.
- Help them to develop effective coping strategies.

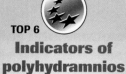

TOP 6

Indicators of polyhydramnios

1. Severe dyspnea
2. Orthopnea
3. Edema of the vulva, legs, and abdomen
4. Significant uterine enlargement
5. Difficulty outlining the fetal parts
6. Difficulty detecting fetal heart tones

Severe signs and symptoms of polyhydramnios

- Dyspnea
- Orthopnea
- Edema of the vulva, legs, and abdomen

Managing polyhydramnios

- High-protein, low-sodium diet
- Mild sedation
- Indomethacin (Indocin)
- Amniocentesis
- Induction of labor (if the fetus is mature and symptoms are severe)

POLYHYDRAMNIOS

● Definition
- Also termed hydramnios
- Refers to an abnormally large amount of amniotic fluid in the uterus
- Normally, amniotic fluid volume ranges from 500 to 1,000 ml at term; with polyhydramnios, the amount typically is greater than 2,000 ml
- Fluid may have increased gradually (chronic type) by the third trimester or rapidly (acute type) between 20 and 24 weeks' gestation

● Pathophysiology
- Exact cause unknown in about 35% of all cases
- It may be associated with diabetes mellitus (about 25%), erythroblastosis (about 10%), multiple gestations (about 10%), and anomalies of the central nervous system, such as neural tube defects, or GI anomalies that prevent ingestion of the amniotic fluid (about 20%)
- Normally, amniotic fluid is produced by the membrane cells and from fetal urine
  - This fluid is swallowed by the fetus and then absorbed through the intestinal membranes, eventually being transferred across the placenta
  - With polyhydramnios, fluid accumulates due to a problem with the fetus's ability to swallow or absorb the fluid or due to overproduction of urine

● Assessment findings
- Signs and symptoms depend on the length of gestation, the amount of amniotic fluid, and whether the disorder is chronic or acute
- Mild signs and symptoms include abdominal discomfort, slight dyspnea, and edema of feet and ankles
- Severe signs and symptoms include severe dyspnea, orthopnea, and edema of the vulva, legs, and abdomen
- Symptoms common to mild and severe cases include uterine enlargement greater than expected for the length of gestation, and difficulty in outlining the fetal parts and in detecting fetal heart tones

● Diagnostic test findings
- Ultrasonography reveals evidence of excess amniotic fluid
- It also reveals underlying conditions

● Management
- High-protein, low-sodium diet
- Mild sedation
- Indomethacin (Indocin), which crosses the placenta to decrease fetal urine production leading to a decrease in amniotic fluid
- Amniocentesis to remove excess fluid
- Induction of labor if the fetus is mature and symptoms are severe

Nursing interventions

- Maintain bed rest to aid in increasing ureteroplacental perfusion and decreasing pressure on the cervix
- Monitor the patient for signs and symptoms of premature labor
- Encourage the patient to avoid straining on defecation, which may increase uterine pressure leading to membrane rupture
- Immediately report any complaints of increasing dyspnea
- Monitor vital signs frequently, including fetal heart rate for changes
- Prepare the woman for amniocentesis and possible labor induction as appropriate; keep in mind that amniocentesis for fluid removal is only temporary and may need to be done repeatedly

Possible complications

- Prolapsed umbilical cord when membranes rupture
- Increased incidence of malpresentations and increased perinatal mortality from fetal malformations and premature deliveries
- Increased incidence of postpartum maternal hemorrhage

OLIGOHYDRAMNIOS

Definition

- Amniotic fluid volume is severely reduced (typically, the amount is less than 500 ml at term) and the fluid is highly concentrated
- May result in prolonged, dysfunctional labor usually beginning before term
- Places the fetus at risk for various conditions
  - Renal anomalies
  - Pulmonary hypoplasia
  - Wrinkled, leathery skin
  - Increased skeletal deformities
  - Fetal hypoxia

Pathophysiology

- Exact cause is unknown
- The condition is associated with obstruction of the fetal urinary tract; in some cases, fetal kidneys fail to develop
- Placental blood flow is inadequate; premature rupture of the membranes may occur

Assessment findings

- Patients are typically asymptomatic

Diagnostic test findings

- Ultrasonography reveals no pocket larger than 1 cm

Management

- Close medical supervision of the mother and fetus
- Fetal monitoring

- Amnioinfusion (infusion of warmed sterile normal saline or lactated Ringer's solution) to treat or prevent variable decelerations

● **Nursing interventions**
- Monitor maternal and fetal status closely
  - Monitor vital signs and fetal heart rate patterns
  - Monitor maternal weight gain pattern, notifying health care provider if weight loss occurs
- Provide emotional support before, during, and after ultrasonography
- Assist parents with coping measures if fetal anomalies are suspected
- Instruct the mother in signs and symptoms of labor, including possible danger signs
- Reinforce the need for close supervision and follow-up
- Assist with amnioinfusion as indicated
  - Encourage the woman to lie on her left side to prevent pressure on the vena cava
  - Ensure that solution is warmed to woman's body temperature to prevent chilling of the mother and fetus
  - Continuously monitor maternal vital signs and fetal heart rate during procedure
  - Note development of any uterine contractions, notify the health care provider, and continue to monitor closely
  - Maintain strict sterile technique during the procedure
  - Watch for continuous fluid drainage via the vagina; report any sudden cessation of fluid flow, which suggests fetal head engagement leading to fluid retention within the uterus and possible development of hydramnios

● **Possible complications**
- Dystocia
- Umbilical cord compression
- Abnormalities in fetal heart rate patterns, such as variable decelerations and reduced variability

ECTOPIC PREGNANCY

● **Definition**
- Refers to the implantation of the fertilized ovum outside the uterine cavity
- Most ectopic pregnancies occur in a fallopian tube; other sites include the cervix, ovary, or abdominal cavity (see *Sites of ectopic pregnancies*)
- Is the second most common cause of vaginal bleeding during pregnancy
- Is a significant cause of maternal death due to hemorrhage

Possible complications of oligohydramnios

- Dystocia
- Umbilical cord compression
- Abnormalities in fetal heart rate patterns

Key facts about ectopic pregnancy

- Implantation of the fertilized ovum outside the uterine cavity
- Most occur in fallopian tube; other sites include the cervix, ovary, or abdominal cavity
- Second most common cause of vaginal bleeding during pregnancy
- Significant cause of maternal death due to hemorrhage

Sites of ectopic pregnancies

In most women with ectopic pregnancies, the ovum implants in the fallopian tube, either in the fimbria, ampulla, or isthmus. Other sites of implantation are possible and include the interstitium, tubo-ovarian ligament, ovary, abdominal viscera, and internal cervical os.

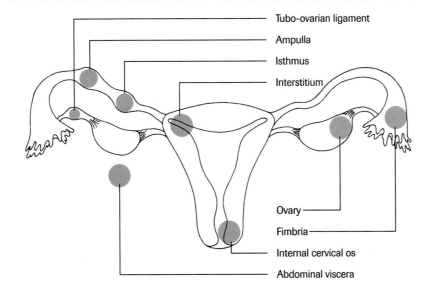

Tubo-ovarian ligament
Ampulla
Isthmus
Interstitium
Ovary
Fimbria
Internal cervical os
Abdominal viscera

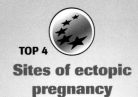

TOP 4

Sites of ectopic pregnancy

1. Fallopian tube (fimbria, ampulla, or isthmus)
2. Ovary
3. Cervical os (internal)
4. Abdominal viscera

Conditions likely to contribute to ectopic pregnancy

- Endosalpingitis
- Diverticula
- Tumors that press against the fallopian tube
- Previous surgery
- Transmigration of the ovum

● Pathophysiology

- Ectopic pregnancies result from any condition that prevents or retards the passage of a fertilized ovum through the fallopian tube, such as hormonal factors, tubal damage from previous pelvic or tubal surgery, damage from pelvic inflammatory disease, tubal atony, tubal spasms, and malformed fallopian tubes
    - Endosalpingitis, an inflammatory reaction that causes folds of the tubal mucosa to agglutinate, narrowing the tube
    - Diverticula, the formation of blind pouches that cause tubal abnormalities
    - Tumors pressing against the tube
    - Previous surgery (tubal ligation or resection, or adhesions from previous abdominal or pelvic surgery)
    - Transmigration of the ovum (from one ovary to the opposite tube), resulting in delayed implantation
- Ectopic pregnancy may also result from congenital defects in the reproductive tract or ectopic endometrial implants in the tubal mucosa
- The increased prevalence of sexually transmitted tubal infection may also be a factor as may the use of an intrauterine device, which causes irritation of the cellular lining of the uterus and the fallopian tubes

Key assessment findings for ectopic pregnancy

- Normal pregnancy symptoms or no symptoms other than mild abdominal pain
- Amenorrhea or abnormal menses
- Slight vaginal bleeding and unilateral pelvic pain over the mass
- Abnormally low hCG titers
- Sudden, severe abdominal pain radiating to the shoulder
- Boggy and tender uterus
- Syncope
- Nausea and vomiting
- Shock (with profuse hemorrhage)

● **Assessment findings**
- Symptoms of normal pregnancy or no symptoms other than mild abdominal pain (the latter especially likely in abdominal pregnancy)
  – Amenorrhea or abnormal menses (after fallopian tube implantation)
  – Slight vaginal bleeding and unilateral pelvic pain over the mass
  – Abnormally low hCG titers
- Rupture of the tube produces sudden, severe abdominal pain often radiating to the shoulder as the abdomen fills with blood
  – Pain is commonly precipitated by activities that increase abdominal pressure, such as a bowel movement
  – Extreme pain with movement of the cervix and adnexal palpation during pelvic examination
  – Uterus boggy and tender
  – Rectal pressure if blood collects in Douglas' cul-de-sac
  – Syncope
  – Nausea and vomiting
  – Shock with profuse hemorrhage

● **Diagnostic test findings**
- Serum pregnancy (hCG) test result shows an abnormally low level of hCG; when repeated in 48 hours, the level remains lower than the levels found in a normal intrauterine pregnancy
- Real-time ultrasonography determination of intrauterine pregnancy or ovarian cyst (performed if serum pregnancy test results are positive)
- Culdocentesis (aspiration of fluid from the vaginal cul-de-sac) detects free blood in the peritoneum (performed if ultrasonography detects absence of a gestational sac in the uterus)
- Laparoscopy may reveal pregnancy outside the uterus (performed if culdocentesis is positive)

● **Management**
- Laparascopic removal of the ruptured tube (salpingectomy); if ovarian pregnancy, oophorectomy
- Incision into the tube to remove the pregnancy (salpingostomy)
- Methotrexate administered to stop division of embryo
- Careful follow-up of hCG levels until not detectable
- Supportive treatment, including transfusion with whole blood or packed RBCs to replace excessive blood loss, administration of a broad-spectrum I.V. antibiotic for sepsis, administration of supplemental iron (given orally or I.M.), and institution of a high-protein diet
- Emotional support for parents grieving over the loss of the pregnancy

Managing ectopic pregnancy

- Laparascopic removal of the ruptured tube; if ovarian pregnancy, oophorectomy
- Salpingostomy
- Methotrexate to stop division of embryo
- Supportive treatment
- Emotional support

● **Nursing interventions**
- Ask the patient the date of her last menses and obtain serum hCG levels as ordered
- Assess vital signs and monitor vaginal bleeding for extent of fluid loss
- Check the amount, color, and odor of vaginal bleeding; monitor pad count
- Withhold oral food or fluid (maintain nothing-by-mouth status) in anticipation of possible surgery; prepare the patient for surgery, as indicated
- Assess the patient for signs and symptoms of hypovolemic shock secondary to blood loss from tubal rupture, and monitor urine output closely for a decrease suggesting fluid volume deficit
- Administer blood transfusions (for replacement) as ordered and provide emotional support
- Record the location and character of the pain, and administer an analgesic as ordered
- Determine if the patient is Rh-negative; if she is, administer $Rh_o(D)$ immune globulin (RhoGAM) as ordered after treatment or surgery
- Provide a quiet, relaxing environment, and offer the patient emotional support
  - Encourage her and her partner to express their feelings of fear, loss, and grief
  - Help her to develop effective coping strategies
  - Refer her to a mental health professional for additional counseling, if necessary
- To prevent recurrent ectopic pregnancy, urge the patient to have pelvic infections treated promptly to prevent diseases of the fallopian tube
- Inform patients who have undergone surgery involving the fallopian tubes or those with confirmed pelvic inflammatory disease that they're at increased risk for another ectopic pregnancy

● **Possible complications**
- Rupture of the tube causes life-threatening complications, including hemorrhage, shock, and peritonitis
- Infertility results if the uterus or both fallopian tubes or both ovaries are removed

ISOIMMUNIZATION

● **Definition**
- Also known as *Rh sensitivity*
- Refers to a condition in which the pregnant woman is Rh negative but her fetus is Rh positive

TOP 4

Things to know about ectopic pregnancy

1. Fertilized ovum is implanted outside the uterus.
2. The most common site is the fallopian tube.
3. Patient may experience normal symptoms of pregnancy.
4. Laparoscopy or oophorectomy may be necessary.

Key facts about isoimmunization

- Also known as *RH sensitivity*
- Condition in which the pregnant woman is Rh negative but her fetus is Rh positive
- Left untreated, can lead to hemolytic disease in the neonate

TOP 3

Test findings in isoimmunization

1. Increased concentration of bilirubin and RBC break-down products in amniotic fluid
2. Anti-D antibody titer of 1:16 or greater
3. Edema revealed in radiologic studies

Managing isoimmunization

- Monitoring of the indirect Coombs' test
- Delta optical density analysis of amniotic fluid at 26 weeks
- Intrauterine transfusion
- Emotional support to parents
- Administration of $Rh_o(D)$ im-munoglobulin

- If left untreated, isoimmunization can lead to hemolytic disease in the neonate
- Before the development of $Rh_o(D)$ immune globulin (human), this condition was a major cause of kernicterus and neonatal death

● **Pathophysiology**
- With isoimmunization, an antigen-antibody immunologic reaction within the body occurs when an Rh-negative pregnant patient carries an Rh-positive fetus
- During the woman's first pregnancy, an Rh-negative female becomes sensitized by exposure to Rh-positive fetal blood antigens inherited from the father
- A female may also become sensitized from receiving blood transfu-sions with alien Rh antigens, causing agglutinins to develop; from in-adequate doses of $Rh_o(D)$; or from failure to receive $Rh_o(D)$ after sig-nificant fetal-maternal leakage from abruptio placentae
- Subsequent pregnancy with an Rh-positive fetus provokes increasing amounts of maternal agglutinating antibodies to cross the placental barrier, attach to Rh-positive cells in the fetus, and cause hemolysis and anemia
- To compensate for this, the fetus steps up the production of RBCs, and erythroblasts (immature RBCs) appear in the fetal circulation
- Extensive hemolysis results in the release of large amounts of uncon-jugated bilirubin, which the liver can't conjugate and excrete, causing hyperbilirubinemia and hemolytic anemia (see *Pathogenesis of Rh iso-immunization*)

● **Assessment findings**
- None (mother asymptomatic)

● **Diagnostic test findings**
- Increased concentration (optical density) of bilirubin and RBC break-down products in the amniotic fluid
- An anti-D antibody titer of 1:16 or greater
- Radiologic studies possibly showing edema and, in those with hy-drops fetalis, the halo sign (edematous, elevated, subcutaneous fat layers) and the Buddha position (fetus' legs are crossed)

● **Management**
- Monitoring of the indirect Coombs' test (measures the amount of an-tibodies in the maternal blood)
- Delta optical density analysis of the amniotic fluid at 26 weeks
- Intrauterine transfusion
- Emotional support to the parents
- Possible early delivery of the fetus

Pathogenesis of Rh isoimmunization

Rh isoimmunization spans pregnancies in Rh-negative mothers who give birth to Rh-positive neonates. The illustrations below outline the process of isoimmunization.

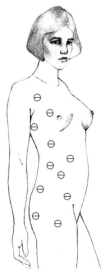

1. Before pregnancy, the woman has Rh-negative blood.

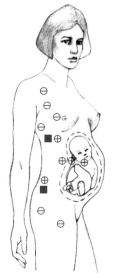

2. She becomes pregnant with an Rh-positive fetus. Normal antibodies appear.

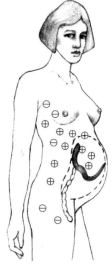

3. Placental separation occurs.

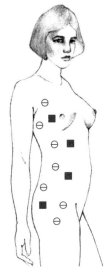

4. After delivery, the mother develops anti–Rh-positive antibodies.

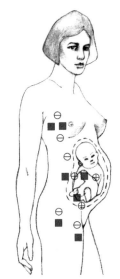

5. With the next Rh-positive fetus, antibodies enter fetal circulation, causing hemolysis.

Key

Rh– blood ⊖

Rh+ blood ⊕

Normal antibodies ■

When to administer RhoGAM to an Rh-negative woman

- After a transfusion reaction
- After an ectopic pregnancy
- After a spontaneous or induced abortion
- After amniocentesis or abruptio placentae
- After abdominal trauma
- At 28 weeks' gestation
- After delivery of a neonate with $Rh_0(D)$-positive blood

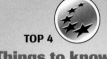

TOP 4

Things to know about isoimmunization

1. The mother is Rh negative but her fetus is Rh positive.
2. An antigen-antibody immunologic reaction results.
3. Large amounts of unconjugated bilirubin are released.
4. Hyperbilirubinemia and hemolytic anemia result.

Administering RhoGAM

RhoGAM is a concentrated solution of immune globulin containing $Rh_0(D)$ antibodies. Intramuscular (I.M.) injection keeps the Rh-negative mother from producing active antibody responses and forming anti-$Rh_0(D)$ to Rh-positive fetal blood cells and endangering future Rh-positive neonates.

RhoGAM is indicated for the Rh-negative mother after abortion, ectopic pregnancy, or delivery of a neonate having $Rh_0(D)$-positive or Du-positive blood and Coombs'-negative cord blood, accidental transfusion of Rh-positive blood, amniocentesis, abruptio placentae, or abdominal trauma. It's given within 72 hours to prevent future maternal sensitization. Administration at about 28 weeks' gestation can also protect the fetus of the Rh-negative mother.

RhoGAM is given I.M. into the gluteal site. When administering RhoGAM, the same steps are followed as for any I.M. injection. However, be sure to also include the following:
- Check the vial's identification numbers with another nurse and sign the triplicate form that comes with the RhoGAM.
- Attach the top copy to the patient's chart.
- Send the remaining two copies along with the empty RhoGAM vial to the laboratory or blood bank.
- Give the woman a card indicating her Rh-negative status and instruct her to carry it with her or keep it in a convenient location.

- Administration of $Rh_0(D)$ immunoglobulin at 28 weeks' gestation and within 72 hours following delivery of Rh-positive neonate to attain passive antibody protection for future pregnancies

● **Nursing interventions**
- Assess all pregnant women for possible Rh incompatibility
- Expect to administer $Rh_0(D)$ I.M. as ordered to all Rh-negative women after transfusion reaction, ectopic pregnancy, or spontaneous or induced abortion, or during the second and third trimester to patients with abruptio placentae, placenta previa, or amniocentesis (see *Administering RhoGAM*)
- Administer RhoGAM as ordered to Rh-negative women at 28 weeks' gestation and within 72 hours after delivery as ordered
- Assist with intrauterine transfusion as indicated
  - Beforehand, obtain a baseline fetal heart rate (FHR) through electronic monitoring, and explain to the patient the procedure and its purpose
  - Afterward, carefully observe the patient for uterine contractions and fluid leakage from the puncture site
  - Monitor FHR for tachycardia or bradycardia
- Prepare the patient for a planned delivery, usually 2 to 4 weeks before term date, depending on maternal history, serologic tests, and amniocentesis

- Assist with labor induction if indicated from the 34th to 38th week of gestation
    - During labor, monitor the fetus electronically and obtain capillary blood scalp sampling to determine acid-base balance
    - An indication of fetal distress necessitates immediate cesarean delivery
- Provide emotional support to the mother and family, encouraging them to express their fears concerning possible complications of treatment

● **Possible complications**
- Hemolytic disease in the neonate

CYSTITIS

● **Definition**
- Refers to an inflammation and infection of the lower urinary tract
- Involves the bladder

● **Pathophysiology**
- Cystitis, in a pregnant woman, is typically the result of vesicoureteral reflux, urinary stasis, and compression of the ureters
- During pregnancy the ureters dilate secondary to the effects of progesterone, which results in urinary stasis
- Additionally, pregnancy results in mild glycosuria, providing a good medium for organism growth

● **Assessment findings**
- Burning on urination
- Urinary urgency and frequency
- Temperature of 101° F (38.3° C)

● **Diagnostic test findings**
- Urine culture positive for the causative organism; greater than 100,000 organisms/ml of urine
- Sensitivity identification of appropriate antibiotic

● **Management**
- Proper perineal hygiene
- Increased fluid intake
- Urine culture to identify organism
- Medication therapy
    - An oral sulfonamide may be used in early pregnancy; use in later pregnancy can cause neonatal hyperbilirubinemia and kernicterus
    - Ampicillin (Amcill), amoxicillin, and cephalosporins are safe for use during pregnancy
    - Tetracyclines are contraindicated because they can slow fetal bone growth and cause staining of the teeth

TOP 3
Causes of cystitis
1. Vesicoureteral reflux
2. Urinary stasis
3. Compression of the ureters

Key assessment findings for cystitis
- Burning on urination
- Urinary urgency and frequency
- Temperature of 101° F (38.3° C)

Managing cystitis
- Proper perineal hygiene
- Increased fluid intake
- Urine culture to identify organism
- Oral sulfonamide in early pregnancy
- Ampicillin, amoxicillin, and cephalosporins (safe for use during pregnancy)

TOP 3

Ways to prevent recurrent cystitis

1. Wipe the perineum from front to back and clean it with soap and water after bowel movements.
2. If infection-prone, urinate immediately after sexual intercourse.
3. Never postpone urination; empty the bladder completely.

Key facts about pyelonephritis

- Inflammation and infection of the upper urinary tract
- Can affect renal pelvis, interstitial tissue, renal tubules, and kidneys
- Commonly an extension of a lower urinary tract infection

● **Nursing interventions**
- Collect all urine specimens for culture and sensitivity testing carefully and promptly
- Explain that an uncontaminated midstream urine specimen is essential for accurate diagnosis (before collection, teach the woman to clean the perineum properly and to keep the labia separated during urination)
- Evaluate the patient's voiding pattern, and monitor urine output (volume and characteristics)
- Urge the patient to drink about 3 to 4 qt (3 to 4 L) of fluids a day during treatment; more or less than this amount may alter the effect of the antimicrobial
- Suggest the woman assume a knee-chest position for about 15 minutes at least once, but ideally twice, per day to help alleviate pressure on the bladder, thus promoting urine drainage
- Explain the nature and purpose of antimicrobial therapy
  – Emphasize the importance of completing the prescribed course of therapy
  – Also emphasize the importance of strictly adhering to the prescribed dosage
- Familiarize the patient with prescribed medications and their possible adverse effects
  – If antibiotics cause GI distress, suggest the taking the medication with milk or a meal if appropriate
  – Monitor the patient for GI disturbances from antimicrobial therapy and for other possible adverse reactions
- To prevent recurrent cystitis, teach the woman steps to prevent it
  – Advise her to carefully wipe the perineum from front to back and to thoroughly clean it with soap and water after bowel movements
  – If she's infection-prone, she should urinate immediately after sexual intercourse
  – Tell her never to postpone urination and to empty her bladder completely
- Warn the patient that infection may recur later in pregnancy when urinary stasis increases due to pressure on the bladder from the enlarging uterus

● **Possible complications**
- Pyelonephritis
- Preterm labor

PYELONEPHRITIS

● **Definition**
- Refers to an inflammation and infection of the upper urinary tract due to bacterial invasion

- Commonly this infection involves the renal pelvis and interstitial tissue; occasionally it can involve the renal tubules
- One or both kidneys may be affected

● **Pathophysiology**
- Pyelonephritis commonly results from the extension of an infection in the lower urinary tract
- Typically the infection spreads from the bladder to the ureters and then to the kidneys, commonly through vesicoureteral reflux
- Bacteria refluxed to intrarenal tissues may quickly create colonies of infection

● **Assessment findings**
- Severe colicky pain
- Vomiting
- Dehydration
- Sudden onset with chills
- Temperature of 103° to 105° F (39.4° to 40.6° C)
- Flank pain, commonly on the right side

● **Diagnostic test findings**
- Pyuria (pus in urine)
- Urine sediment revealing leukocytes singly, in clumps, and in casts and possibly a few RBCs
- Significant bacteriuria; urine culture revealing more than 100,000 organisms/µl of urine
- Low specific gravity and osmolality and slightly alkaline urine pH
- Complete blood count revealing elevations in white blood cell count (up to 40,000/µl), neutrophil count, and erythrocyte sedimentation rate

● **Management**
- Urine culture
- Hospitalization
- I.V. antibiotics
- Monitoring of fluid intake and output
- Vital signs
- Laboratory reports
- Monitoring fetal status

● **Nursing interventions**
- Administer an antipyretic for fever as ordered; offer comfort measures to decrease temperature such as cool washcloths
- Administer plenty of fluids to achieve a urine output of more than 2,000 ml/day
    – This helps empty the bladder of contaminated urine
    – It's also the best way to prevent calculus formation
- Obtain urine cultures as ordered; ensure specimen gets to the laboratory within 30 minutes of collection to prevent overgrowth of bacteria

Key assessment findings for pyelonephritis

- Severe colicky pain
- Vomiting
- Dehydration
- Sudden onset with chills
- Temperature of 103° to 105° F (39.4° to 40.6° C)
- Flank pain, commonly on the right side

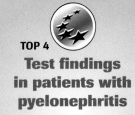

TOP 4

Test findings in patients with pyelonephritis

1. Pyuria
2. Elevated white blood cell count
3. Elevated neutrophil count
4. Elevated erythrocyte sedimentation rate

Managing pyelonephritis

- Hospitalization
- I.V. antibiotics
- Monitoring of maternal vital signs and intake and output
- Monitoring of fetal status

- Assess the patient's vital signs, including temperature, regularly to determine response to therapy; assess fetal heart rate pattern for changes
- Check the patient's voiding pattern and urine characteristics for evidence of improvement or complications; closely measure intake and output
- Instruct patient to avoid bacterial contamination by wiping the perineum from front to back after bowel movements and to void when the urge occurs
- Teach proper technique for collecting a clean-catch urine specimen
- Stress the need to complete the prescribed antibiotic regimen even after symptoms subside; encourage long-term follow-up care

● **Possible complications**
- Preterm labor
- Premature rupture of membranes
- Fetal death

CANDIDAL INFECTIONS

● **Definition**
- Refers to a vaginal yeast infection
- Is commonly considered a sexually transmitted disease

● **Pathophysiology**
- The causative organism is *Candida albicans*
- Candidiasis is common during pregnancy due to changes in vaginal pH from increased estrogen level
- It usually occurs in women receiving antibiotic therapy for another infection and in women with gestational diabetes or HIV infection
- If infection present at the time of delivery, the neonate may become infected

● **Assessment findings**
- Thick, white, cheeselike pruritic vaginal discharge
- Dysuria and dyspareunia
- Intense pruritus
- Vaginal redness and irritation

● **Diagnostic test findings**
- Wet mount slide positive for organism

● **Management**
- Drug therapy with an antifungal, such as miconazole cream (Monostat) or oral fluconazole (Diflucan)
- Review of personal hygiene
- Condom use or abstinence from intercourse until infection is cured

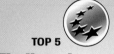

TOP 5
Findings in candidiasis

1. Thick, white, cheeselike pruritic vaginal discharge
2. Dysuria and dyspareunia
3. Intense pruritus
4. Vaginal redness and irritation
5. Wet mount slide positive for *Candida albicans*

● **Nursing interventions**
  • Instruct the woman in use of drug therapy such as cream application
  • Urge the woman to check with her health care provider before purchasing over-the-counter products to ensure the product is safe to use during pregnancy
  • Provide comfort measure to help with pruritus and irritation
  • Encourage adherence to therapy program to ensure complete irradication of infection before delivery
● **Possible complications**
  • If infection is present at delivery, candidal infection or thrush is possible in the neonate because of direct contact with organism in vagina

SPONTANEOUS ABORTION

● **Definition**
  • Refers to the spontaneous expulsion of the products of conception from the uterus before fetal viability (fetal weight of less than 17½ oz [496 g] and gestation of less than 20 weeks)
  • Also known as *miscarriage*
  • Up to 15% of all pregnancies and about 30% of first pregnancies end in spontaneous abortion
  • At least 75% of spontaneous abortions occur during the first trimester
  • Several different types of spontaneous abortion exist (see *Types of spontaneous abortion,* page 122)
● **Pathophysiology**
  • More than 50% are caused by abnormalities in fetoplacental development
  • Fetal factors usually cause such abortions at 6 to 10 weeks' gestation
    – Defective embryologic development from abnormal chromosome division (the most common cause of fetal death)
    – Faulty implantation of fertilized ovum
    – Failure of the endometrium to accept the fertilized ovum
  • Placental factors usually cause spontaneous abortion around the 14th week, when the placenta takes over the hormone production necessary to maintain the pregnancy
    – Premature separation of the normally implanted placenta
    – Abnormal placental implantation
    – Abnormal platelet function
  • Maternal factors usually cause spontaneous abortion between 11 and 19 weeks
    – Maternal infection
    – Severe malnutrition

Managing candidal infection

• Antifungal
• Review of personal hygiene
• Condom use or abstinence from intercourse until infection is cured

---

Key facts about spontaneous abortion

• Spontaneous expulsion of the products of conception from the uterus before fetal viability
• Up to 15% of all pregnancies and about 30% of first pregnancies end in spontaneous abortion
• At least 75% of spontaneous abortions occur during the first trimester

---

Maternal factors contributing to spontaneous abortion

• Infection
• Severe malnutrition
• Abnormalities of the reproductive organs
• Endocrine problems
• Trauma
• Blood group incompatibility and Rh isoimmunization
• Drug ingestion

Types of spontaneous abortion

Spontaneous abortions occur without medical intervention. They can occur in various ways:

- Complete abortion — Uterus passes all products of conception. Minimal bleeding usually accompanies complete abortion because the uterus contracts and compresses the maternal blood vessels that fed the placenta.
- Habitual abortion — Spontaneous loss of three or more consecutive pregnancies constitutes habitual abortion.
- Incomplete abortion — Uterus retains part or all of the placenta. Before 10 weeks' gestation, the fetus and placenta are usually expelled together; after the 10th week, they're expelled separately. Because part of the placenta may adhere to the uterine wall, bleeding continues. Hemorrhage is possible because the uterus doesn't contract and seal the large vessels that fed the placenta.

- Inevitable abortion — Membranes rupture and the cervix dilates. As labor continues, the uterus expels the products of conception.
- Missed abortion — Uterus retains the products of conception for 2 months or more after the fetus has died. Uterine growth ceases; uterine size may even seem to decrease. Prolonged retention of the dead products of conception may cause coagulation defects such as disseminated intravascular coagulation.
- Septic abortion — Infection accompanies abortion. This may occur with spontaneous abortion, but usually results from a lapse in sterile technique during therapeutic abortion.
- Threatened abortion — Bloody vaginal discharge occurs during the first half of pregnancy. About 20% of pregnant women have vaginal spotting or actual bleeding early in pregnancy. Of these, about 50% abort.

    – Abnormalities of the reproductive organs (especially incompetent cervix, in which the cervix dilates painlessly and without blood in the second trimester)
- Other maternal factors that can cause spontaneous abortion
    – Endocrine problems, such as thyroid dysfunction or lowered estriol secretion
    – Trauma, including any type of surgery that necessitates manipulation of the pelvic organs
    – Blood group incompatibility and Rh isoimmunization
    – Drug ingestion

● Assessment findings
- Symptom severity depends on the gestational age at the time of spontaneous abortion
- Signs and symptoms include uterine cramping and vaginal bleeding

● Diagnostic test findings
- Presence of hCG in the blood or urine confirms pregnancy, with decreased hCG levels suggesting spontaneous abortion

Managing spontaneous abortion

TYPE OR STAGE	MANAGEMENT
Threatened abortion	• Limitation of the patient's activities for 24 to 48 hours • Bed rest • Pad count • Restriction of coitus for about 2 weeks
Imminent and incomplete abortion	• Dilatation and curettage or vacuum and aspiration to ensure emptying of the uterus
Complete abortion	• Rest • Monitoring for temperature elevation and bleeding • If the uterus emptied on its own and the patient has no signs of infection, no further intervention is needed

- Pelvic examination reveals size of the uterus, which is inconsistent with the length of the pregnancy
- Tissue cytology indicates evidence of products of conception
- Laboratory tests reflect decreased hemoglobin levels and hematocrit from blood loss
- Ultrasonography positive for presence or absence of fetal heartbeats or an empty amniotic sac

Management
(See *Managing spontaneous abortion.*)

Nursing interventions
- Do *not* allow bathroom privileges because the patient may expel uterine contents without knowing it
- After she uses the bedpan, inspect the contents carefully for intrauterine material
- Note the amount, color, and odor of vaginal bleeding
- Save all pads the patient uses for evaluation
- Administer an analgesic and oxytocin as ordered
- Assess vital signs every 4 hours for 24 hours or more frequently, depending on the extent of bleeding
- Monitor urine output closely
- Provide good perineal care
- Check the patient's blood type and administer RhoGAM as ordered
- Provide emotional support and counseling during the grieving process
- Encourage the patient and her partner to express their feelings
  - Some couples may want to talk to a member of the clergy
  - Others, depending on their religion, may wish to have the fetus baptized
- Help the patient and her partner to develop effective coping strategies

Key interventions for spontaneous abortion

- Do *not* allow bathroom privileges.
- After bedpan use, inspect contents carefully for intrauterine material.
- Note the amount, color, and odor of vaginal bleeding.
- Assess vital signs every 4 hours for 24 hours or more frequently, depending on the extent of bleeding.
- Monitor urine output closely.
- Check the patient's blood type and administer RhoGAM as ordered.
- Provide emotional support and counseling during the grieving process.
- Encourage the patient and her partner to express their feelings.

TIME-OUT FOR TEACHING

After a miscarriage

If your patient experiences a spontaneous abortion, be sure to include these instructions in her teaching plan:

- Expect vaginal bleeding or spotting to continue for several days.
- Immediately report bleeding that lasts longer than 10 days, is excessive, or appears bright red.
- Watch for signs of infection, such as a temperature higher than 100° F (37.8° C) and foul-smelling vaginal discharge.

- Gradually increase your daily activities to include whatever tasks you feel comfortable doing as long as these activities don't increase vaginal bleeding or cause fatigue.
- Abstain from sexual intercourse for about 2 weeks.
- Use a contraceptive when you and your partner resume intercourse.
- Avoid the use of tampons for 1 to 2 weeks.
- Arrange for a follow-up visit with your physician in 2 to 4 weeks.

- Explain all procedures and treatments to the patient and provide teaching about aftercare and follow-up (see *After a miscarriage*)

PREGNANCY-INDUCED HYPERTENSION

● **Definition**
- Also called *hypertension of pregnancy* or *gestational hypertensive disorder*
- A potentially life-threatening disorder that usually develops after the 20th week of pregnancy
- Most common in nulliparous women
- Two categories of PIH
  - Preeclampsia
    · Nonconvulsive form of the disorder
    · Develops in about 7% of pregnancies and may be mild or severe
    · Marked by the onset of hypertension after 20 weeks' gestation
    · The incidence is significantly higher in low socioeconomic groups
  - Eclampsia
    · Convulsive form of the disorder
    · Occurs between 24 weeks' gestation and the end of the first postpartum week
    · Incidence increases among women who are pregnant for the first time, have multiple fetuses, and have a history of vascular disease
- Currently, PIH and its complications are the current most common cause of maternal death in developed countries

TOP 4

Things to know about pregnancy-induced hypertension

1. It can be life-threatening.
2. It usually develops after the 20th week.
3. It's most common in nulliparous women.
4. It's typically classified as preeclampsia or eclampsia.

Key facts about preeclampsia

- Nonconvulsive form
- Occurs after 20 weeks' gestation
- May be mild or severe
- Higher incidence in low socioeconomic groups

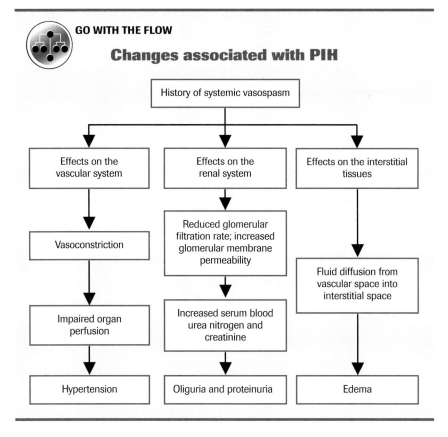

GO WITH THE FLOW

Changes associated with PIH

History of systemic vasospasm

Effects on the vascular system → Vasoconstriction → Impaired organ perfusion → Hypertension

Effects on the renal system → Reduced glomerular filtration rate; increased glomerular membrane permeability → Increased serum blood urea nitrogen and creatinine → Oliguria and proteinuria

Effects on the interstitial tissues → Fluid diffusion from vascular space into interstitial space → Edema

Pathophysiology
- Exact cause is unknown
- Systemic peripheral vasospasm occurs, affecting every organ system (see *Changes associated with PIH*)
- Geographic, ethnic, racial, nutritional, immunologic, and familial factors may contribute to preexisting vascular disease, which, in turn, may contribute to its occurrence
- Age is also a factor; adolescents younger than age 19 and primiparas older than age 35 are at higher risk

Assessment findings
- Blood pressure over 140/90 mm Hg or an increase of 30 mm Hg systolic and 15 mm Hg diastolic over baseline obtained on two occasions at least 4 to 6 hours apart
- Increase in generalized edema associated with a sudden weight gain of more than 5 lb (2.3 kg) per week
- Usually appears between the 20th and 24th weeks of gestation and disappears within 42 days after delivery
- A final diagnosis usually deferred until blood pressure returns to normal after delivery; if blood pressure remains elevated, chronic hypertension, either alone or superimposed on PIH, may be the cause

Key facts about eclampsia

- Convulsive form
- Occurs between 24 weeks' gestation and the end of the first postpartum week
- Higher incidence with first pregnancies, multiple gestations, and history of vascular disease

TOP 3

Findings in pregnancy-induced hypertension

1. Blood pressure over 140/90 mm Hg or an increase of 30 mm Hg systolic and 15 mm Hg diastolic over baseline obtained on two occasions at least 4 to 6 hours apart
2. Increase in generalized edema associated with a sudden weight gain of more than 5 lb (2.3 kg) per week
3. Proteinuria

Managing pregnancy-induced hypertension

- High-protein, low-salt diet
- Adequate fluid intake
- Bed rest
- Antihypertensive
- Magnesium sulfate

Key signs and symptoms of magnesium sulfate toxicity

- Decreased deep tendon reflexes
- Muscle flaccidity
- Central nervous system depression
- Decreased respiratory rate
- Decreased renal function

- Additional signs and symptoms with severe preeclampsia include increased blood urea nitrogen, creatinine, and uric acid levels; frontal headaches; blurred vision; hyperreflexia; nausea; vomiting; irritability; cerebral disturbances; and epigastric pain

● **Diagnostic test findings**
  - Proteinuria
    – In preeclampsia, more than 300 mg/24 hours [1+]
    – In eclampsia, 5 g/24 hours [5+] or more

● **Management**
  - High-protein diet with adequate fluid intake with restriction of excessively salty foods
  - Bed rest in a lateral position
  - Close observance of blood pressure, fetal heart rate, edema, proteinuria, and signs of pending eclampsia
  - Administration of an antihypertensive, such as methyldopa and hydralazine
  - Administration of magnesium sulfate, a neuromuscular sedative that reduces the amount of acetylcholine that the motor nerves produce, thus preventing seizures (urine output must be at least 30 ml/hour because 99% of the drug is excreted by the kidneys)
    – Signs and symptoms of magnesium sulfate toxicity must be promptly identified and management initiated
    – Signs and symptoms include elevated serum levels, decreased deep tendon reflexes, muscle flaccidity, central nervous system depression, and decreased respiratory rate and renal function
    – The antidote to magnesium sulfate is calcium gluconate kept at the bedside
  - Nonstress tests every one to two times per week; biophysical profile every 3 weeks

● **Nursing interventions**
  - Monitor the patient regularly for changes in blood pressure, pulse rate, respiratory rate, fetal heart rate, vision, level of consciousness, and deep tendon reflexes and for headache unrelieved by medication; report changes immediately
  - Do the following before administering medication
    – Observe the patient for signs of fetal distress by closely monitoring the results of stress and nonstress tests
    – Keep emergency resuscitative equipment and an anticonvulsant readily available in case of seizures and cardiac or respiratory arrest
    – Maintain a patent airway and have oxygen readily available
    – Prepare for emergency cesarean delivery if indicated

Safety with magnesium

If your patient requires I.V. magnesium therapy, be cautious when administering the drug. Follow these guidelines to ensure safety during administration:

- Always administer the drug as a piggyback infusion so that if the patient develops signs and symptoms of toxicity, the drug can be discontinued immediately.
- Monitor serum magnesium levels, obtaining a baseline level before initiating therapy and then frequently thereafter.
- Keep in mind that to be effective as an anticonvulsant, serum magnesium levels should be between 5 and 8 mg/dl. Levels above 8 mg/dl indicate toxicity and place the patient at risk for respiratory depression, cardiac arrhythmias, and cardiac arrest.

- Assess the patient's deep tendon reflexes. Ideally this should be the patellar reflex. However, if the patient has received epidural anesthesia, test the biceps or triceps reflex. Diminished or hypoactive reflexes suggest magnesium toxicity.
- Assess for ankle clonus by rapidly dorsiflexing the patient's ankle three times in succession and then remove your hand, observing foot movement. If no further motion is noted, ankle clonus is absent; if the foot continues to move voluntarily, clonus is present. Moderate (3 to 5) or severe (6 or more) movements may suggest magnesium toxicity.
- Have calcium gluconate readily available at the patient's bedside. Anticipate administering this antidote for magnesium toxicity.

- Maintain seizure precautions to protect the patient from injury; never leave unattended any patient whose condition is unstable
- If the woman is receiving magnesium sulfate I.V., administer the loading dose over 15 to 30 minutes and then maintain the infusion at a rate of 1 to 2 g/hour (see *Safety with magnesium*)
  - Carefully monitor the I.V. infusion of magnesium sulfate, watching for signs and symptoms of toxicity such as absence of patellar reflexes, flushing, muscle flaccidity, decreased urine output, a significant drop in blood pressure (more than 15 mm Hg) and respiratory rate less than 12 breaths/minute
  - Keep calcium gluconate readily available at the bedside to counteract the toxic effects of magnesium sulfate
- Monitor the extent and location of edema, and take the necessary precautions
  - Elevate affected extremities to promote venous return
  - Avoid constricting hose, slippers, or bed linens
- Assess fluid balance by measuring intake and output and by checking daily weight; insert an indwelling urinary catheter if necessary to provide a more accurate measurement of output
- Provide a quiet, darkened room until the patient's condition stabilizes and enforce absolute bed rest

Key interventions for pregnancy-induced hypertension

- Monitor the patient regularly for changes in blood pressure, pulse rate, respiratory rate, fetal heart rate, vision, level of consciousness, and deep tendon reflexes and for headache.
- Closely monitor the results of stress and nonstress tests.
- Keep emergency resuscitative equipment and an anticonvulsant readily available.
- Maintain a patent airway and have oxygen readily available.
- Prepare for emergency cesarean delivery, if indicated.
- Maintain seizure precautions.
- If the woman is receiving magnesium sulfate I.V., administer the loading dose over 15 to 30 minutes and then maintain the infusion at a rate of 1 to 2 g/hour.
- Monitor the extent and location of edema.
- Assess fluid balance.

- Provide emotional support for the patient and her family
  - Encourage them to verbalize their feelings
  - If the patient's condition necessitates premature delivery, point out that infants of mothers with PIH are usually small for gestational age but sometimes fare better than other premature infants of the same weight, possibly because they have developed adaptive responses to stress in utero
- Help the patient and her family to develop effective coping strategies

● Possible complications
- Seizures (eclampsia)
- Maternal mortality in eclampsia is 10% to 15%, usually resulting from intracranial hemorrhage and heart failure
- Severe complications of eclampsia include cerebral edema, stroke, abruptio placentae with or without disseminated intravascular coagulation, and fetal death

HELLP SYNDROME

● Definition
- Refers to a category of PIH that primarily involves changes in blood components and liver function
- HELLP stands for hemolysis, elevated liver enzymes, and low platelets
- As many as 12% of women with PIH develop HELLP syndrome, occurring in both primigravidas and multigravidas
- Women with severe preeclampsia are at high risk for developing this syndrome
- When it does occur, maternal and infant mortality is high (about one-fourth of the women and one-third of infants die of this disorder)
- However, after birth, laboratory results return to normal usually within 1 week and the mother experiences no further problems

● Pathophysiology
- Exact cause is unknown
- Beliefs about the development of the underlying signs have been proposed
  - Hemolysis is believed to result from damage to erythrocytes as they pass through small damaged blood vessels
  - Elevated liver enzyme levels are believed to result from obstruction in liver flow by fibrin deposits
  - Low platelet count is believed to be the result of vascular damage secondary to vasospasm

---

Severe complications of eclampsia

- Cerebral edema
- Stroke
- Abruptio placentae
- Fetal death

Key facts about HELLP syndrome

- Refers to a category of PIH that primarily involves changes in blood components and liver function
- Stands for **h**emolysis, **e**levated **l**iver enzymes, and **l**ow **p**latelets
- Women with severe preeclampsia are at high risk for HELLP syndrome
- Maternal and infant mortality is high
- Exact cause is unknown

Assessment findings
- Pain, most commonly in the right upper quadrant, epigastric area, or lower chest
- Nausea and vomiting
- General malaise
- Severe edema
- Right upper quadrant possibly tender on palpation because of a distended liver
- Signs and symptoms of preeclampsia

Diagnostic test findings
- Hemolysis of RBCs (appearing fragmented and irregular on a peripheral blood smear)
- Thrombocytopenia (a platelet count below 100,000/µl)
- Elevated liver enzyme levels—alanine aminotransferase and serum aspartate aminotransferase

Management
- Intensive care management for the woman and her fetus
- Drug therapy, such as magnesium sulfate to reduce blood pressure and prevent seizures
- Transfusions of fresh frozen plasma or platelets to reverse the thrombocytopenia
- Delivery of the fetus, either vaginally or by cesarean delivery, as soon as possible once the fetus is determined to be mature

Nursing interventions
- Assess maternal vital signs and fetal heart rate frequently; be alert for signs and symptoms of complications including hemorrhage, hypoglycemia, hyponatremia, subcapsular liver hematoma, and renal failure
- Maintain a quiet, calm, dimly lit environment to reduce the risk of seizures; institute seizure precautions
- Avoid palpating the abdomen because this increases intra-abdominal pressure, which could lead to rupture of a subcapsular liver hematoma
- Institute bleeding precautions
  - Monitor the patient for signs and symptoms of bleeding
  - Administer blood transfusions and medications as ordered
- If the patient develops hypoglycemia, expect to administer I.V. dextrose solutions
- Prepare the patient for delivery
  - Explain all events and procedures being done
  - Assist with evaluations for fetal maturity
- Be aware that because of the increased risk of bleeding due to thrombocytopenia, the woman may not be a candidate for epidural anesthesia

---

Key assessment findings for HELLP syndrome

- Pain (most common in the right upper quadrant, epigastric area, or lower chest)
- Nausea and vomiting
- General malaise
- Severe edema
- Signs and symptoms of preeclampsia

Key test findings for HELLP syndrome

- Hemolysis of RBCs
- Thrombocytopenia
- Elevated liver enzyme levels

Key interventions for HELLP syndrome

- Assess maternal vital signs and fetal heart rate frequently.
- Maintain a quiet, calm, dimly lit environment.
- Institute bleeding precautions.
- If the patient develops hypoglycemia, expect to administer I.V. dextrose solutions.
- Prepare the patient for delivery.
- Assess the patient carefully for hemorrhage throughout labor and delivery.

Complications of HELLP syndrome

- Fetal or maternal death
- Hemorrhage
- Hypoglycemia
- Hyponatremia
- Subcapsular liver hematoma
- Renal failure

Factors associated with an incompetent cervix

- Congenital structural defects
- Previous cervical trauma resulting from surgery or delivery
- Increasing maternal age

Managing an incompetent cervix

- Placement of cerclage in the cervix
- Bed rest after surgery
- Removal of sutures at 37 to 39 weeks' gestation
- Emotional support

- Assess the patient carefully throughout labor and delivery for possible hemorrhage

● **Possible complications**
- Fetal or maternal death
- Hemorrhage
- Hypoglycemia
- Subcapsular liver hematoma
- Renal failure

INCOMPETENT CERVIX

● **Definition**
- Also called *premature cervical dilation*
- Refers to a painless premature dilation of the cervix
- It generally occurs in the 4th to 5th month of gestation, most commonly around the 20th week of gestation

● **Pathophysiology**
- This condition is associated with congenital structural defects or previous cervical trauma resulting from surgery or delivery
- It's also associated with increasing maternal age

● **Assessment findings**
- History of repeated second trimester spontaneous abortions
- Cervical dilation in the absence of contractions or pain
- Pink-stained vaginal discharge
- Increased pelvic pressure with possible ruptured membranes and release of amniotic fluid

● **Diagnostic test findings**
- Ultrasound revealing defect
- Nitrazine test result indicates rupture of membranes (if occurred)

● **Management**
- Placement of a purse-string suture, known as a *cerclage,* in the cervix to help keep the cervix closed until term or the patient goes into labor
    - McDonald's procedure using nylon sutures horizontally and vertically to close off cervix to only a few millimeters in size
    - Shirodkar procedure using sterile tape in a purse-string fashion to close off cervix entirely
- Bed rest after surgery
- Removal of sutures at 37 to 39 weeks' gestation
- Emotional support

● **Nursing interventions**
- Assess complaints of vaginal drainage and investigate history for previous cervical surgeries

- Prepare woman for cervical cerclage under regional anesthesia as indicated; monitor maternal vital signs and fetal heart rate patterns closely
- Instruct woman in signs and symptoms of labor with the need to notify health care provider if any occur
- Maintain bed rest after surgery as ordered; if necessary, place the woman in a slight or modified Trendelenburg position to alleviate pressure of the uterus on the sutured area
- Encourage follow-up to evaluate progress of pregnancy
- Advise the woman that the sutures will be removed around the 37th to 39th week of pregnancy

● **Possible complications**
  - Spontaneous abortion
  - Preterm birth

DIABETES

● **Definition**
  - Metabolic disorder characterized by hyperglycemia (elevated serum glucose level) resulting from lack of insulin, lack of insulin effect, or both
  - A disorder of carbohydrate, protein, and fat metabolism
  - Three general classifications are recognized
    - Type 1, absolute insulin insufficiency
    - Type 2, insulin resistance with varying degrees of insulin secretory defects (insulin resistance with an inadequate compensatory secretory response)
    - Gestational diabetes, which emerges during pregnancy

● **Pathophysiology**
  - Evidence indicates that diabetes mellitus has diverse causes
    - Heredity
    - Environment (infection, diet, toxins, stress)
    - Lifestyle changes in genetically susceptible people
  - In people genetically susceptible to type 1 diabetes, a triggering event causes production of autoantibodies against the beta cells of the pancreas
    - The resulting destruction of the beta cells leads to a decline in and ultimate lack of insulin secretion
    - Insulin deficiency leads to hyperglycemia, enhanced lipolysis (decomposition of fat), and protein catabolism
    - These characteristics occur when more than 90% of the beta cells have been destroyed

Complications associated with an incompetent cervix

- Spontaneous abortion
- Preterm birth

Types of diabetes

- **Type 1 diabetes mellitus:** an absolute insulin insufficiency
- **Type 2 diabetes mellitus:** an insulin resistance with varying degrees of insulin secretory defects
- **Gestational diabetes:** diabetes that emerges during pregnancy

Factors that contribute to diabetes

- Heredity
- Environment
- Lifestyle

- Type 2 diabetes mellitus is a chronic disease caused by one or more of the following factors: impaired insulin production, inappropriate hepatic glucose production, or peripheral insulin receptor insensitivity
  - Genetic factors are significant
  - Onset is accelerated by obesity and a sedentary lifestyle
  - Added stress can be a pivotal factor
- Gestational diabetes mellitus occurs when a woman not previously diagnosed with diabetes shows glucose intolerance during pregnancy
  - It isn't known whether gestational diabetes results from an inadequate insulin response to carbohydrates, if it's due to excessive insulin resistance, or if both factors play a role in its development
  - Risk factors include obesity; history of delivering large infants (usually more than 10 lb [4.5 kg]); unexplained fetal or perinatal loss; evidence of congenital anomalies in previous pregnancies; over age 25, and family history of diabetes

Assessment findings

- Hyperglycemia
- Glycosuria
- Polyuria
- Increased incidence of candidal infections
- Hydramnios
- Signs and symptoms of macrovascular and microvascular changes
  - Peripheral vascular disease
  - Retinopathy
  - Nephropathy
  - Neuropathy

Diagnostic test findings

- Screening with an oral glucose challenge test (a fasting plasma glucose level)
- 100-g glucose load is used at 24 to 28 weeks' gestation
- If 1 hour glucose level is greater than 180 mg/dl, a 3-hour glucose tolerance test using a 100-g glucose load is scheduled
- Two abnormal levels or a fasting glucose level greater than 95 mg/dl confirms diagnosis of gestational diabetes (see *Oral glucose challenge test values for pregnancy*)

Management

- Gestational diabetes mellitus
  - Blood glucose levels monitoring; fasting blood sugar (FBS) and 2-hour postprandial
  - Target glucose levels for FBS less than 100 mg and postprandial less than 120 mg
  - Careful monitoring of diet, exercise, and insulin administration and patient education

Oral glucose challenge test values for pregnancy*

TEST TYPE	GLUCOSE LEVEL DURING PREGNANCY (MG/DL)
Fasting	95
1 hour	180
2 hour	155
3 hour	140

* Following a 100-g glucose load. Rate is abnormal if two values are exceeded.

– Oral antidiabetics are contraindicated during pregnancy because of their adverse effects on the fetus and neonate; may be used in second or third trimester if the patient is noncompliant with her insulin regimen

- Type 1 diabetes mellitus
  – Close monitoring of glucose levels because of tendency for wide fluctuations in blood glucose levels
  – In general, insulin requirements decrease during the first trimester and increase during second and third trimesters
  – Evaluation of glycosylated hemoglobin levels every 3 months as an overall indicator of blood glucose control

Nursing interventions

- Monitor the woman's status carefully throughout the pregnancy; assess weight gain, blood glucose levels, nutritional intake, and fetal growth parameters
- Review results of fingerstick blood glucose monitoring; assess the patient for signs and symptoms of hypoglycemia and hyperglycemia
- Assist with arranging follow-up laboratory studies, including glycosylated hemoglobin levels, and urine studies as necessary
- Encourage a consistent exercise program, including the use of snacks
- Instruct the woman in all aspects of diabetic care management, including insulin, injection administration technique, self monitoring, nutrition, and danger signs and symptoms (see *Pregnant patient with diabetes,* page 134)
- Assist with preparations for labor, including explanations about possible labor induction and required monitoring
- Closely assess the woman in the postpartum period for changes in blood glucose levels and insulin requirements
  – Typically the woman with preexisting diabetes will require no insulin in the immediate postpartum period (because insulin resis-

Managing type 1 diabetes mellitus

- Monitoring of glucose levels (tendency for wide fluctuations)
- Evaluation of glycosylated hemoglobin levels every 3 months

Key interventions for diabetes

- Monitor the woman's status carefully throughout the pregnancy.
- Review results of fingerstick blood glucose monitoring.
- Assist with arranging follow-up laboratory studies.
- Encourage a consistent exercise program.
- Instruct the woman in all aspects of diabetic care management.
- Assist with preparations for labor.
- Closely assess the woman in the postpartum period for changes in blood glucose levels and insulin requirements.

TIME-OUT FOR TEACHING

Pregnant patient with diabetes

Be sure to include these topics in your teaching plan for the pregnant patient with diabetes:

- explanation of diabetes
- procedure for fingerstick blood glucose monitoring
- frequency of blood glucose monitoring
- insulin requirements
- insulin administration technique
- insulin action, dosage, frequency, and possible effects
- possible danger signs
- implications for mother and fetus
- dietary restrictions
- activity and exercise precautions
- regular checkups and diagnostic testing
- need for compliance and follow-up.

Negative effects of type 1 diabetes

- Increased risk of congenital anomalies
- Hydramnios
- Macrosomia
- Pregnancy-induced hypertension
- Spontaneous abortion
- Fetal death

Key facts about sickle cell anemia

- Recessive autosomal disorder in which RBCs become sickle shaped
- Occurs primarily in people of African and Mediterranean descent
- Most common in tropical Africans
- Pregnant women with the sickle cell trait experience increased incidence of pyelonephritis

---

tance is gone), eventually returning to her prepregnancy insulin requirements in several days
  – The woman with gestational diabetes usually exhibits normal blood glucose levels within 24 hours after delivery, requiring no further insulin or diet therapy
- Encourage the woman with gestational diabetes to adhere to follow-up health maintenance visits to obtain glucose testing to allow for early detection of possible type 2 diabetes

● **Possible complications**
- The patient with gestational diabetes has a 30% to 40% chance of developing diabetes mellitus in 1 to 25 years
- Type 1 diabetes is associated with an increased risk of congenital anomalies, hydramnios, macrosomia, PIH, spontaneous abortion, and fetal death
- A condition unique to the infant of a mother with type 1 diabetes mellitus is sacral agenesis, a congenital anomaly characterized by incomplete formation of the spinal column

SICKLE CELL ANEMIA

● **Definition**
- A recessive autosomal disorder in which RBCs become sickle shaped
- Occurs primarily in people of African and Mediterranean descent
- Most common in tropical Africans; may also occur in people from Puerto Rico, Turkey, India, the Middle East, and the Mediterranean
- Pregnant women with the sickle cell trait seem to experience an increased incidence of asymptomatic bacteriuria, resulting in an increased incidence of pyelonephritis

Pathophysiology

- Sickle cell anemia results from substitution of the amino acid valine for glutamic acid in the hemoglobin S gene encoding the beta chain of hemoglobin
- Abnormal hemoglobin S, found in the RBCs of patients, becomes insoluble during hypoxia
    - These cells become rigid, rough, and elongated, forming a crescent or sickle shape
    - The sickling produces hemolysis
    - The altered cells also pile up in the capillaries and smaller blood vessels, making the blood more viscous
    - Normal circulation is impaired, causing pain, tissue infarction, and swelling
    - Vascular obstruction in the capillaries leads to anemia
- Each patient with sickle cell anemia has a different hypoxic threshold and different factors that trigger a sickle cell crisis
    - Illness, exposure to cold, stress, acidotic states or a pathophysiologic process that causes water to move out of the sickle cells precipitates a crisis in most patients
    - The blockages then cause anoxic changes that lead to further sickling and obstruction

Assessment findings

- Anemia
- Fatigue
- Complaints of burning and pain on urination
- Pooling of blood in lower extremities
- Severe pain (if crisis develops)

Diagnostic test findings

- Positive family history and typical clinical features
- Hemoglobin electrophoresis reveals hemoglobin S
- Stained blood smear shows sickled cells
- Hemoglobin level of 6 mg/dl or less (may decrease to as low as 5 mg/dl during a crisis)
- Decreased RBC count and erythrocyte sedimentation rate
- Increased indirect bilirubin level (during a crisis)
- Clean-catch urine specimen positive for bacteria

Management

- Evaluation of blood studies, including hemoglobin levels and hematocrit
- Avoidance of contributing factors, such as dehydration, stress, hypoxia, infection, acidosis, and sudden cooling
- Prevention of thrombophlebitis (positive Homans' sign)

Sickle cell crisis triggers

- Illness
- Exposure to cold
- Stress
- Acidotic states
- Pathophysiologic processes that cause water to move out of the sickle cells

Key assessment findings for sickle cell anemia

- Anemia
- Fatigue
- Complaints of burning and pain on urination
- Pooling of blood in lower extremities
- Severe pain

Key test findings in sickle cell anemia

- Hemoglobin electrophoresis reveals hemoglobin S
- Sickled cells on stained blood smear
- Hemoglobin level of 6 mg/dl or less
- Decreased RBC count and erythrocyte sedimentation rate
- Increased indirect bilirubin level (during a crisis)

Managing sickle cell anemia

- Evaluation of blood studies
- Avoidance of contributing factors
- Prevention of thrombophlebitis
- Folic acid supplementation
- Blood transfusion therapy
- Oxygen therapy and fluids during labor
- Analgesic during crisis

Key interventions for sickle cell anemia

- Assess hydration.
- Monitor vital signs and fetal heart rate.
- Monitor the patient's weight gain and fundal height.
- Assess the patient's lower extremities for venous pooling.
- Encourage the patient to avoid standing for long periods.
- Encourage chair rest with legs elevated.
- Assess for signs and symptoms of infection.
- Provide comfort and emotional support.

- Folic acid supplement to decrease erythropoietic demands and capillary stasis
- Blood transfusion therapy
- Oxygen therapy and fluids during labor
- An analgesic for relief of pain during crisis

● **Nursing interventions**
- Monitor the patient's complete blood count regularly
- Assess the patient's hydration status
  - Monitor her intake and output
  - Check for signs of dehydration
  - Urge her to drink at least eight 8-ounce glasses of fluid each day
- Monitor vital signs and fetal heart rate and pattern as indicated
- Monitor weight gain and assess fundal height for changes indicating adequate fetal growth
- Assess the patient for signs and symptoms of sickle cell crisis and chronic complications; administer an analgesic and I.V. fluids if crisis develops
- Expect to administer hypotonic saline solution I.V. for fluid replacement because the woman's kidneys have difficulty concentrating urine to remove large amounts of fluid
- Obtain a clean-catch urine specimen for culture to assess for possible bacteriuria
- Assess lower extremities for venous pooling; encourage the woman to avoid standing for long periods of time and to rest in a chair with legs elevated or in side-lying position to promote venous return to the heart
- Prepare the patient for ultrasound at 16 to 24 weeks and weekly nonstress tests beginning at about 30 weeks' gestation
- Be aware that blood flow velocity tests may be ordered to evaluate blood flow through the uterus and placenta; reduced blood flow may suggest intrauterine growth retardation
- Anticipate the patient's desire to determine if the fetus has the disease; assist with percutaneous umbilical blood sampling to obtain a sample for RBC electrophoresis
- Watch for signs and symptoms of infection, such as fever, chills, or purulent drainage
- Assess the patient's respiratory status
  - Perform a respiratory assessment including auscultation of breath sounds regularly
  - Expect to administer oxygen if the woman develops a crisis
- Provide comfort and emotional support to the patient and her family
- Assist with measures to maintain hydration during labor and delivery

● **Possible complications**
- Pregnant women experience an increased incidence of PIH, urinary tract infections, heart failure, pneumonia, pulmonary infarction, crisis, and postpartum hemorrhage
- Risk for intrauterine growth retardation results in low-birth-weight infants
- Perinatal fetal death may results from spontaneous abortion and prematurity

FOLIC ACID–DEFICIENCY ANEMIA

● **Definition**
- A common, slowly progressive megaloblastic anemia (enlarged RBCs)
- Folic acid, or folacin, is one of the B vitamins important for the normal formation of RBCs and the synthesis of deoxyribonucleic acid
- Folic acid plays a major role in preventing neural tube defects in the fetus

● **Pathophysiology**
- Folic acid is found in most body tissues where it acts as a coenzyme in metabolic processes
  - Although its body stores are comparatively small, this vitamin is plentiful in most well-balanced diets
  - However, folic acid is water-soluble and heat-labile, and is easily destroyed by cooking
  - About 20% of folic acid intake is excreted unabsorbed
  - An insufficient intake, usually less than 50 mcg/day, generally results in folic acid–deficiency anemia within 4 months
- During pregnancy, folic acid–deficiency anemia usually occurs in women with multiple gestations, believed to be the result of the increased demand for folic acid by the fetuses
- It's also seen in women who have underlying hemolytic illness that results in rapid destruction and production of RBCs
- Certain drugs, such as hydantoin (an anticonvulsant that interferes with folate absorption), and hormonal contraceptives may also play a causative role

● **Assessment findings**
- Severe, progressive fatigue (the hallmark of folic acid deficiency)
- Pallor or jaundice
- Shortness of breath
- Palpitations
- Diarrhea
- Nausea or anorexia
- Headaches, weakness, or light-headedness

Key facts about folic acid

- B vitamin
- Involved in normal formation of RBCs and the synthesis of deoxyribonucleic acid
- Found in most body tissues
- Acts as a coenzyme in metabolic processes
- Insufficient intake results in folic acid–deficiency anemia

Signs and symptoms of folic acid–deficiency anemia

- Severe, progressive fatigue
- Pallor, jaundice
- Shortness of breath
- Palpitations
- Diarrhea
- Nausea or anorexia
- Headaches, weakness, or light-headedness
- Forgetfulness
- Irritability

Tips for increasing folic acid intake

- Eat green leafy vegetables, wheat products, peanut butter, and liver.
- Eat foods high in vitamin C to encourage folic acid absorption.

Negative effects of folic acid–deficiency anemia

- Early spontaneous abortion
- Premature separation of the placenta
- Fetal neural tube defects

- Forgetfulness
- Irritability

● **Diagnostic test findings**
- Macrocytic RBCs
- Decreased reticulocyte count
- Increased mean corpuscular volume
- Abnormal platelet count
- Decreased serum folate levels (below 4 mg/ml)

● **Management**
- Folic acid supplementation, orally (1 to 5 mg/day) or parenterally (to patients who are severely ill, have malabsorption, or can't take oral medication)
- Diet high in folic acid

● **Nursing interventions**
- Strongly urge women expecting to become pregnant to begin a vitamin supplement (over-the-counter) or be conscious about eating folic acid–rich foods, such as green leafy vegetables, wheat products, peanut butter and liver, during this time
- Assist with planning a well-balanced diet, including foods high in folic acid and between-meal snacks
- Encourage the woman to eat a rich source of vitamin C at each meal to enhance absorption of folic acid
- Administer folic acid supplement as ordered; throughout pregnancy assess the patient's compliance with therapy
- If the patient has severe anemia and requires hospitalization, plan activities, rest periods, and diagnostic tests to conserve energy
    - Monitor pulse rate often
    - If tachycardia occurs, the patient's activities are too strenuous
- Monitor the patient's complete blood count, platelet count, and serum folate levels as ordered
- Assess maternal vital signs and fetal heart rate as indicated
- Instruct the woman in the use of prescribed folic acid supplement and need to continue supplement throughout pregnancy

● **Possible complications**
- Early spontaneous abortion
- Premature separation of the placenta
- Fetal neural tube defects

IRON DEFICIENCY ANEMIA

● **Definition**
- A disorder of oxygen transport in which hemoglobin synthesis is deficient

- Most common anemia during pregnancy, affecting up to 25% of all pregnancies
- Associated with low fetal birth weight and preterm birth

Pathophysiology

- During pregnancy, the development of iron deficiency anemia is directly related to the pregnancy, which results in the maternal iron stores being used for fetal RBC production
- Many women enter pregnancy with a deficit of iron stores, resulting from a diet low in iron (inadequate intake), heavy menstrual periods (blood loss), or unwise weight-reducing programs
- Iron stores are apt to be low in women experiencing a short period (under 2 years) between pregnancies or those from low socioeconomic communities
- Iron deficiency anemia is considered a microcytic (small-sized RBC), hypochromic (less hemoglobin than the average RBC) anemia
  - When iron intake is inadequate, it's unavailable for incorporation into RBCs
  - As a result, cells aren't as large or as rich in hemoglobin as they normally are

Assessment findings

- Fatigue
- Listlessness
- Pallor
- Exercise intolerance
- Pica
- Exertional dyspnea, tachycardia (if severe)

Diagnostic test findings

- Low hemoglobin level (females, less than 10 g/dl)
- Low hematocrit (females, less than 33%)
- Low serum iron level (less than 30 mcg/dl) with high binding capacity (over 400 mcg/dl)
- Low serum ferritin level (less than 100 mg/dl)
- Low RBC count, with microcytic and hypochromic cells (in early stages, RBC count may be normal)
- Decreased mean corpuscular hemoglobin (less than 30) in severe anemia
- Depleted or absent iron stores (by specific staining) and hyperplasia of normal precursor cells (by bone marrow studies)

Management

- Prevention with the incorporation of iron supplementation in all prenatal vitamins

TOP 4

Things to know about iron deficiency anemia

1. It's characterized by deficient hemoglobin synthesis.
2. It's the most common anemia during pregnancy.
3. It affects 25% of all pregnancies.
4. It can cause low fetal birth weight and preterm birth.

Key assessment findings in iron deficiency anemia

- Pallor
- Fatigue
- Pica
- Exertional dyspnea
- Listlessness

TOP 4

Test findings in iron deficiency anemia

1. Low hemoglobin level
2. Low hematocrit
3. Low serum iron level
4. Low serum ferritin level

- Oral iron supplements, such as ferrous sulfate or ferrous or parenteral iron therapy if anemia is severe
- Well-balanced diet

● **Nursing interventions**
- Instruct all pregnant women to use prenatal vitamins as prescribed
- Administer oral iron supplement with an acid, for example, orange juice, to enhance absorption; advise women to take prescribed iron supplements with orange juice or a vitamin C supplement to enhance absorption
- Monitor the patient's complete blood count and serum iron and ferritin levels regularly
- Assess the family's dietary habits for iron intake, noting the influence of childhood eating patterns, cultural food preferences, and family income on adequate nutrition
- Monitor the woman's vital signs, especially heart rate, noting any tachycardia, which suggests that activities are too strenuous
- Evaluate the patient for signs and symptoms of decreased perfusion to vital organs—dyspnea, chest pain, dizziness, and symptoms of neuropathy such as tingling in the extremities
- Assess fetal heart rate at each visit; if the patient is hospitalized, monitor fetal heart rate frequently, at least every 4 hours
- Provide frequent rest periods to decrease physical exhaustion and assist the woman with planning activities so that she has sufficient rest between them
- If anemia is severe, expect to administer oxygen as ordered to help prevent and reduce hypoxia
- Administer an iron supplement as ordered
    - Use the Z-track injection method when administering iron I.M. to prevent skin discoloration, scarring, and irritating iron deposits in the skin
    - If the patient receives iron I.V., monitor the infusion rate carefully
        - Stop the infusion and begin supportive treatment immediately if the patient shows signs of an allergic reaction
        - Watch for dizziness and headache and for thrombophlebitis around the I.V. site
- Assist with planning a well-balanced diet with an increased intake of foods high in vitamins and iron; consult nutritional therapy as indicated
- Provide patient education about therapy
    - Offer suggestions for high-fiber foods to prevent constipation from iron therapy
    - Warn the patient that the medication may cause stool be appear black and tarry

● **Possible complications**
  • Low-birth-weight neonates
  • Preterm birth

CARDIAC DISEASE

● **Definition**
  • Remains a problem for women who become pregnant despite advances in therapy
  • Women with cardiac disease who otherwise may not have thought of becoming pregnant are now becoming pregnant because of medical improvements
  • Involves some type of impaired cardiac function
  • Can occur primarily from congenital or rheumatic heart disease
    – Congenital heart disease: atrial septal defect, ventricular septal defect, pulmonary stenosis, coarctation of the aorta
    – Rheumatic heart disease: endocarditis with scar-tissue formation on the mitral, aortic, or tricuspid valves with resulting stenosis or regurgitation
    – Women with mitral valve prolapse may require prophylactic antibiotic therapy during labor to protect the valve
  • Determining the degree of risk, that is whether a woman with cardiac disease can complete a pregnancy successfully, is based upon the type and extent of her disease
    – Criteria developed by the New York State Heart Association is often used to predict the outcome of a pregnancy
    – These criteria classify the woman into one of four categories based on the degree of compromise (see *Heart disease and pregnancy*, page 142)

● **Pathophysiology**
  • The underlying problem depends on the location and severity of the defect
  • Valvular stenosis decreases blood flow through the valve, increasing the workload on heart chambers located before the stenotic valve
  • Regurgitation permits blood to leak through an incompletely closed valve, increasing the workload on heart chambers on either side of the affected valve
  • The normal heart can compensate for increased demands, but if myocardial or valvular disease develops, or if the patient has a congenital heart defect, cardiac decompensation may occur
  • A patient with a cardiac disorder is at greatest risk when hemodynamic changes reach their maximum, between the 28th and 32nd week of gestation

---

Key facts about cardiac disease in pregnancy

• Involves impaired cardiac function
• Can occur from congenital or rheumatic heart disease

Congenital heart diseases

• Atrial septal defect
• Ventricular septal defect
• Pulmonary stenosis
• Coarctation of the aorta

Pathophysiology of cardiac disease in pregnancy

• Valve stenosis decreases blood flow.
• Workload on heart chambers increases.
• Regurgitation occurs through incompletely closed valves.
• Workload on heart chambers increases.

Heart disease and pregnancy

A patient with heart disease may experience a difficult pregnancy; success depends on the type and extent of the disease. A patient in class I or II usually completes a successful pregnancy and delivery without major complications. A woman in class III must maintain complete bed rest to complete the pregnancy. A patient in class IV is a poor candidate for pregnancy.

CLASS	DESCRIPTION
I	The patient has unrestricted physical activity. Ordinary activity causes no discomfort, cardiac insufficiency, or angina.
II	The patient has a slight limitation on physical activity. Ordinary activity causes excessive fatigue, palpitations, dyspnea, or angina.
III	The patient has a moderate to marked limitation on activity. With less than ordinary activity she experiences excessive fatigue, palpitations, dyspnea, or angina.
IV	The patient can't engage in any physical activity without discomfort. Cardiac insufficiency or angina occurs even at rest.

Key assessment findings in cardiac disease

- Tachycardia
- Dyspnea
- Diastolic murmur
- Crackles at lung bases
- Hemoptysis
- Orthopnea

Managing cardiac disease

- Activity limitation
- Close medical supervision
- Rest
- Limited sodium intake
- Prophylactic antibiotics
- Serial ultrasounds, nonstress tests, and biophysical profile

● **Assessment findings**
- Dyspnea
- Tachycardia
- Fatigue
- Orthopnea
- Edema of hands, face, and feet
- Palpitations
- Diastolic murmur at the heart's apex
- Cough
- Hemoptysis
- Crackles at the bases of the lungs

● **Management**
- Activity limitation
- Close medical supervision with more frequent prenatal visits and adjustments in prepregnancy drug therapy
- Rest
- Limited sodium intake
- Prophylactic antibiotic as indicated
- Serial ultrasounds, nonstress tests, and biophysical profile to evaluate fetal status

● **Nursing interventions**
- Assess maternal vital signs and cardiopulmonary status closely for changes
  - Question the patient about any complaints of increasing shortness of breath, dyspnea, palpitations, or edema
  - Monitor fetal heart rate for changes

- Monitor weight gain throughout pregnancy
  - Assess the patient for edema
  - Note any pitting
- Reinforce the use of prescribed medications to control heart disease
- Alert the patient to danger signs and symptoms that need to be reported immediately
- Reinforce the need for more frequent prenatal visits and assist with arranging follow-up testing
- Anticipate the need for increased doses of maintenance medications; explain to the woman the rationale for this increase
- Assess nutritional pattern
  - Work with the patient to develop a workable meal plan that is high in protein
  - Stress the need for prenatal vitamins and stool softeners if ordered
- Encourage frequent rest periods throughout the day, with activity pacing and energy-conservation measures
- Advise the woman to report any signs and symptoms of infection, such as upper respiratory tract or urinary tract infection, as soon as noticed, to prevent overtaxing the heart
- Advise the woman to rest in the lateral recumbent position to prevent supine hypotension syndrome; if necessary, use the semi-Fowler's position to aid dyspnea
- Prepare the woman for labor, anticipating the use of epidural anesthesia
- Monitor fetal heart rate, uterine contractions, and maternal vital signs closely for changes during labor
- Assess vital signs closely after delivery
- Anticipate anticoagulant and cardiac glycoside therapy for the woman with severe heart failure immediately after delivery
- Encourage ambulation, as ordered, as soon as possible after delivery
- Anticipate administration of a prophylactic antibiotic, if not already ordered, after delivery to prevent subacute bacterial endocarditis

● **Possible complications**
- Maternal cardiac decompensation, including myocardial failure and cardiomyopathy
- Intrauterine growth retardation
- Fetal distress
- Prematurity

SUBSTANCE ABUSE

● **Definition**
- Refers to the misuse or overuse of substances, including alcohol, prescription, over-the-counter, and illicit drugs

Key interventions in cardiac disease

- Assess maternal vital signs and cardiopulmonary status.
- Monitor weight gain.
- Encourage frequent rest periods.
- Assess nutritional status.
- Educate the patient about the signs and symptoms of infection.

Negative effects of cardiac disease

- Maternal cardiac decompensation
- Intrauterine growth retardation
- Fetal distress
- Prematurity

- During pregnancy, most commonly associated with alcohol and illicit drugs
- The number of substance abusers has increased during the last decade
- Most substance abusers are polysubstance abusers, making it difficult to predict maternal-fetal-neonatal implications resulting from synergistic effects

Pathophysiology
- Substance abuse leads to fetal harm
- Substance abuse is most detrimental when used during the first trimester when fetal organs are being formed

Assessment findings
- Most pregnant women who abuse substances don't seek prenatal care
- Substance abuse may be compounded by malnutrition, sexually transmitted diseases, or poor self-image

Management
- Therapy depends on the substance being abused
- Long-term counseling and rehabilitation (social, medical, psychiatric, and vocational) is necessary

Nursing interventions
- Provide the patient with support and guidance
- Assist with measures to obtain necessary support services, such as adequate nutrition and housing
- Encourage participation in an active treatment program
- Monitor the woman as closely as possible during the pregnancy for adequate progression, fetal growth and development, and signs and symptoms of complications
- Enlist the aid of social services and other supportive agencies as necessary
- Prepare for the delivery of a substance-dependent neonate; anticipate drug screening on the neonate's urine and stools
- Anticipate the possible placement of the neonate in foster care if the mother is unable to adequately care for the neonate

Possible complications
- Increased risk of maternal infection with hepatitis B or human immunodeficiency virus
- Maternal cellulitis, septic phlebitis, superficial abscesses, or acute pulmonary edema
- Delivery of drug addicted neonate
- Fetal alcohol syndrome
- Congenital anomalies

SEXUALLY TRANSMITTED DISEASES

Definition
- Spread through sexual contact with an infected partner
- Although all sexually transmitted diseases (STDs) can be serious, during pregnancy certain STDs place the woman at greater risk for problems because of their potential effect on the pregnancy, fetus, or neonate (see *Selected STDs and pregnancy*, pages 146 to 149)

Pathophysiology
- STDs can be caused by numerous organisms
  - Fungi
  - Bacteria
  - Protozoas
  - Parasites
  - Viruses
- Regardless of the cause, the organism invades the body, placing the mother and fetus at risk for problems

Assessment findings
- The signs and symptoms exhibited by the patient with an STD typically involve some type of vaginal discharge or lesion
- Vulvar or vaginal irritation, such as itching or pruritus, commonly accompany the discharge or lesion

Management
- Pharmacologic therapy with antifungal or antimicrobial
- Safe-sex practices
- Treatment of partner

Nursing interventions
- Explain the mode of transmission of the STD and educate the patient about measures to reduce the risk of transmission
- Administer drug therapy as ordered
  - Instruct the patient in drug therapy regimens as appropriate
  - Advise the patient to comply with therapy, completing the entire course of drug therapy
- Urge the patient to refrain from sexual intercourse until the active infection is completely gone
- Instruct the patient to have her partner examined so that treatment can be initiated, thus preventing the risk of reinfection
- Provide comfort measures for the patient to reduce vulvar and vaginal irritation
  - Encourage the woman to keep the vulvar area clean and dry
  - Advise her to avoid using strong soaps, creams, or ointments unless prescribed

(Text continues on page 148.)

Key interventions for STDs
- Explain STD transmission to the patient.
- Administer drug therapy as ordered.
- Provide comfort measures to reduce vulvar and vagina irritation.
- Encourage follow-up care.

TOP 2

Ways to reduce vulvar and vaginal irritation
1. Keep vulvar area clean and dry.
2. Avoid using strong soaps, creams, or ointments unless prescribed.

Selected STDs and pregnancy

This chart lists several sexually transmitted diseases (STDs), their causative organisms, assessment findings, and appropriate treatment for pregnant patients.

STD	CAUSATIVE ORGANISM	ASSESSMENT FINDINGS
Trichomoniasis	Single-cell protozoan infection	• Yellow-gray, frothy, odorous vaginal discharge • Vulvar itching, edema, and redness • Vaginal secretions on a wet slide treated with potassium hydroxide positive for organism
Bacterial vaginosis	*Gardnerella vaginalis* infection (most commonly)	• Thin, gray vaginal discharge with a fishlike odor • Intense pruritus • Wet mount slide positive for clue cells (epithelial cells with numerous bacilli clinging to the cells' surface)
Chlamydia	*Chlamydia trachomatis*	• Commonly produces no symptoms; suspicion raised if partner treated for nongonococcal urethritis • Heavy, gray-white vaginal discharge • Painful urination • Positive vaginal culture using special chlamydial test kit
Syphilis	*Treponema pallidum*	• Painless ulcer on vulva or vagina (primary syphilis) • Hepatic and splenic enlargement, headache, anorexia, and maculopapular rash on the palms of the hands and soles of the feet (secondary syphilis; occurring about 2 months after initial infection) • Cardiac, vascular, and central nervous system changes (tertiary syphilis; occurring after an undetermined latent phase) • Positive Venereal Disease Research Laboratory (VDRL) serum test; confirmed with positive rapid plasma reagin and fluorescent treponemal antibody absorption tests • Dark-field microscopy positive for spirochete

TREATMENT	SPECIAL CONSIDERATIONS
• Topical clotrimazole (Gyne-Lotrimin) instead of metronidazole (Flagyl) because of its possible teratogenic effects if used during the first trimester of pregnancy	• Possibly associated with preterm labor, premature rupture of membranes, and postcesarean infection • Treatment of partner required, even if asymptomatic
• Topical vaginal metronidazole after the first trimester, usually late in pregnancy	• Rapid growth and multiplication of organisms, replacing the normal lactobacilli organisms that are found in the healthy woman's vagina • Treatment goal of reestablishing the normal balance of vaginal flora • Untreated infections associated with amniotic fluid infections and, possibly, preterm labor and premature rupture of membranes
• Amoxicillin (Amoxil)	• Screening for infection at first prenatal visit because it's one of the most common types of vaginal infection seen during pregnancy • Repeated screening in the third trimester if the woman has multiple sexual partners • doxycycline (Vibramycin) – drug of choice for treatment if the woman isn't pregnant – contraindicated during pregnancy due to association with fetal long bone deformities • Concomitant testing for gonorrhea due to high incidence of concurrent infection • Possible premature rupture of the membranes, preterm labor, and endometritis in the postpartum period resulting from infection • Possible development of conjunctivitis or pneumonia in neonate born to mother with infection present in the vagina
• Penicillin G benzathine (Bicillin L-A) I.M. (single dose)	• Possible transmission across placenta after approximately 18 weeks' gestation, leading to spontaneous miscarriage, preterm labor, stillbirth, or congenital anomalies in the neonate • Standard screening for syphilis at the first prenatal visit, screening at 36 weeks' gestation for women with multiple partners, and possible rescreening at beginning of labor, with neonates tested for congenital syphilis using a sample of cord blood • Jarisch-Herxheimer reaction (sudden hypotension, fever, tachycardia, and muscle aches) after medication administration, lasting for about 24 hours, and then fading because spirochetes are destroyed

(continued)

Selected STDs and pregnancy *(continued)*

STD	CAUSATIVE ORGANISM	ASSESSMENT FINDINGS
Genital herpes	Herpes simplex virus, type 2	• Painful, small vesicles with erythematous base on vulva or vagina rupturing within 1 to 7 days to form ulcers • Low-grade fever • Dyspareunia • Positive viral culture of vesicular fluid • Positive enzyme linked immunosorbent assay
Gonorrhea	*Neisseria gonorrhoeae*	• May not produce symptoms • Yellow-green vaginal discharge • Male partner who experiences severe pain on urination and purulent yellow penile discharge • Positive culture of vaginal, rectal, or urethral secretions
Condyloma acuminata	Human papillomavirus	• Discrete papillary structures that spread, enlarge, and coalesce to form large lesions; increasing in size during pregnancy • Possible secondary ulceration and infection with foul odor
Group B streptococci infection	Spirochete	• Usually produces no symptoms

• Suggest the use of cool or tepid sitz baths to relieve itching
• Encourage the woman to wear cotton underwear and avoid tight-fighting clothing as much as possible
• Instruct the patient in safer sex practices, including the use of condoms and spermicides such as nonoxynol 9
• Encourage follow-up to ensure complete resolution of the infection (if possible)

● **Possible complications**
• Preterm labor
• Premature rupture of membranes
• Neonatal conjunctivitis or pneumonia from chlamydia
• Congenital herpes in the neonate
• Ophthalmia neonatorum
• Respiratory distress syndrome

Negative effects of STDs

• Preterm labor
• Premature rupture of membranes
• Neonatal conjunctivitis or pneumonia
• Neonatal congenital herpes
• Ophthalmia neonatorum
• Respiratory distress syndrome

TREATMENT	SPECIAL CONSIDERATIONS
• Acyclovir (Zovirax) orally or in ointment form	• Reduction or suppression of symptoms, shedding, or recurrent episodes only with drug therapy, not a cure for infection • Abstinence urged until vesicles completely heal • Primary infection transmission possible across the placenta, resulting in congenital infection in the neonate • Transmission to neonate possible if active lesions are present in the vagina or on the vulva at birth, which can be fatal • Cesarean delivery recommended if patient has active lesions
• Cefixime (Suprax) as a one-time I.M. injection	• Associated with spontaneous miscarriage, preterm birth, and endometritis in the postpartum period • Treatment of sexual partners required to prevent reinfection • Major cause of pelvic infectious disease and infertility • Severe eye infection leading to blindness in the neonate (ophthalmia neonatorum) if infection present at birth
• Topical application of trichloroacetic acid or bichloroacetic acid to lesions • Lesion removal with laser therapy, cryocautery, or knife excision	• Serious infections associated with the development of cervical cancer later in life • Lesions left in place during pregnancy unless bothersome and removed during the postpartum period
• Broad-spectrum penicillin such as ampicillin	• Occurs in as many as 15% to 35% of pregnant women • May lead to urinary tract infection, intra-amniotic infection leading to preterm birth, and postpartum endometritis • Screening for all pregnant women recommended by The Centers for Disease Control and Prevention at 35 to 38 weeks' gestation

HUMAN IMMUNODEFICIENCY VIRUS INFECTION

Definition
- Human immunodeficiency virus (HIV) is the causative organism for acquired immunodeficiency syndrome (AIDS)
- Considered an STD, it can have serious implications for the pregnant woman and her fetus

Pathophysiology
- HIV infection is caused by a retrovirus that targets the helper T-lymphocytes that contain the CD4+ antigen
  - The virus integrates itself into the cell's genetic makeup, ultimately causing cellular dysfunction

Key signs and symptoms of HIV infection

- Lymphadenopathy
- Bacterial pneumonia
- Fevers
- Nights sweats
- Weight loss

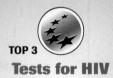

TOP 3

Tests for HIV

1. Enzyme-linked immunosorbent assay
2. Western blot test
3. CD4+ lymphocyte count

Key interventions for HIV infection

- Educate the mother about prevention.
- Institute standard precautions for the mother and neonate.
- Monitor CD4+ T-lymphocyte counts and viral loads as indicated.
- Assess for signs and symptoms of infection.

– The cells are no longer able to function in mounting an appropriate immune response, leaving the patient vulnerable to opportunistic infections
- The virus may be contracted through sexual intercourse, exposure to infected blood, vertical transmission across the placenta to the fetus during pregnancy, labor and delivery birth, or by breast milk to the neonate

Assessment findings
- Lymphadenopathy
- Bacterial pneumonia
- Fevers
- Nights sweats
- Weight loss
- Dermatologic problems
- Thrush
- Thrombocytopenia
- Diarrhea
- Severe vaginal yeast infection that is difficult to treat
- Abnormal Papanicolaou smear
- Frequent humanpapilloma virus infections, frequent and recurrent bacterial vaginosis, trichomonas and genital herpes infections

Diagnostic test findings
- Two positive enzyme-linked immunosorbent assays confirmed with the Western blot test identifies the woman as being positive for HIV
- CD4+ T lymphocyte count is less than 200 cells/µl

Management
- Combination antiretroviral therapy in an attempt to reduce the mother's viral load and thus minimize the risk of vertical transmission of the infection to the fetus
- Supportive care

Nursing interventions
- Institute standard precautions when caring for the mother throughout the pregnancy and after delivery and when caring for the neonate
- Teach the pregnant woman measures to minimize the risk of virus transmission
- Provide emotional support and guidance for the woman who is HIV positive and considering pregnancy
- Allow the pregnant woman who's discovered to be HIV positive to verbalize her feelings and provide support for her
- Monitor CD4+ T-lymphocyte counts and viral loads as indicated
- Assess the patient for signs and symptoms of opportunistic infections

- Encourage the patient to maintain prenatal follow up to evaluate the status of the pregnancy
- Administer antiretroviral therapy as ordered
  - Instruct the patient in the same
  - Assist with scheduling medications
  - Evaluate the patient for compliance on return visits
- Institute measures during labor and delivery to minimize the fetus's risk of exposure to maternal blood or body fluids
- Avoid the use of internal fetal monitors, scalp blood sampling, forceps, and vacuum extraction to prevent the creation of an open lesion on the fetal scalp
- Advise the mother that breast-feeding isn't recommended because of the risk of possible virus transmission
- Withhold blood sampling and injections on the neonate until maternal blood has been removed with the first bath
- Educate the mother about the mode of HIV transmission and safer sex practices

MULTIPLE GESTATIONS

● **Definition**
- Also known as *multiple pregnancy*
- Refers to a pregnancy involving more than one fetus
- Considered a complication of pregnancy because the woman's body must adjust to the effects of the multiple fetuses
- The increased use of fertility drugs has lead to a dramatic doubling of the incidence of multiple gestations

● **Pathophysiology**
- Multiple gestations are the result of the fertilization of one ova forming a zygote that divides into two identical ones or the fertilization of two or more ova
- The increasing use of fertility drugs for assisted reproductive methods has lead to a rise in the number of multiple gestations

● **Assessment findings**
- Increased size of uterus at a rate faster than usual
- Complaints of feeling fluttering actions at different areas of the abdomen with quickening rather than at one specific, consistent spot
- Increased amount of fetal activity than expected for the date
- Multiple sets of fetal heart sounds
- Increased fatigue and backache

● **Diagnostic test findings**
- Elevation of alpha-fetoprotein levels

Signs and symptoms of multiple gestations

- Increase in uterus size at a rate faster than usual
- Quickening at different areas of the abdomen
- More fetal activity than expected
- Multiple sets of fetal heart sounds
- Increased fatigue and backache
- Elevated alpha-fetoprotein levels
- Evidence of multiple gestational sacs or amniotic sacs

- Evidence of multiple gestational sacs on ultrasound and possibly evidence of multiple amniotic sacs early in the pregnancy

● **Management**
- Close maternal and fetal monitoring and surveillance

● **Nursing interventions**
- Assist the woman with understanding her current condition and the need for close, frequent follow-up
- Encourage frequent rest periods throughout the day to help relieve fatigue
- Urge the woman to rest in the side-lying position to prevent supine hypotension syndrome
- Monitor maternal vital signs, weight gain, and fundal height at every visit; assess fetal heart rates and position at every visit
- Arrange for follow-up testing, such as ultrasounds and nonstress tests
- Urge the woman to take a prenatal vitamin and to eat a well-balanced diet high in vitamins and iron
- Alert the woman of the signs and symptoms that she would need to report immediately, especially those of preterm labor
- Provide emotional support to the woman and her family
  - Allow the pregnant woman to verbalize her fears and anxieties about the pregnancy and fetuses
  - Correct any misconceptions that the woman voices

● **Possible complications**
- PIH
- Hydramnios
- Placenta previa
- Preterm labor
- Anemia
- Postpartum bleeding
- Preterm births
- Velamatous cord insertion (the cord inserted into the fetal membranes [with twins])
- Twin-to-twin transfusion

NCLEX CHECKS

It's never too soon to begin your NCLEX preparation. Now that you've reviewed this chapter, carefully read each of the following questions and choose the best answer. Then compare your responses to the correct answers.

Multiple gestation complications

- Pregnancy-induced hypertension
- Hydramnios
- Placenta previa
- Preterm labor
- Anemia
- Postpartum bleeding
- Preterm births
- Velamatous cord insertion
- Twin-to-twin transfusion

1. A pregnant woman experiencing severe abruptio placentae would most likely exhibit:

- ☐ **A.** fetal bradycardia.
- ☐ **B.** painless vaginal bleeding.
- ☒ **C.** rigid, boardlike abdomen.
- ☐ **D.** vague abdominal discomfort.

2. What is the most common site for an ectopic pregnancy?

- ☒ **A.** Fallopian tube
- ☐ **B.** Tubo-ovarian ligament
- ☐ **C.** Ovary
- ☐ **D.** Cervical os

3. Which drug would be used to treat a pregnant woman with a candidal infection?

- ☐ **A.** Doxycycline (Vibramycin)
- ☐ **B.** Azithromycin (Zithromax)
- ☐ **C.** Acyclovir (Zovirax)
- ☒ **D.** Miconazole (Monistat)

4. Which of the following substances is the antidote for magnesium sulfate toxicity?

- ☐ **A.** Protamine sulfate
- ☐ **B.** Vitamin K
- ☐ **C.** Naloxone hydrochloride
- ☒ **D.** Calcium gluconate

5. HELLP syndrome is associated with:

- ☒ **A.** hemolysis.
- ☒ **B.** elevated liver enzymes.
- ☐ **C.** decreased liver enzymes.
- ☐ **D.** increased platelets.
- ☒ **E.** decreased platelets.

6. At which time during pregnancy would a woman with cardiac disease be at greatest risk for problems?

- ☐ **A.** 8 to 12 weeks
- ☐ **B.** 16 to 24 weeks
- ☒ **C.** 28 to 32 weeks
- ☐ **D.** 36 to 40 weeks

TOP 8

Items to study for your next test on prenatal complications and high-risk conditions

1. Maternal risk factors
2. The three types of placenta previa
3. Signs and symptoms of abruptio placentae
4. Common sites of ectopic pregnancy
5. Complications of isoimmunization
6. Categories of pregnancy-induced hypertension
7. HELLP syndrome
8. Management of diabetes during pregnancy

ANSWERS AND RATIONALES

1. CORRECT ANSWER: C

With severe abruptio placentae, the woman would most likely exhibit a rigid, boardlike abdomen with moderate vaginal bleeding and signs and symptoms of shock. Fetal bradycardia is associated with moderate abruptio placentae. Painless vaginal bleeding is associated with placenta previa. Vague abdominal discomfort is associated with mild abruptio placentae.

2. CORRECT ANSWER: A

The most common site of an ectopic pregnancy is the fallopian tube, either in the fimbria, ampulla, or isthmus. Other less-common sites include the tubo-ovarian ligament, ovary, internal cervical os, abdominal viscera, and interstitium.

3. CORRECT ANSWER: D

Miconazole is used to treat candidal (fungal) infections. Chlamydia infection in the pregnant woman is treated with azithromycin or amoxicillin (Amoxil). Doxycycline is used to treat women with chlamydia who aren't pregnant. Acyclovir is used to treat genital herpes.

4. CORRECT ANSWER: D

Calcium gluconate is the antidote for magnesium sulfate toxicity. Protamine sulfate is the antidote for heparin overdose; vitamin K is the antidote for warfarin toxicity. Naloxone reverses the effects of opioids.

5. CORRECT ANSWERS: A, B, AND E

HELLP syndrome is an acronym that refers to a category of PIH that primarily involves changes in blood components and liver function, which include hemolysis, elevated liver enzymes, and a low or decreased platelet count.

6. CORRECT ANSWER: C

Although the risks for the pregnant woman with heart disease and her fetus are always present, the most dangerous time is between 28 to 32 weeks, when hemodynamic changes reach their maximum and the mother's heart may be unable to compensate adequately for these changes.

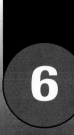

Normal labor and delivery

LEARNING OBJECTIVES

After studying this chapter, you should be able to:

- Differentiate among the four stages of labor.
- State the nurse's role when caring for a patient in labor.
- Describe a pregnant patient's physiologic and psychological responses to labor.
- Identify methods of assessing fetal status during labor.
- Describe current theories of pain.
- Identify potential sources of pain during labor and delivery.
- Name the pharmacologic and nonpharmacologic methods used to relieve pain during labor and delivery.
- Discuss the nurse's role in caring for a patient who has received an analgesic or anesthesia during labor and delivery.
- Describe potential maternal, fetal, and neonatal adverse reactions to pharmacologic measures used during labor and delivery.

CHAPTER OVERVIEW

Throughout labor, many physiologic events occur, resulting in the delivery of the neonate. Specific signs indicate the onset of labor; as the patient progresses, various physiologic and psychosocial responses occur. Throughout labor and delivery, the patient and fetus are monitored closely to ensure the optimal outcome for both. If necessary, obstetric procedures, analgesia, and an anesthetic may be used.

LABOR INITIATION AND COMPONENTS

● **Overview**
- Typically labor begins when the fetus is mature enough to be able to sustain life outside of the uterus while being small enough not to pose difficulty when passing through the birth canal
- The exact mechanism that triggers the onset of labor is unknown
- Current beliefs focus on a combination of occurrences as responsible for initiating labor
    - Uterine stretching
    - Changes in estrogen and progesterone balance
    - Oxytocin stimulation
    - Cervical pressure
    - Prostaglandin production by the fetus
    - Aging of the placenta
    - Increased fetal cortisol levels
- Researchers have attempted to explain the onset of labor with various theories
    - Oxytocin stimulation
        · Researchers haven't proven that either maternal or fetal oxytocin initiates labor
        · Research supports that oxytocin increases after labor has begun, although it doesn't initiate labor
        · It's believed that the myometrium of a patient at term is increasingly sensitive to oxytocin
            - Increased myometrial sensitivity may be a result of estrogen's stimulatory effects
            - Subsequently, the uterus contracts, which works toward the end of labor
    - Progesterone withdrawal
        · Human labor isn't associated with significant changes in the level of major steroid hormones or in the ratio of estrogen to progesterone
        · Marked diurnal variations in progesterone levels have been observed in monkeys and may occur in humans
        · The decrease in progesterone metabolism in the fetus (and possibly the pregnant woman) may stimulate prostaglandin synthesis in the chorioamnion
        · The result is an increase in uterine contractility

Key facts about labor initiation

- Typically begins when the fetus is mature enough to be able to sustain life outside of the uterus
- Exact mechanism that triggers onset is unknown

Occurrences that may initiate labor

- Uterine stretching
- Changes in estrogen and progesterone balance
- Oxytocin stimulation
- Cervical pressure
- Prostaglandin production by the fetus
- Aging of the placenta
- Increased fetal cortisol levels

– Fetal-maternal communication
  · Estrogen acts as an irritant to the myometrium and endometrium
  · The result is the promotion of prostaglandin synthesis
  · Subsequently, myometrial muscle contraction increases
    - These contractions help to transmit impulses over the uterine muscles after the muscle cells have been irritated
    - As a result, the muscle fibers contract

Components of labor

- Four important components of labor (4 Ps) must work together for labor to progress normally
  – Passage
  – Passenger
  – Power
  – Psyche
- If any component is altered, the outcome of labor can be adversely affected

PASSAGE

Description

- Passage refers to the route that the fetus must travel when leaving the uterus, ultimately arriving at the external perineal area for birth
- The route includes the maternal pelvis and soft tissues
- The maternal pelvis must be of adequate size for the fetus to pass through

Shape of the pelvis

- Shape of the pelvis also can determine the ability and ease with which the fetus can pass (see *Types of pelves*, page 158)
  – Gynecoid-shaped pelvis is the most common type of pelvis
    · It occurs in about 50% of females
    · It's a round shape with adequate diameters to allow easy passage of fetal skull and shoulders
  – Anthropoid-shaped pelvis occurs in about 25% of females
    · It's oval with longer anteroposterior diameter
    · This type of pelvis may pose difficulty in passage except when fetus is in occiput posterior position
  – Android-shaped pelvis occurs in about 20% of females
    · It's heart-shaped, like the normal male pelvis
    · Diameter is somewhat narrowed, making fetal passage difficult
  – Platypelloid-shaped pelvis occurs in about 5% of females
    · It's oval or flat
    · The fetus may have difficulty rotating sufficiently to match the shape of the pelvis at the appropriate diameters

The four Ps of labor

1. Passage
2. Passenger
3. Power
4. Psyche

Key facts about passage

- Refers to the route that the fetus travels when leaving the uterus
- Route includes the maternal pelvis and soft tissues
- Maternal pelvis must be large enough for the fetus to pass through

Types of female pelves

- Gynecoid – round shape; most common
- Anthropoid – oval with longer anteroposterior diameter
- Android – heart-shaped; like normal male pelvis
- Platypelloid – oval or flat

Types of pelves

The illustrations below show four types of pelves. Each pelvis varies in size, allowing for an ideal — or in some cases a difficult — delivery of the fetus.

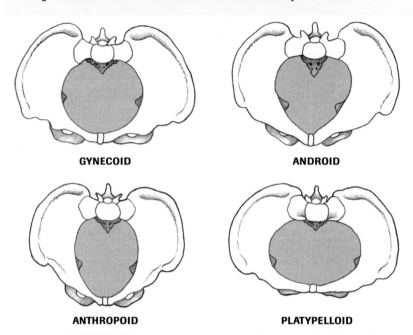

GYNECOID   ANDROID

ANTHROPOID   PLATYPELLOID

The four pelvic joints

1. Symphysis pubis
2. Right sacroiliac joint
3. Left sacroiliac joint
4. Sacrococcygeal joint

False pelvis vs. true pelvis

- False pelvis — portion above the pelvic inlet; supports internal organs and upper body
- True pelvis — includes pelvic inlet, outlet, and cavity
- The false pelvis is separated from the true pelvis by the linea terminalis (runs from the sacral prominence at the posterior pelvis to the superior portion of the symphysis pubis)

● **Bony structures**
- The bony structures of the pelvis, including the pelvic joints and bones, also are important during labor and delivery
- Pelvic joints provide stability to the pelvis
  - Symphysis pubis
  - Right sacroiliac joint
  - Left sacroiliac joint
  - Sacrococcygeal joint
- Pelvic bones give the pelvis its shape
  - Two hip bones, consisting of the ilium, ischium, and pubis, form the front and side aspects of the pelvis
  - Sacrum and coccyx form the posterior portion of the pelvis
- For pregnancy purposes, the pelvis can be divided into two parts
  - False pelvis
    · The portion above the pelvic inlet
    · Considered the superior half of the pelvis
    · Provides support for the internal organs and upper part of the body

– True pelvis
  • Consists of the pelvic inlet, pelvic outlet, and pelvic cavity
    - The pelvic inlet is the entrance to the true pelvis; it's widest from side to side
    - The pelvic outlet is the inferior part of the pelvis encompassed posteriorly by the coccyx, laterally by the ischial tuberosities, and anteriorly by the inferior portion of the symphysis pubis; it's widest from the front to the back
    - The pelvic cavity is the curved area between the pelvic inlet and pelvic outlet
  • Considered the inferior half of the pelvis
– An imaginary line (linea terminalis) separates the false pelvis from the true pelvis
  • The line runs from the sacral prominence at the posterior pelvis to the superior portion of the symphysis pubis at the anterior
  • Area above the line is considered the false pelvis and the area below the line, the true pelvis

Pelvic diameters

• For the fetus to pass through the pelvis during labor and delivery, the woman's pelvic diameters must be adequate
• Typically, several pelvic diameters are measured
  – Anteroposterior diameters of the pelvic inlet considered adequate for vaginal delivery
    • True conjugate — $4\frac{3}{8}$" (11 cm) or greater
    • Diagonal conjugate — $4\frac{7}{8}$" to $5\frac{1}{8}$" (12.5 to 13 cm)
    • Obstetric conjugate — $4\frac{7}{8}$" to $5\frac{1}{8}$"
  – The transverse diameter of the inlet measures $5\frac{3}{8}$" (13.5 cm) or greater
  – The oblique diameter of the inlet is 5" (12.7 cm) or greater
  – Diameters of the pelvic outlet considered adequate for vaginal delivery are as follows:
    • Anteroposterior diameter is about $4\frac{5}{8}$" (11.7 cm)
    • Transverse or intertuberous diameter ranges from $3\frac{7}{8}$" to $5\frac{3}{8}$" (10 to 13.5 cm)
    • Posterior sagittal diameter is about $3\frac{1}{2}$" (9 cm)

Soft tissues

• Soft tissues of the pelvis play a role in labor and delivery
• The lower segment of the uterus expands to accommodate intrauterine contents as the walls of the upper segment thicken
• The cervix is drawn up and over the presenting part as it descends
• The vaginal canal distends to accommodate the passage of the fetus

Head diameters at term

The illustration below depicts three commonly used measurements of fetal head diameters. The measurements are averages for term neonates. Individual measurements vary with fetal size, attitude, and presentation.

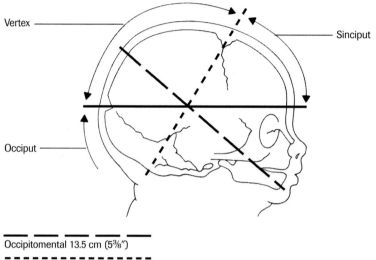

Vertex

Sinciput

Occiput

Occipitomental 13.5 cm (5⅜″)

Suboccipitobregmatic 9.5 cm (3¾″)

Occipitofrontal 11.75 cm (4⅝″)

PASSENGER

● **Description**
- Refers to the fetus and its ability to move through the passage
- Affected by several fetal features

● **Fetal skull**
- Its size is important as the fetus travels through the birth canal
- Contains eight bones
  - The two fused frontal bones in the forehead, the two parietal bones at the crown of the head, and the occipital bone at the back of the head are important during childbirth
  - The bones meet at suture lines composed of strong, flexible, fibrous tissues, which allow the cranial bones to move and overlap, making it possible for the skull to decrease in size for easier passage through the birth canal
- Typically, the smallest diameter of the fetal skull enters the pelvis first
- The head can flex or extend 45 degrees and rotate 180 degrees, which allows its smallest diameters to move down the birth canal and pass through the maternal pelvis (see *Head diameters at term*)

Key facts about the fetal skull

- Size is important (fetus must be able to travel through the birth canal).
- It contains eight bones, which meet at suture lines composed of strong, flexible, fibrous tissues that allow the bones to move and overlap, making it possible for the skull to decrease in size for easier passage through the birth canal.
- Typically, the smallest diameter of the fetal skull enters the pelvis first.
- The head can flex or extend 45 degrees and rotate 180 degrees, which allows its smallest diameters to move down the birth canal and pass through the maternal pelvis.
- The ability of the skull to change shape also eases passage during labor and delivery (sutures of skull allow cranial bones to shift, resulting in molding of the fetal head during labor and delivery).

Molding of the head: Cephalic presentations

In a cephalic presentation, the skull molds to adapt to an unyielding maternal pelvis. The degree of head flexion or extension dictates which head diameter enters the pelvis first. The illustrations below show possible cephalic presentations; dotted lines indicate molding.

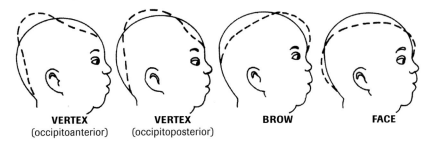

VERTEX
(occipitoanterior)

VERTEX
(occipitoposterior)

BROW

FACE

- Its ability to change its shape is also important
  - Eases its passage during labor and delivery
  - In response to the pressure exerted by the maternal pelvis and birth canal during labor and delivery, the sutures of the skull allow the cranial bones to shift, resulting in molding of the fetal head (see *Molding of the head: Cephalic presentations*)

● **Presentation**
- Describes the fetal body part that will be first to pass through the cervix and be delivered
- Primarily determined by fetal attitude, lie, and position
- Affects the duration and difficulty of labor
  - The uterine contractions that work to open the cervix and push the fetus through the birth canal can be ineffective if they aren't working against the proper forces
  - For example, if the fetus is in a breech position with the soft buttocks pressing against the cervix as the presenting part, the force exerted against the cervix is less than it would be with the firm head as the presenting part
- Affects the method of delivery
  - If the presenting part of the fetus is too large to pass through the mother's pelvis or if the fetus is lying in a position that's undeliverable, a surgical delivery may be necessary
  - Besides the usual risks associated with surgery, an abnormal presentation places the mother and fetus at greater risk for many complications associated with childbirth
- Typically described as cephalic, breech, or shoulder
  - Cephalic presentation occurs when the head presents first
    · The most common type of presentation

Types of fetal presentation

- Cephalic — head presents first; most common type
- Breech — buttocks or feet present first
- Shoulder — shoulder, iliac crest, hand, or elbow presents first

Types of cephalic presentation

- Vertex — head sharply flexed; parietal bones or space between the fontanels presents first
- Brow — head moderately flexed
- Face — head poorly flexed
- Mentum — hyperextension of head; chin presents first

Types of breech presentation

- Complete — thighs of the fetus are tightly flexed on the abdomen, causing the buttocks and flexed feet to present first
- Frank — fetal hips are flexed but the legs are extended and resting on the chest, causing the buttocks to present first
- Footling — in absence of hip or thigh flexion, one or both feet present first; most difficult of the breech deliveries; cord prolapse is common; cesarean birth may be necessary

- Vertex presentation occurs when the head is flexed sharply so that the parietal bones or the space between the fontanels is the presenting part
- A brow presentation occurs when the head is moderately flexed, causing the brow to enter first
- A face presentation occurs when the fetus is poorly flexed, causing the face to present first
- A mentum presentation occurs when the fetal head is hyperextended, causing the chin to present first
– Breech presentation occurs when the buttocks or feet present first
  - A complete breech presentation occurs when the thighs of the fetus are tightly flexed on the abdomen, causing the buttocks and flexed feet to present first
  - A frank breech presentation occurs when the fetal hips are flexed but the legs are extended and resting on the chest, causing the buttocks to present first
  - A footling breech presentation occurs in the absence of hip or thigh flexion of one (single) or both (double) extremities such that one or both feet are the presenting part
    - The most difficult of the breech deliveries
    - Cord prolapse is common because of the space that the extended leg creates
    - Cesarean birth may be necessary to reduce the risk of fetal or maternal mortality
– Shoulder presentation occurs when the presenting part is the shoulder, iliac crest, hand, or elbow
  - Fetus is lying horizontally in the pelvis
  - In the multiparous woman there may be various causes
    - Relaxation of the abdominal walls (the uterus is unsupported and falls forward, causing the fetus to turn horizontally)
    - Pelvic contraction (the vertical space in the pelvis is smaller than the horizontal space)
    - Placenta previa (the low-lying placenta decreases the vertical space in the uterus)
  - Early identification and intervention is critical; from a visual standpoint, the mother's abdomen may have an abnormal or distorted shape — wider horizontally and shorter vertically
  - The fetus must be turned before delivery
    - Attempts to turn the fetus are usually unsuccessful unless the fetus is small or preterm
    - Cesarean birth is almost always necessary to reduce the risk of fetal or maternal mortality (see *Classifying fetal presentation*)

Classifying fetal presentation

Fetal presentation may be broadly classified as cephalic, breech, shoulder, or compound. Cephalic presentations comprise almost all deliveries. Of the remaining three, breech deliveries are most common.

CEPHALIC

In the cephalic (or head-down) presentation, the position of the fetus may be further classified by the presenting skull landmark, such as vertex, brow, sinciput, or mentum (chin).

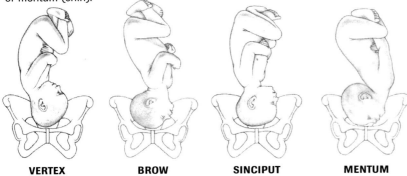

VERTEX   **BROW**   **SINCIPUT**   **MENTUM**

BREECH

In the breech (or head-up) presentation, the position of the fetus may be further classified as *complete,* where the knees and hips are flexed; *frank,* where the hips are flexed and knees remain straight; *kneeling,* where the knees are flexed and the hips remain extended; and *incomplete,* where one or both hips remain extended and one or both feet or knees lie below the breech.

COMPLETE   **FRANK**   **INCOMPLETE**

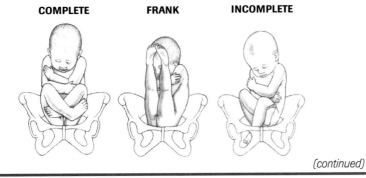

(continued)

● **Lie**
  • Refers to the relationship of the long axis (spine) of the fetus to the long axis of the mother
  • Can be described as longitudinal, transverse, or oblique
    – Longitudinal lie
      · The long axis of the fetus is parallel to the long axis of the mother
      · The fetus is lying vertically, or top-to-bottom, in the uterus
      · Nearly all (99%) fetuses are in a longitudinal lie at the onset of labor

Types of fetal lie

- Longitudinal — fetus is lying vertically in the uterus; further classified as cephalic or breech; nearly all fetuses are in longitudinal lie at onset of labor
- Transverse — fetus is lying horizontally in the uterus; occurs in less than 1% of cases
- Oblique — fetal spine and maternal spine are at 45-degree angles (midway between transverse and longitudinal lies); rare

---

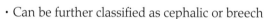

Classifying fetal presentation *(continued)*

SHOULDER

Although a fetus may adopt one of several shoulder presentations, examination can't differentiate among them; thus, all transverse lies are considered shoulder presentations.

COMPOUND

In compound presentation, an extremity prolapses alongside the major presenting part so that two presenting parts appear in the pelvis at the same time.

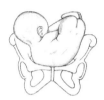

- Can be further classified as cephalic or breech
  - In a cephalic longitudinal lie, a location on the fetal head—determined by attitude and position—is the presenting part
  - In a breech longitudinal lie, the fetal buttocks or foot (possibly feet) is the presenting part
- Transverse lie
  - The long axis of the fetus is perpendicular to the long axis of the mother
  - The fetus is lying horizontally, or side-to-side, in the uterus
  - Less than 1% of fetuses are in transverse lie at the onset of labor
  - If labor progresses, the presenting part may be a shoulder, iliac crest, hand, or elbow
- Oblique lie
  - The fetal spine and the maternal spine are at 45-degree angles to each other
  - This lie is midway between the transverse and longitudinal lies
  - A rare occurrence, it's considered abnormal if the fetus maintains this position after the onset of labor

● **Attitude**
- The relationship of the fetal body parts to one another
- Denotes whether the presenting parts of the fetus are in flexion or extension
- Complete flexion is the most common fetal attitude
  - The traditional position referred to when describing a fetus in utero—fetal position
    - The neck is completely flexed, with the head tucked down onto the chest and the chin touching the sternum

TOP 4

Things to know about fetal attitude

1. Refers to the relationship of fetal body parts to one another
2. Denotes whether presenting parts are in flexion or extension
3. Most common—complete flexion
4. Second most common—moderate flexion

- The arms are folded over the chest with the elbows flexed
- The lower legs are crossed and the thighs are drawn up onto the abdomen, with the calf of each leg pressed against the thigh of the opposite leg
  - Involves a vertex presentation through the birth canal
  - The ideal attitude for gestation and for birth because the fetus occupies the smallest space possible in the uterus
  - Makes for the easiest delivery because the smallest anteroposterior diameter of the fetal skull is presented to pass through the pelvis
- Moderate flexion is the second most common fetal attitude
  - Commonly known as the military position because the straightness of the head makes the fetus appear to be "at attention"
    - The neck is slightly flexed
    - The head is held straight but the chin doesn't touch the chest
  - Involves sinciput (forehead) presentation through the birth canal
  - Many fetuses assume this attitude early in labor but convert to a complete flexion (vertex presentation) as labor progresses
  - Birth usually isn't difficult because the second smallest anteroposterior diameter of the skull is presented through the pelvis during delivery
- Partial extension is an uncommon fetal attitude
  - Involves brow presentation through the birth canal
    - The neck is extended
    - The head is moved backward slightly so that the brow becomes the first part of the fetus to pass through the pelvis during delivery
  - Can cause a difficult delivery, because the anteroposterior diameter of the skull may be equal to or larger than the opening in the pelvis
- Complete extension is relatively rare and is considered abnormal
  - Can result from any one of various factors
    - Oligohydramnios (less-than-normal amniotic fluid)
    - Neurologic abnormalities
    - Multiparity or a large abdomen with decreased uterine tone
    - Nuchal cord with multiple coils around the neck
    - Fetal malformation (found in as many as 60% of cases)
  - Involves a face presentation through the birth canal
    - The head and neck of the fetus are hyperextended with the occiput touching the upper back
    - The back is usually arched, increasing the degree of hyperextension
  - For every 1 in 500 births, the fetus will maintain this attitude as it begins its decent through the pelvis

Types of fetal attitude

- **Complete flexion** — most common fetal attitude; referred to as *fetal position;* neck completely flexed, head tucked down, and chin touching sternum; arms folded over the chest with elbows flexed; lower legs crossed and thighs drawn up to abdomen; ideal attitude for birth
- **Moderate flexion** — second most common fetal attitude; commonly known as *military position* (straightness of head makes fetus appear to be "at attention"); neck slightly flexed; head held straight but chin doesn't touch chest; many fetuses assume this attitude early in labor but convert to a complete flexion as labor progresses; doesn't usually complicate birth
- **Partial extension** — uncommon fetal attitude; neck extended; head moved backward slightly so that the brow becomes the first part of the fetus to pass through the pelvis during delivery; can cause difficult delivery
- **Complete extension** — relatively rare; head and neck hyperextended with occiput touching the upper back; back usually arched; can be caused by oligohydramnios, neurologic abnormalities, multiparity, nuchal cord, and fetal malformation; requires cesarean delivery

Defining fetal presenting parts

- Occiput — vertex presentation
- Mentum — face presentation
- Sacrum — breech presentation
- Scapula or acromion process — shoulder presentation

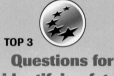

TOP 3

Questions for identifying fetal position

1. Is the presenting part facing the mother's right (R) or left (L)?
2. Is the presenting part the occiput (O), the mentum (M), the sacrum (Sa), or the scapula or acromion process (A)?
3. Is the presenting part pointing to the anterior (A) or posterior (P) section of the mother's pelvis or to the center, or transverse (T)?

– With complete extension, the occipitomental diameter of the head is presented to pass through the pelvis during delivery; commonly this skull diameter is too large to pass through the pelvis, necessitating a cesarean delivery

● **Position**

- The relationship of the presenting part of the fetus to a specific section of the mother's pelvis
- Important to define because it can influence the progression of labor and the possible need for surgical intervention
- The patient's pelvis is divided into four sections, based on her right and left and front and back: right anterior, left anterior, right posterior, and left posterior
- Four parts of the fetus are used to define the presenting part in relation to one of the mother's pelvic sections: occiput (O), vertex presentation; mentum (M), face presentation; sacrum (Sa), breech presentation; and scapula or acromion process (A), shoulder presentation
- Fetal position is described by using three letters
    - The first letter designates whether the presenting part is facing to the mother's right (R) or left (L)
    - The second letter is the presenting part of the fetus (O, M, Sa, or A)
    - The third letter designates whether the presenting part is pointing to the anterior (A) or posterior (P) section of the mother's pelvis or to the center (transverse [T])
- Various combinations are possible
    - The most common are left occiput anterior (LOA) and right occiput anterior (ROA) — both cephalic vertex presentations (see *Fetal positions*)
    - Positions in vertex presentations include ROA, ROT, ROP, LOA, LOT, LOP
    - Positions in face presentation include RMA, RMT, RMP, LMA, LMT, LMP
    - Positions in breech presentation include RSaA, RSaT, RSaP, LSaA, LSaT, LSaP

● **Station**

- The relationship of the presenting part of the fetus to the ischial spines of the mother's pelvis
    - Station 0 is at the level of the ischial spines
    - When the fetus reaches this point in its descent, engagement occurs
- Measured in centimeters
    - When the presenting part is above the level of the ischial spines, station is referred to as "minus"
    - When the presenting part is below the level of the ischial spines, station is referred to as "plus"

Fetal positions

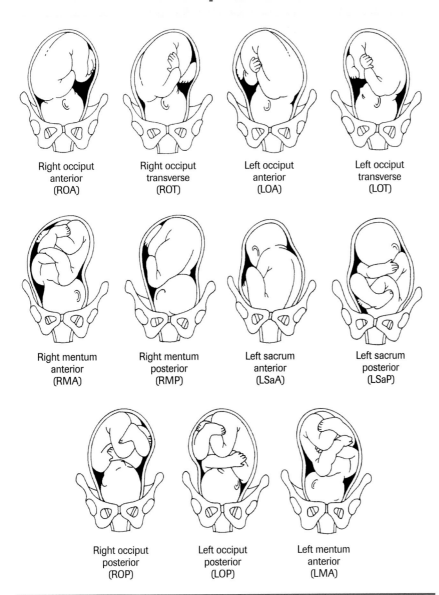

Right occiput anterior (ROA)

Right occiput transverse (ROT)

Left occiput anterior (LOA)

Left occiput transverse (LOT)

Right mentum anterior (RMA)

Right mentum posterior (RMP)

Left sacrum anterior (LSaA)

Left sacrum posterior (LSaP)

Right occiput posterior (ROP)

Left occiput posterior (LOP)

Left mentum anterior (LMA)

- Measurements range from −1 to −4 cm (minus station) and +1 to +4 cm (plus station)
- When the station is measured at +4 cm, the presenting part of the fetus is at the perineum; this is commonly known as "crowning" (see *Measuring fetal station,* page 168)

TOP 4

Facts about station

1. Station 0 is at the level of the ischial spines
2. Minus station measurements range from −1 to −4 cm
3. Plus station measurements range from +1 to +4 cm
4. Station +4 cm is at the perineum and is known as "crowning"

Measuring fetal station

Fetal station, determined by vaginal examination, is the relationship of the presenting part to the ischial spines. In *engagement*, the presenting part of the fetus is at the level of the mother's ischial spines. In *crowning*, the presenting part of the fetus is at the perineum.

- **Engagement** – presenting part of the fetus is at the level of the mother's ischial spines
- **Crowning** – presenting part of the fetus is at the perineum

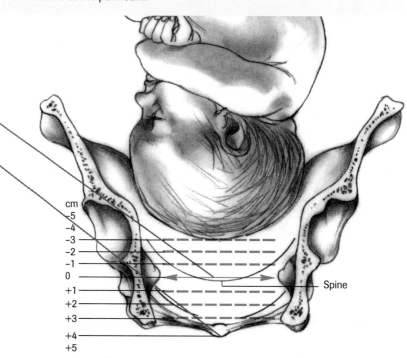

```
cm
-5
-4
-3
-2
-1
 0                    Spine
+1
+2
+3
+4
+5
```

Key facts about power

- Refers to the force of uterine contractions
- Contractions result in cervical effacement and dilation
- Contraction of abdominal muscles provides a secondary source of power

The pattern of contractions

- Normally occur in a wavelike manner
- Begin at a point in the upper segment of the uterus, build and intensify, and then sweep down over the uterus
- Uterine relaxation occurs in the same manner
- After a brief rest period, another contraction begins

POWER

- **Description**
  - Refers to the force of uterine contractions
  - Uterine contractions ultimately result in complete cervical effacement and dilation (see discussion later in this chapter)
  - Contraction of the abdominal muscles such as with pushing and bearing down provides a secondary source of power
- **Contraction pattern**
  - Normal uterine contractions occur in a wavelike manner
  - They begin at a point in the upper segment of the uterus, build and intensify, and then sweep down over the uterus
  - Relaxation of the uterus occurs in the same manner
  - After a brief period of rest, during which blood flow returns to supply oxygen and vital nutrients to the uterus and placenta, another contraction begins

- When contractions begin in the lower segment of the uterus they're ineffective and actually cause tightening of the cervix

PSYCHE

- **Description**
  - Refers to the feelings that the woman brings to labor
  - For some, feelings may include apprehension and fear; for others, excitement and wonderment are common
  - A major component is the woman's psychological readiness for labor
- **Factors affecting psychological readiness**
  - Presence of a support person and support systems positively affects the woman's ability to manage labor
  - The degree of preparation for childbirth is important; asking questions during prenatal visits and attending childbirth education classes can help the woman prepare for the events of labor
  - Past experiences and coping measures can be used as a basis for managing the events of labor
  - Accomplishment of the tasks of pregnancy provide the woman and her partner with the necessary knowledge base for the labor and birth experience, having accepted the pregnancy and being prepared for the birth
  - Ideally, the outcome is to provide the woman with as much control over the situation as possible

PRELIMINARY SIGNS OF LABOR

- **Lightening**
  - The descent of the fetal head into the pelvis
    - The uterus becomes lower and more anterior and the contour of the abdomen changes because of the change in the shape of the uterus
    - Commonly occurs 2 to 4 weeks before birth in primiparas—probably due to the tone of the abdominal muscles
    - It can occur the day labor begins or after the start of labor in multiparas
  - Increases pressure on the bladder, which may cause urinary frequency
  - Allows the mother to breathe easier because pressure on the diaphragm is decreased
  - Increased abdominal pressure from shifting of the fetus and uterus may cause pressure on the sciatic nerve with resultant leg pains
  - The mother may also notice an increase in vaginal discharge due to the pressure of the fetus on the cervix
- **Braxton Hicks contractions**
  - Mild contractions of the uterus that occur throughout pregnancy

---

Factors that affect psychological readiness for labor and birth

- Presence of support system
- Degree of preparation
- Childbirth education classes
- Past experiences
- Coping measures
- Accomplishment of pregnancy tasks
- Feeling of control over situation

Quick guide to preliminary signs of labor

- **Lightening** – descent of fetal head into the pelvis; occurs 2 to 4 weeks before birth in primiparas; can occur the day of birth or after start of labor in multiparas
- **Braxton Hicks contractions** – mild, irregular contractions of the uterus that occur throughout pregnancy
- **Cervical changes** – ripening, effacement, and dilation; occurs several days before initiation of labor
- **Energy** – bursts of energy before onset of labor
- **Weight loss** – 1 to 3 lb up to 3 days before labor begins; may be accompanied by flulike symptoms, diarrhea, and freqent voiding

Spotlight on Braxton Hicks contractions

- Mild contractions of the uterus that occur throughout pregnancy
- Irregular (unlike labor contractions); time between contractions and their strength vary
- Gradually increase in frequency and intensity throughout pregnancy
- Relieved by increased activity, eating, drinking, or changing position
- Typically painless, especially early in pregnancy
- Pain felt only in the abdomen and groin — never in the back
- Don't cause progressive cervical effacement or dilation
- May become extremely strong a few days to 1 month before labor begins, causing genuine discomfort
- Commonly misinterpreted as true labor, especially by the primipara

- Unlike contractions of labor, Braxton Hicks contractions are irregular
  - The length of time between them and strength vary widely
  - A gradual increase in frequency and intensity occurs through the pregnancy
- Can be diminished with increased activity, eating, drinking, or changing position, something that can't be done with the contractions of labor
- Braxton Hicks contractions are typically painless — especially early in pregnancy
  - Many women feel only a tightening of the abdomen in the first or second trimester
  - If the woman feels pain from these contractions, it's felt only in the abdomen and the groin — never in the back
- Braxton Hicks contractions don't cause progressive effacement or dilation of the cervix
  - The uterus can still be indented with a finger during a contraction, which indicates that the contractions aren't performing with the efficiency necessary to bring about these changes
  - Braxton Hicks contractions may become extremely strong a few days to a month before labor begins
  - When they strengthen they can cause genuine discomfort and are commonly misinterpreted as true labor, especially by the primipara (see *Distinguishing between true and false labor*)

Cervical changes

- Usually occur several days before initiation of labor
- Cervix softens (ripens), begins to efface, and dilates slightly
  - Ripening of the cervix can only be determined during a pelvic examination performed by the health care provider, usually in the last weeks of the third trimester
  - When the cervix ripens, the cervix undergoes a change in position, tipping forward in the vagina

Burst of energy

- Patient may experience a sudden burst of energy before the onset of labor after having experienced increased fatigue for most of the third trimester
- Patient may perform housecleaning activities; this is called the "nesting" instinct

Loss of weight

- The pregnant woman may lose 1 to 3 lb (0.5 to 1.4 kg) up to 3 days before labor begins
- The hormone, relaxin, is released causing flulike signs and symptoms and diarrhea
- The levels of estrogen and progesterone are altered, possibly resulting in an increase in voiding and subsequent fluid loss

Distinguishing between true and false labor

Knowing how to recognize the primary characteristics of true and false labor can help you distinguish between the two conditions.

TRUE LABOR	FALSE LABOR
Regular contractions	Irregular contractions
Back discomfort that spreads to the abdomen	Discomfort that's localized in the abdomen
Progressive cervical dilation and effacement	No cervical change
Gradually shortened intervals between contractions	No change or irregular change
Increased intensity of contractions with ambulation	Contractions may be relieved with ambulation
Contractions that increase in duration and intensity	Usually no change in contractions

- Loss of more than 3 lb (1.4 kg) in 1 week due to fluid and excrement loss requires immediate notification of the health care provider

SIGNS OF TRUE LABOR

● **Uterine contractions**
- Involuntary but specific in their action to bring about the effacement and dilation of the cervix
- Ultimately responsible for pushing the fetus through the birth canal
- Initially irregular but soon become regular with a predictable pattern, as labor progresses
    - Early contractions occur anywhere from 5 to 30 minutes apart and last 30 to 45 seconds
    - The interval between the contractions allows blood flow to resume to the placenta thereby supplying oxygen to the fetus and removing waste products
- Increase in frequency, duration, and intensity; during the transition phase of the first stage of labor, when contractions reach their maximum frequency, duration, and intensity, they each last 60 to 90 seconds and recur every 2 to 3 minutes
- Painful and wavelike, building and receding
    - Begin in the lower back and move around to the abdomen and, possibly, the legs
    - Stronger in the upper uterus (to push the fetus downward) than in the lower uterus (to thin the walls and allow for dilation), sweeping down over the uterus in this manner

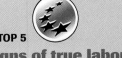

TOP 5

Signs of true labor

1. Uterine contractions — responsible for pushing the fetus through the birth canal; cause effacement and dilation of the cervix
2. Uterus becomes hard on palpation; indentation with a finger not possible
3. Cervical thinning and dilation, resulting in show
4. Expulsion of cervical mucus plug
5. Rupture of membranes

TOP 5

Facts about uterine contractions

1. Involuntary
2. Initially irregular but soon become regular
3. Increase in frequency, duration, and intensity
4. Painful and wavelike
5. Unaffected by activity, eating, drinking, or changing position

What happens when membranes rupture

- The membrane sac that contains and supports the fetus and the amniotic fluid ruptures
- May occur spontaneously at the beginning of labor or remain intact, necessitating rupture by the health care provider
- May occur as a sudden gush or a slow leakage of fluid
- May cause the fetal head to engage in the pelvis, possibly shortening labor
- Labor begins within 24 hours of rupture for most women
- Changes pH of amniotic secretions that can be detected by litmus paper test
- Causes appearance of ferning as seen in fluid specimen viewed under a microscope

– The uterus becomes hard on palpation; indentation with a finger isn't possible
- Unaffected by activity, eating, drinking, or changing position
- Cause progressive effacement and dilation of the cervix
- As labor progresses, a visible bulging of intact membranes can be observed

● **Show**
- Commonly termed bloody show, this occurs as the cervix thins and begins to dilate
  – The mucus plug that has sealed the cervical canal during pregnancy is expelled
  – The mucus from the plug mixes with blood from the cervical capillaries because of the pressure of the fetus on the canal and other changes in the cervix
  – Pink-tinged, blood-tinged, or brownish secretions result
- In some primiparas, the mucus plug may be passed up to 2 weeks before labor begins

● **Rupture of fetal membranes**
- The fetal membranes, composed of the amniotic and chorionic membranes, cover the fetal surface of the placenta and form a sac that contains and supports the fetus and the amniotic fluid
  – The fluid is produced by the amniotic membrane
  – The fluid acts as a cushion throughout gestation, protects the fetus from temperature changes, protects the umbilical cord from pressure, and probably aids in fetal muscular development by allowing the fetus to move freely
- The membranes may rupture spontaneously at the beginning of labor, or they may remain intact throughout active labor, until the health care provider ruptures them or the fetus is delivered
  – Spontaneous rupture of the membranes isn't painful because the membranes have no nerve supply
  – Even if most of the fluid is lost when the membranes rupture, the fetus will always be surrounded by fluid because it continues to be produced until after the fetus is delivered
- The rupture may occur as a sudden gush of fluid or as a steady or intermittent, slow leakage of fluid
- The amniotic fluid that's lost after the rupture of the membranes should be clear, odorless, and milky; any variation requires prompt reporting and further evaluation
  – The fluid passed is tested to confirm spontaneous rupture of membranes
  – The nitrazine test involves the use of litmus paper to detect the pH of the secretions; change in the paper color to bright blue indi-

cates a change in pH from amniotic fluid with rupture of membranes

- – A vaginal examination with a speculum may be used when visualization is necessary but cervical manipulation is contraindicated; pooling of fluid at the base of the cervix indicates rupture of membranes
- – A sample of fluid can be applied to a slide and viewed under a microscope; appearance of ferning indicates rupture of membranes
- Rupture of the membranes may cause the fetal head to engage in the pelvis, possibly shortening labor
- Labor begins within 24 hours for most women
  - – Membrane rupture more than 24 hours before labor begins is called a "premature rupture of membranes"
  - – Premature rupture of membranes is associated with an increased risk of infection and umbilical cord prolapse

STAGES OF LABOR

● First stage

- Measured from the onset of true labor to complete dilation of the cervix
- Duration usually ranges from 6 to 18 hours in a primipara and from 2 to 10 hours in a multipara
- Divided into three phases—latent, active, and transitional
  - – During the latent phase, cervical dilation measures 0 to 3 cm and contractions are irregular and short and last 20 to 40 seconds
    - · This phase lasts about 6 hours in a primipara and 4½ hours in a multipara
    - · If the cervix isn't "ripe" when entering this phase, it may be prolonged
    - · Any analgesia given early in labor may prolong this phase
  - – During the active phase, cervical dilation measures 4 to 7 cm; contractions are 5 to 8 minutes apart, last 45 to 60 seconds, and are moderate to strong in intensity
    - · This phase lasts about 3 hours in a primipara and 2 hours in a multipara
    - · Typically, membranes rupture during this phase if they haven't already done so
  - – During the transitional phase, cervical dilation measures 8 to 10 cm and contractions are 1 to 2 minutes apart, last 60 to 90 seconds, and are strong in intensity
    - · With complete cervical dilation, membranes rupture if they haven't already done so
    - · A feeling of loss of control commonly occurs during this phase
    - · At the end of this phase, the patient feels the urge to push

Cardinal movements of labor

ENGAGEMENT, DESCENT, FLEXION

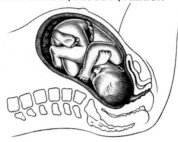

INTERNAL ROTATION

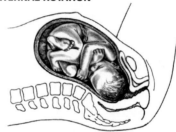

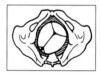

EXTENSION BEGINNING (ROTATION COMPLETE)

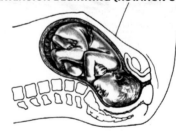

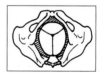

Key facts about stage 2 of labor

- Extends from complete dilation to delivery of the neonate
- Lasts from 2 to 60 minutes, with 40 minutes the average
- Occurs in seven cardinal movements

Second stage

- Extends from complete cervical dilation to delivery of the neonate
- Duration usually ranges from 2 to 60 minutes, averaging about 40 minutes (20 contractions) for the primipara and 20 minutes (10 contractions) for the multipara
- The fetus is moved along the birth canal by mechanisms of labor, positional changes occurring during the second stage of labor; commonly referred to as the "cardinal movements of labor"
    – The cardinal movements are necessary because of the size of the fetal head in relation to the irregularly shaped pelvis

Cardinal movements of labor *(continued)*

EXTENSION COMPLETE

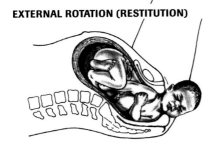
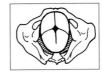

EXTERNAL ROTATION (RESTITUTION)

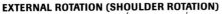
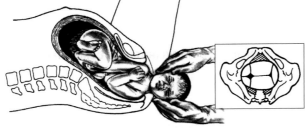

EXTERNAL ROTATION (SHOULDER ROTATION)

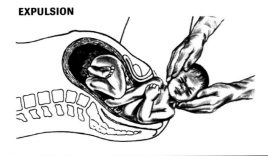

EXPULSION

- Specific, deliberate, and precise, the movements change from one to the next to allow the smallest diameter of the fetus to pass through a corresponding diameter of the woman's pelvis
- Seven movements occur — engagement, descent, flexion, internal rotation, extension, external rotation, and expulsion (see *Cardinal movements of labor*)

Seven cardinal movements of labor

1. **Engagement** — presenting part of the fetus is level with the mother's ischial spines
2. **Descent** — downward movement of the fetus
3. **Flexion** — movement of the fetal head forward so that chin is pressed to chest
4. **Internal rotation** — rotation of head that enables passage through the ischial spines
5. **Extension** — occiput is delivered; the head extends; and the head, face, and chin are delivered
6. **External rotation** — head rotates from anteroposterior position back to diagonal or transverse position
7. **Expulsion** — delivery of the remainder of the fetal body

– Engagement occurs when the presenting part of the fetus has passed far enough into the pelvis so that it's level with the ischial spines
  · The biparietal diameter of the fetal head passes the pelvic inlet
  · An engaged fetus indicates that the pelvic inlet is large enough for the fetus to pass through, because the widest part of the fetus has passed through the narrowest part of the pelvis
– Descent is the downward movement of the fetus
  · Determined when the biparietal diameter of the head passes the ischial spines and moves into the pelvic inlet
  · Progresses intermittently with contractions and occurs because of several forces: direct pressure on the fetus by the contracting uterine fundus, pressure from amniotic fluid, pressure from Valsalva's maneuver with the abdominal muscles, and straightening and extension of the fetal body
  · Full descent is accomplished when the fetal head passes beyond the dilated cervix and contacts the posterior vaginal floor
– Flexion occurs during descent and is caused by the resistance of the fetal head against the pelvic floor
  · The combined pressure from uterine and abdominal muscle contractions and this resistance forces the head of the fetus to bend forward so that the chin is pressed to the chest
  · This allows the smallest diameter of the fetal head to descend through the pelvis
  · The movement of flexion causes the presenting diameter to change from occipitofrontal (nasal bridge to the posterior fontanel) to suboccipitobregmatic (posterior fontanel to sub-occiput) in an occiput anterior position
  · In an occiput posterior position, flexion is incomplete, causing a larger presenting diameter and a prolonged labor
– Internal rotation refers to the rotation of the head to pass through the ischial spines
  · The fetal head typically enters the pelvis with the anteroposterior head diameter in a transverse (right to left) position because the diameter at the pelvic inlet is widest from right to left; the shoulders of the fetus must also pass through the pelvic inlet
  · If the head were to remain in the transverse position, the shoulders would be too wide to pass through
  · Subsequently, the head rotates about 45 degrees as it meets the resistance of the pelvic floor
  · As a result, the anteroposterior diameter of the head is in the anteroposterior plane of the pelvis (front to back), which places the widest part of the shoulders in line with the widest part of the pelvic inlet

What happens during internal rotation

- The fetal head rotates to allow passage of the shoulders through the ischial spines.
- The fetal head typically enters the pelvis in a transverse position because the diameter at the pelvic inlet is widest from right to left.
- The head rotates about 45 degrees as it meets the resistance of the pelvic floor.
- As a result, the anteroposterior diameter of the head is in the anteroposterior plane of the pelvis, which places the widest part of the shoulders in line with the widest part of the pelvic inlet.
- This movement also aligns the fetus in the optimum position to continue descent through the pelvic outlet.

- This movement also aligns the fetus in the optimum position to continue its descent with the widest part of the fetal head at the widest diameter of the pelvic outlet because the diameter at the pelvic outlet is widest from front to back
- At this point, the face of the fetus is usually against the back of the mother and the back of the fetal head is against the front of her pelvis

– Extension occurs after internal rotation is complete
  - As the head passes through the pelvis, the occiput emerges from the vagina and the back of the neck is stopped under the symphysis pubis (pubic arch)
  - Further descent is temporarily halted; the shoulders are too wide to pass through the pelvis or under the pubic arch in this position
  - With the back of the neck resting against the pubic arch, the structure acts as a pivot
  - The upward resistance from the pelvic floor causes the head to extend
  - As this occurs, the brow, nose, mouth, and chin present successively

– External rotation, also called *restitution,* refers to the external rotation of the head and the subsequent rotation of the shoulders into the anteroposterior position in the pelvis
  - After the head presents, the neonate must rotate so that the face, which at the completion of extension is facedown, is turned facing one of the mother's inner thighs
  - The head rotates about 45 degrees, back to the position assumed earlier during descent — with the anteroposterior head diameter in a transverse (right to left) position
  - This movement is necessary because the shoulders, which previously turned to fit through the pelvic inlet, must now turn again to fit through the pelvic outlet and under the pubic arch
  - The anterior shoulder (closest to the front of the mother) is delivered first with the possible assistance of downward flexion on the neonate's head
  - After the anterior shoulder is delivered, a slight upward flexion may be necessary to deliver the posterior shoulder
  - During this movement in the birth process, neonates weighing more than 9.9 lb (4,490 g) are more likely to experience shoulder dystocia than neonates weighing less; it occurs when the shoulders are stopped at the pelvic outlet because there isn't enough space for them to pass through

– Expulsion refers to delivery of the remainder of the body, signifying the end of the second stage of labor

What happens during extension

- As the head passes through the pelvis, the occiput emerges from the vagina and the back of the neck is stopped by the symphysis pubis.
- Further descent is temporarily halted because the shoulders are too wide to pass through the pelvis or under the pubic arch in this position.
- Upward resistance from the pelvic floor causes the head to extend against the pubic arch.
- As this occurs, the brow, nose, mouth, and chin present successively.

What happens during external rotation

- After the head presents, the body must rotate (facing toward one of the mother's inner thighs).
- The head rotates 45 degrees, with the anteroposterior diameter in a transverse position.
- The shoulders turn again, allowing them to fit through the pelvic outlet and under the pubic arch.
- The anterior shoulder is delivered first with the possible assistance of downward flexion on the neonate's head.
- Slight upward flexion may be necessary to deliver the posterior shoulder.

Key facts about stage 3 of labor

- Extends from the delivery of the neonate to delivery of the placenta
- Lasts from 5 to 30 minutes
- Divided into the placental separation and the placental expulsion phases

Spotlight on placental separation

- Separation of the placenta from the uterus
- Occurs after the uterus resumes contractions
- With the fetus no longer in the uterus, the walls of the uterus contract on an almost empty space
- The placenta folds and begins to separate
- As the placenta pulls away from the uterine wall, bleeding begins and aids expulsion of the placenta
- The placenta falls to the upper vagina or lower uterine segment
- Signs include umbilical cord lengthening, gush of vaginal blood, and change in uterine shape

● **Third stage**

- Also called the *placental stage;* the time between the delivery of the neonate and delivery of the placenta
  – After delivery of the neonate, uterine contractions commonly cease for several minutes
  – The uterus can be felt as a round mass, firm to the touch, just below the level of the umbilicus
  – After the brief period of rest, when the contractions resume, the uterus takes on a discoid shape and remains that way until the placenta has separated from the uterus
- Duration ranges from 5 to 30 minutes
- Can be divided into two phases — placental separation and placental expulsion
  – Separation of the placenta from the uterus occurs after the uterus resumes contractions
    · The uterine contractions continue in wavelike fashion
    · During the contractions of the other stages, the fetus exerted pressure on the placenta, which prevented it from separating prematurely; with the fetus no longer in place, the walls of the uterus contract on an almost empty space, and nothing is left to exert reverse pressure on the placenta
    · The placenta folds and begins to separate
    · As the placenta pulls away from the uterine wall, bleeding begins and further pushes the placenta away
    · During this process, the placenta falls to the upper vagina or lower uterine segment
      - About 80% of all placentas begin separation at the center and fold onto themselves, ready to be delivered with the fetal surface exposed
        ·· Called a Schultze placenta
        ·· Appears shiny and glistening from the fetal membranes (see *Picturing the placenta*)
      - If the placenta separates first at its edges, it slides down the surface of the uterus where it's delivered with the maternal surface exposed
        ·· Called a Duncan placenta
        ·· Appears red, raw, and irregular from the ridges that separate the blood collection spaces
    · The outer area of the endometrium (decidua) — the lining of the uterus — is expelled at the same time as the placenta
      - The remainder of the decidua separates into two layers

Picturing the placenta

At term, the placenta (the spongy structure within the uterus from which the fetus derives nourishment) is flat, cakelike, round or oval, measuring 6″ to 7¾″ (15 to 19.5 cm) in diameter and ¾″ to 1¼″ (2 to 3 cm) in breadth at its thickest part. The maternal side is lobulated; the fetal side, shiny.

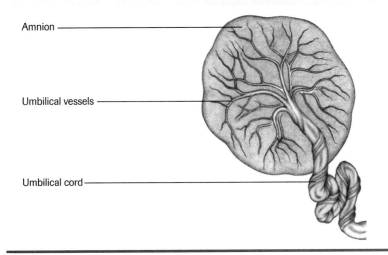

Amnion

Umbilical vessels

Umbilical cord

- The superficial layer, which is shed in the lochia during the postpartum period, and the basal layer, which remains to regenerate new endothelium
   – Signs that the placenta has separated and is ready to be delivered include the lengthening of the umbilical cord, a sudden gush of vaginal blood, and a change in the shape of the uterus
- Placental expulsion and delivery is accomplished with the natural bearing down by the mother or gentle pressure on the fundus of the contracting uterus (Credé's maneuver); if the placenta doesn't deliver spontaneously, it may need to be removed manually
- Pressure should never be applied to the uterus in a noncontracted state to avoid possible eversion of the uterus and resultant gross hemorrhage

● **Fourth stage**
- Time immediately after the delivery of the placenta
   – Typically, it encompasses the first hour after delivery
   – It's commonly referred to as the recovery period
- Although it's the beginning of the postpartum period, this stage is commonly considered part of the labor and delivery process
- Primary activity is stabilizing the status of the neonate and helping him get acclimated to extrauterine life
- Then the focus is on the promoting maternal-neonatal bonding

The placenta at term

- Flat
- Cakelike
- Round or oval
- 6″ to 7¾″ (15 to 19.5 cm) in diameter and ¾″ to 1¼″ (2 to 3 cm) in breadth
- Lobulated maternal side
- Shiny fetal side

Spotlight on placental expulsion

- With separation and movement into the upper vagina or lower uterine segment, placenta is ready for expulsion
- Accomplished by natural bearing down or Credé's maneuver
- Pressure should never be applied to a noncontracted uterus

Key facts about stage 4 of labor

- Covers the time immediately after delivery of the placenta
- Typically, the first hour after delivery
- Referred to as the recovery period

Typical maternal responses to labor

- Intrathoracic pressure increases during pushing in the second stage.
- Cardiac output increases.
- Water loss increases.
- Oxygen consumption increases (hyperventilation may occur).
- Leukocytosis occurs.
- Plasma fibrinogen levels increase.
- Blood coagulation and blood glucose levels decrease.
- Gastric motility and absorption decrease.
- Gastric emptying time is prolonged.
- Forward and upward displacement of the bladder base occurs.
- Proteinuria may occur.
- Urine becomes concentrated.
- Softening at the symphysis pubis and sacral and coccyx joints occurs.
- Stimulation of uterine and cervical nerve plexuses occurs.

MATERNAL PHYSIOLOGIC RESPONSES TO LABOR

- **Cardiovascular system**
  - Intrathoracic pressure increases during pushing in the second stage
  - Peripheral resistance increases during contractions, subsequently elevating blood pressure and decreasing pulse rate
  - Cardiac output increases during labor

- **Fluid and electrolytes**
  - Diaphoresis and hyperventilation during labor leads to increased water loss
  - Increased respiratory rate increases evaporative water volume

- **Respiratory system**
  - Increased respiratory rate leads to increased oxygen consumption
  - Hyperventilation may occur in response to increased oxygen needs

- **Hematopoietic system**
  - Leukocytosis occurs during birth, possibly due to the stress and heavy exertion that occurred during labor
  - Plasma fibrinogen levels increase
  - Blood coagulation time and blood glucose levels decrease

- **GI system**
  - GI tract is primarily inactive during labor
    - May be due to the shunting of blood to vital organs
    - May also be due to the pressure exerted on the stomach and intestine from the contracting uterus
  - Gastric motility and absorption decrease
  - Gastric emptying time is prolonged

- **Renal system**
  - Fetal engagement results in forward and upward displacement of the bladder base
  - Proteinuria from muscle breakdown is possible
  - Impairment of blood and lymph drainage from the bladder base, resulting from edema caused by the presenting part, may occur
  - Urine becomes concentrated as the body attempts to conserve fluid and electrolytes being lost through insensible sources

- **Musculoskeletal system**
  - Continued cartilage softening occurs
    - Softening is primarily at the symphysis pubis and sacral and coccyx joints
    - Stretching occurs to aid in passage of the fetus
  - The woman may notice increased back pain or nagging achy pubic pain when walking or turning during labor

● **Neurologic system**
- The neurologic system response involves pain perception
- Uterine and cervical nerve plexuses are stimulated during early labor by uterine contractions and cervical dilation
- Perineal nerves are stimulated at birth secondary to stretching caused by the passage of the fetus

MATERNAL PSYCHOLOGICAL RESPONSES DURING LABOR

● **First stage**
- The patient may feel anticipation, excitement, or apprehension
- During the active phase, the patient becomes serious and concerned about the progress of labor; she may ask for pain medication or use breathing techniques
- During the transitional phase, the patient may lose control, thrash in bed, groan, or cry out

● **Second stage**
- Maternal behavior changes from coping with contractions to actively pushing
- The patient may become exhausted

● **Third stage**
- The patient typically focuses on the neonate's condition
- Patient may feel discomfort from uterine contractions before expelling the placenta

● **Fourth stage**
- The patient focuses on the neonate
- The patient begins to adjust to the role of mother
- The primary activity is promoting maternal-neonatal bonding

NURSING CARE DURING LABOR AND DELIVERY

● **Care during all four stages**
- Monitor and record I.V. fluid intake, urine output, and vital signs according to facility policy, Association of Women's Health, Obstetric and Neonatal Nurses (AWHONN) and American College of Obstetricians and Gynecologists (ACOG)
- Assess the need for pain medication, and evaluate the effectiveness of medication administered
- Provide emotional support to the patient and her partner
- Maintain sterile technique
- Explain the purpose of all nursing actions and equipment used
- Maintain the patient's comfort by offering mouth care, ice chips, and a change of bed linen

Maternal psychological responses to labor

- **Stage 1:** anticipation, excitement, or apprehension
- **Stage 2:** exhaustion
- **Stage 3:** concern for the neonate's condition
- **Stage 4:** attention focused on neonate

Care checklist for all stages of labor

- Monitor fluid intake, urine output, and vital signs.
- Assess the need for pain medication and evaluate the effectiveness of any given.
- Provide emotional support.
- Maintain patient comfort.

Care checklist for first stage of labor

- **Latent phase:** Provide emotional support, offer clear liquids or ice chips, encourage ambulation and bladder emptying, and obtain blood samples and urine specimens.
- **Active phase:** Encourage proper breathing, place patient in upright or side-lying position, and frequently perform perineal care.
- **Transition phase:** Stay with patient at all times because birth may be imminent.

TOP 3

Steps for treating hypotensive supine syndrome

1. Position the patient on her left side.
2. Increase the primary I.V. flow rate.
3. Administer oxygen through a face mask at 6 to 10 L/ minute.

Monitoring checklist for first two stages of labor

- Frequency of contractions
- Duration of contractions
- Intensity of contractions
- FHR

● **First stage**
- Latent phase
  - Provide the mother with a calm environment and psychological support for conflicting emotions (excitement, anxiety and, possibly, depression)
  - Offer clear liquids or ice chips as tolerated
  - Encourage her to ambulate and empty her bladder frequently
  - Involve the woman's partner or support person in her care as much as possible
  - Obtain the required blood samples and urine specimens
- Active phase
  - Anticipate mood swings and difficulty coping and offer support
  - Encourage proper breathing techniques
  - Continue to involve the woman's partner or support person in her care
  - Place the woman in an upright or side-lying position to help provide additional comfort
  - Frequently perform perineal care, especially after each voiding and bowel movement, to reduce the risk of infection
- Transition phase
  - Stay with the woman at all times because birth may be imminent

● **First and second stages**
- Inform the patient of labor progress: dilation, station, effacement, and fetal well-being (see maternal evaluation in labor later in this chapter for more information)
- Monitor the frequency, duration, and intensity of contractions according to facility policy, AWHONN, and ACOG
- Monitor fetal heart rate (FHR) during and between contractions according to facility policy, AWHONN, and ACOG; note rate, accelerations, decelerations, and variability
- Check for rupture of membranes, noting the time, color, odor, amount, and consistency of amniotic fluid
- Check for prolapsed cord, and check FHR immediately after rupture of membranes
- Assess the patient for signs of hypotensive supine syndrome
  - If blood pressure falls, position the patient on her left side
  - Increase the primary I.V. flow rate
  - Administer oxygen through a face mask at 6 to 10 L/minute

● **First, second, and third stages**
- Assist with breathing techniques
- Encourage rest between contractions
- Provide comfort and support to the patient and her partner or support person

● **Second stage**
  - Assist the patient with effective second-stage pushing
  - Observe the perineum for show and bulging
  - Prepare the birthing area as appropriate
  - Help the patient to the preferred birthing position
  - Inform the health care provider of imminent delivery
  - Prepare for delivery, ensuring that emergency equipment is readily available and operational
  - Clean the perineum as ordered, based on facility policy and health care provider's preference
  - Assist with delivery and cutting and clamping of the cord; allow the partner or support person to participate if desired

● **Third stage**
  - Assist with delivery of placenta as necessary
  - Expect to administer oxytocin if ordered, to minimize uterine bleeding
  - Introduce the neonate to the patient and her partner or support person; allow the mother to breast-feed the neonate if desired
  - Administer eye prophylaxis as ordered, after the patient and her partner or support person have held the neonate

● **Fourth stage**
  - Assess lochia and location and consistency of fundus; inspect perineum and episiotomy site if appropriate
  - Monitor maternal vital signs according to facility policy, AWHONN, and ACOG
  - Assess the neonate, including Apgar scoring, to ensure that the neonate is adapting to the extrauterine environment
  - Promote maternal–neonatal bonding
  - Initiate emergency procedures if the patient's or neonate's condition doesn't stabilize

MATERNAL EVALUATION DURING LABOR

● **External assessment in labor progression**
  - The position and presenting part of the fetus is determined by abdominal palpation using Leopold's maneuvers (see *Performing Leopold's maneuvers,* page 184)
    – The first maneuver involves palpating the fundus to identify the occupying fetal part
      · The fetus's head is firm and rounded and moves freely
      · The breech is softer and less regular and moves with the trunk
    – The second maneuver involves palpating the abdomen to identify the location of the fetus's back

---

Care checklist for second stage of labor

- Assist patient with second-stage pushing.
- Observe perineum for show and bulging.
- Prepare birthing area.
- Help patient into birthing position.
- Prepare for delivery.
- Clean the perineum as ordered.
- Assist with delivery and cutting and clamping of the cord; allow the partner or support person to participate if desired.

Care checklist for third stage of labor

- Assist with delivery of placenta.
- Administer oxytocin, if ordered.
- Introduce the neonate to the parents, and allow the mother to breast-feed, if desired.
- Administer eye prophylaxis, as ordered.

Monitoring checklist for fourth stage of labor

- Lochia
- Location and consistency of fundus
- Perineum and episiotomy site
- Maternal vital signs, as ordered
- Neonatal adaptation to extrauterine environment (Apgar)

Key facts about Leopold's maneuvers

- Help determine position and presenting part of fetus
- First maneuver: Palpate fundus to identify the occupying fetal part (head is firm and moves freely, breech is softer and moves with trunk)
- Second maneuver: Palpate abdomen to identify location of fetus's back (back feels firm, smooth, and convex)
- Third maneuver: Grasp lower portion of abdomen above the symphysis pubis to identify the fetal part presenting over the inlet; helps determine attitude
- Fourth maneuver: Move your fingers down both sides of the uterus to assess descent of the presenting part into the pelvis; helps determine whether fetal head is flexed or extended

Performing Leopold's maneuvers

You can determine fetal position, presentation, and attitude by performing Leopold's maneuvers. Ask the patient to empty her bladder, assist her to a supine position, and expose her abdomen. Then perform the four maneuvers in order.

FIRST MANEUVER

Face the patient and curl your fingers around the fundus. With the fetus in vertex position, the buttocks feel irregularly shaped and firm. With the fetus in breech position, the head feels hard, round, and movable.

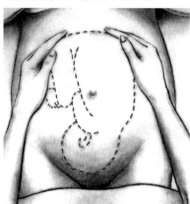

SECOND MANEUVER

Move your hands down the sides of the abdomen, and apply gentle pressure. If the fetus lies in vertex position, you'll feel a smooth, hard surface on one side — the fetal back. Opposite, you'll feel lumps and knobs — the knees, hands, feet, and elbows. If the fetus lies in breech position, you may not feel the back at all.

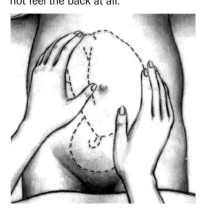

THIRD MANEUVER

Spread apart the thumb and fingers of one hand. Place them just above the patient's symphysis pubis. Bring your fingers together. If the fetus lies in vertex position (and hasn't descended), you'll feel the head. If the fetus lies in vertex position (and has descended), you'll feel a less distinct mass.

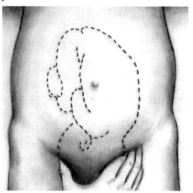

FOURTH MANEUVER

Use this maneuver in late pregnancy. To determine flexion or extension of the fetal head and neck, place your hands on both sides of the lower abdomen. Apply gentle pressure with your fingers as you slide your hands downward, toward the symphysis pubis. If the head presents, one hand's descent will be stopped by the cephalic prominence. The other hand will be unobstructed.

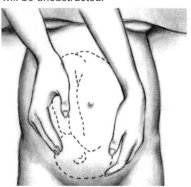

Cervical effacement and dilation

As labor advances, so do cervical effacement and dilation, which promote delivery. During effacement, the cervix shortens and its walls become thin, progressing from 0% effacement (palpable and thick) to 100% effacement (fully indistinct, or effaced, and paper thin). Full effacement obliterates the constrictive uterine neck to create a smooth, unobstructed passageway for the fetus.

At the same time, dilation occurs. This progressive widening of the cervical canal — from the upper internal cervical os to the lower external cervical os — advances from 0 to 10 cm. As the cervical canal opens, resistance decreases. This further eases fetal descent.

NO EFFACEMENT OR DILATION

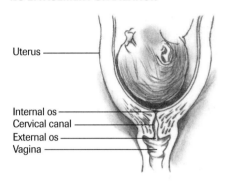

Uterus

Internal os
Cervical canal
External os
Vagina

FULL EFFACEMENT AND DILATION

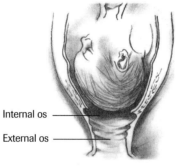

Internal os

External os

      · The back feels firm, smooth, and convex
      · The front is soft, irregular, and concave
   – The third maneuver involves grasping the lower portion of the abdomen above the symphysis pubis to identify the fetal part presenting over the inlet
      · An unengaged head can be rocked from side to side
      · This maneuver helps determine the attitude of the head
   – The fourth maneuver involves moving the fingers down both sides of the uterus to assess the descent of the presenting part into the pelvis
      · As the fingers move downward, greater resistance is met on the cephalic prominence (brow) side
      · This maneuver helps determine whether the head is flexed
- Rupture of membranes is evaluated by testing the pH of the vaginal fluid using the nitrazine test and by the appearance of ferning

● **Internal assessment in labor progression**
- Cervical dilation is evaluated; opening of the external cervical os progresses from 0 to 10 cm (see *Cervical effacement and dilation*)
- Cervical effacement, cervical thinning and shortening, is measured from 0% (thick) to 100% (paper thin)

- Station is determined to establish the relationship of the presenting part to the pelvic ischial spines (see *Measuring fetal station,* which appeared earlier in this chapter)
  - Presenting part even with the ischial spines is at 0 station
  - Presenting part above the ischial spines is −3, −2, or −1
  - Presenting part below the ischial spines is +1, +2, or +3

● **Patient monitoring**
- Encourage the patient to void every 2 hours
  - A full bladder can impede fetal descent and cause dysfunctional labor
  - If the woman can't void or a distended bladder is palpable, the health care provider should be notified
  - Catheterization may be necessary
- Monitor the patient for signs of dehydration, such as poor skin turgor, decreased urine output, and dry mucous membranes
- Use an external pressure transducer to monitor the patient for tetanic contractions (sustained contractions lasting longer than 90 seconds, prolonged contractions with little rest between—occurring more often than every 60 seconds)

FETAL EVALUATION DURING LABOR

● **External electronic fetal monitoring**
- Indirect, noninvasive procedure to evaluate the FHR
- May be accomplished intermittently using a handheld device or continuously with a large fetal monitor
- When continuous monitoring is performed, contraction intensity and frequency are evaluated with a tokodynamometer, a pressure device that, in response to uterine contractions, transfers an electrical impulse to the monitor and creates a readout
  - The ultrasound transducer transmits high-frequency sound waves to the fetal heart
  - The tocotransducer, in turn, responds to the pressure exerted by uterine contractions and simultaneously records their duration and frequency (see *Performing external fetal monitoring*)
  - The monitoring apparatus traces FHR and uterine contraction data onto the same printout paper
- External monitoring is indicated during the first and second stages of labor (when membranes are intact) and when the mother has a communicable disease
- Advantages
  - It can evaluate FHR for decreased variability and periodic changes
  - It also provides a gross evaluation of contractions and a permanent record of contractions

Key facts about external electronic fetal monitoring

- Indirect, noninvasive procedure to evaluate FHR
- May be intermittent (using handheld device) or continuous (using large fetal monitor)
- When continuous monitoring is performed, contraction intensity and frequency are evaluated with a tokodynamometer
- Indicated during first and second stages of labor and when the mother has a communicable disease

Performing external fetal monitoring

When performing external fetal monitoring, follow these steps:

- Explain the procedure to the patient, and make sure she has signed a consent form, if required by your facility.
- Label the monitor strip with the patient's identification number or birth date and her name, the date, maternal vital signs and position, the paper speed, and the number of the strip paper.
- Assist the patient to the semi-Fowler or left-lateral position with her abdomen exposed.
- Apply conduction gel to the ultrasound transducer, and use Leopold's maneuvers to palpate the fetal back, through which fetal heart tones resound most audibly.
- Start the monitor, and apply the ultrasound transducer directly over the site having the strongest heart tones, as shown below.

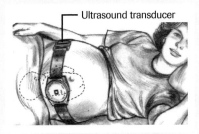

Ultrasound transducer

- Palpate the abdomen to locate the fundus—the area of greatest muscle density in the uterus.
- Using the transducer straps or an elastic stockinette, secure the tocotransducer over the fundus, as shown at top right. Adjust the pen set tracer controls so that the baseline values read between 5 and

15 mm Hg on the monitor strip or as indicated by the model.

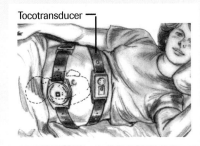

Tocotransducer

- Activate the control that begins the printout.
- Observe the tracings to identify the frequency and duration of uterine contractions, but palpate the uterus to determine intensity of contractions.
- Note the baseline fetal heart rate and assess periodic accelerations or decelerations from the baseline. Compare the fetal heart rate patterns with those of the uterine contractions.
- Move the tocotransducer and the ultrasound transducer to accommodate changes in maternal or fetal position. Readjust both transducers every hour, and assess the patient's skin for reddened areas caused by the strap pressure.
- Clean the ultrasound transducer periodically with a damp cloth to remove dried conduction gel and apply fresh gel as necessary. After using the ultrasound transducer, place the cover over it.
- If the patient reports discomfort in the position that provides the clearest signal, try to obtain a satisfactory 5- or 10-minute tracing with the patient in this position before assisting her to a more comfortable position.

Benefits of external fetal monitoring

- Noninvasive
- Monitors FHR
- Can check for decreased variability
- Provides a gross evaluation of contractions
- Provides a permanent record of contractions

Drawbacks of external fetal monitoring

- May have distortions (artifacts)
- May be uncomfortable for patient
- Can only assess decreased variability
- May divert attention from the patient

- Disadvantages
  - Distortions in the readout (artifacts) occur
  - The patient may find it uncomfortable
  - Only decreased variability can be assessed
  - It may divert the nurse's attention from the patient

Performing internal fetal monitoring

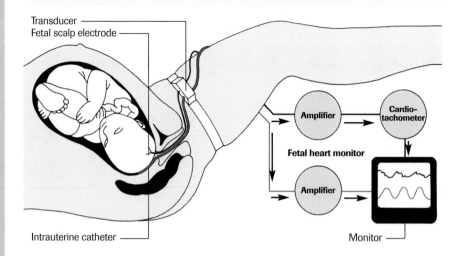

To perform internal fetal monitoring follow these steps:

- Explain the procedure to the patient.
- Label the printout paper with the patient's identification number or name and birth date, the date, the paper speed, and the number on the monitor strip.
- Help the patient into the lithotomy position for a vaginal examination.
- Attach the connection cable to the outlet on the monitor marked UA (uterine activity); connect the cable to the intrauterine catheter, and then zero the catheter with a gauge on the distal end of the catheter.
- Cover the patient's perineum with a sterile drape and clean the perineum according to facility policy.
- Assist the health care provider in performing a vaginal examination to insert the intrauterine catheter into the uterine cavity and to attach the fetal scalp electrode to the fetus. Secure the catheter and electrode to the leg plate transducer.
- Observe the monitoring strip to verify proper placement and a clear tracing.
- Periodically evaluate the strip to determine amount of pressure exerted with each contraction. Note all such

data on the strip and the patient's medical record.
- To monitor the fetal heart rate (FHR), apply conduction gel to the leg plate transducer and secure to the patient's inner thigh with Velcro straps or 2″ tape; connect the leg plate cable to the electrocardiogram outlet on the monitor.
- Assist with continued examination to identify fetal presenting part and level of descent. The health care provider will place the spiral electrode in a drive tube and advance it through the vagina to the presenting part; expect mild pressure to be applied and the drive tube turned clockwise 360 degrees to secure it.
- Connect the color-coded electrode wires to the corresponding color-coded leg plate posts after the electrode is in place and the drive tube has been removed.
- Turn on the recorder and note the time on the printout paper.
- Help the patient to a comfortable position and evaluate the strip to verify proper placement and a clear FHR tracing.

Internal electronic fetal monitoring

- Also called *direct fetal monitoring;* an invasive procedure that uses an internal spiral electrode (ISE) attached to the presenting fetal part (usually the scalp) and a fluid-filled intrauterine pressure catheter (IUPC) inserted into the uterine cavity alongside the fetus
  - The spiral electrode detects the FHR and transmits it to the monitor, which converts the signals to a fetal electrocardiogram waveform
  - The ISE is applied to the epidermis of the presenting part
  - It provides a continuous recording of the FHR
  - Accurate baseline, true baseline variability, and periodic changes (transient and recurrent changes from baseline rates that are associated with uterine contractions) are demonstrated
- Provides information for assessing fetal response to uterine contractions, measuring intrauterine pressure, tracking labor progress, and allowing evaluation of short- and long-term FHR variability.
- Is indicated for high-risk pregnancies (see *Performing internal fetal monitoring*)
- Performed only if the amniotic sac has ruptured, the cervix is dilated at least 3 cm, and the presenting part of the fetus is at least at the −1 station
- The intrauterine catheter is usually removed during the second stage of labor
- Advantages
  - It provides the most precise assessment of the FHR and uterine contractions
  - It's unaffected by changes in maternal or fetal position
- Disadvantages
  - It can't be performed until membranes rupture, the cervix dilates at least 2 cm, and the fetus descends
  - It may cause maternal infection or uterine perforation
  - It may limit maternal movement
  - It may cause fetal hematoma or infection
  - It may cause fetal laceration or abscess if the catheter is inserted into the fetal presenting part
  - It may divert the nurse's attention from the pregnant patient

UTERINE CONTRACTIONS

Phases

- Increment — the building-up phase and longest phase
- Acme — the peak of the contraction
- Decrement — the letting-down phase

Uterine contraction characteristics

- **Duration** – beginning of increment to end of decrement; averages 30 seconds in early labor and 60 seconds in later labor
- **Frequency** – beginning of one contraction to the beginning of the next; averages 5 to 30 minutes apart in early labor and 2 to 3 minutes apart in later labor
- **Intensity** – measured during the acme phase using intrauterine catheter (30 to 50 mm Hg during acme) or by palpation

FHR patterns and their causes

- Early decelerations – from head compression
- Late decelerations – from uteroplacental insufficiency
- Variable decelerations – from umbilical cord compression
- Accelerations – from fetal movement or contractions
- Baseline variability – from interplay of the parasympathetic and sympathetic nervous systems
- Decreased variability – from hypoxia, acidosis, CNS depression medications
- Increased variability – from early mild hypoxia and fetal stimulation

Uterine contractions

As shown below, uterine contractions occur in three phases: increment (building up), acme (peak), and decrement (letting down). Between contractions is a period of relaxation. The two most important features of contractions are duration and frequency. Duration is the elapsed time from the start to the end of one contraction. Frequency refers to the elapsed time from the start of one contraction to the start of the next contraction.

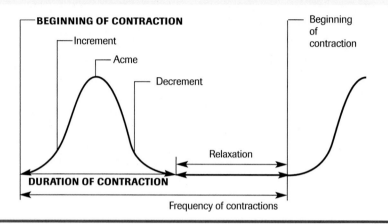

Duration
- Is measured from the beginning of the increment to the end of the decrement (see *Uterine contractions*)
- Averages 30 seconds in early labor and 60 seconds in later labor

Frequency
- Is measured from the beginning of one contraction to the beginning of the next
- Averages 5 to 30 minutes apart in early labor and 2 to 3 minutes apart in later labor

Intensity
- Is measured during the acme phase
- Can be measured with an intrauterine catheter or by palpation (normal resting pressure when using an intrauterine catheter is 5 to 15 mm Hg; pressure increases to 30 to 50 mm Hg during the acme)

FETAL HEART RATE PATTERNS

Early decelerations
- Caused by head compression
- Shape
  - Early decelerations appear as uniform, smooth waveforms (see *Fetal heart rate decelerations*)

Fetal heart rate decelerations

The monitor strips below show early, late, and variable decelerations of fetal heart rate, along with corresponding uterine contractions.

EARLY DECELERATIONS

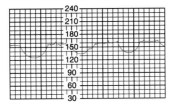

Contractions

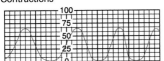

LATE DECELERATIONS

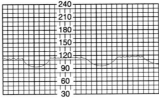

Contractions

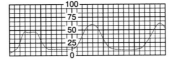

VARIABLE DECELERATIONS

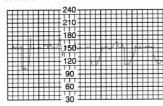

Contractions

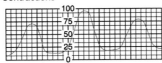

– The waveforms inversely mirror the corresponding contractions
- Range is normally 120 to 160 beats/minute
- Significance
  – Early decelerations are a reassuring pattern indicating fetal head compression
  – They aren't associated with any fetal difficulties
- Nursing interventions
  – Keep in mind that no treatment is required
  – Reassure the patient that the fetus isn't at risk
  – Continue to observe the FHR
  – Document the frequency of decelerations

Key facts about late decelerations in FHR

- Caused by uteroplacental insufficiency
- Appear as uniform, smooth waveforms that inversely mirror the corresponding contractions
- Have late onset in relation to the acmes of contractions
- May drop to below 100 beats/minute when severe
- Considered an ominous sign if persistent and uncorrected

Key nursing interventions for late decelerations

- Place patient in left-lateral position.
- Increase primary I.V. flow rate.
- Administer oxygen via face mask at least 10 L/minute.
- Assess patient for signs of underlying cause.
- Discontinue oxytocin infusion, if applicable.
- Assist with fetal blood sampling, if ordered.

Key facts about variable decelerations in FHR

- Caused by umbilical cord compression
- Have no uniform appearance
- In severe cases, may be below 70 beats/minute for more than 30 seconds
- May be periodic or nonperiodic
- Usually transient and correctable
- Amnioinfusion may be indicated for repetitive variable decelerations

● **Late decelerations**
- Caused by uteroplacental insufficiency
- Shape
  - Late decelerations are smooth, uniform waveforms that inversely mirror the contractions
  - Their onset is late in relation to the acme of the corresponding uterine contractions
- Range
  - Late decelerations are usually within the normal range with a high baseline
  - They may drop to below 100 beats/minute when severe
- Significance
  - Late decelerations are considered an ominous sign if persistent and uncorrected
  - Pattern is associated with decreased Apgar scores, fetal hypoxia, and acidosis
- Nursing interventions (see *Evaluating fetal heart rate decelerations*)
  - Place the patient in the left-lateral position
  - Increase the primary I.V. flow rate
  - Administer oxygen through a face mask at a rate of at least 10 L/minute
  - Assess the patient for signs of the underlying cause
  - Discontinue oxytocin infusion if it's being administered to induce or augment labor
  - Assist with fetal blood sampling, if ordered

● **Variable decelerations**
- Caused by umbilical cord compression
- Shape
  - Variable decelerations have no uniform appearance
  - They vary in onset, occurrence, and waveform
- Range
  - In severe cases, the FHR may decelerate below 70 beats/minute for more than 30 seconds, with a slow return to baseline
  - They may be periodic or nonperiodic
- Significance
  - Variable decelerations occur in about 50% of labors and are usually transient and correctable
  - Occurrences aren't associated with low Apgar scores
- Nursing interventions
  - Continue to monitor and record FHR and contraction duration, frequency, and intensity

GO WITH THE FLOW

Evaluating fetal heart rate decelerations

Use the flowchart below to determine how to proceed when you identify fetal heart rate (FHR) decelerations.

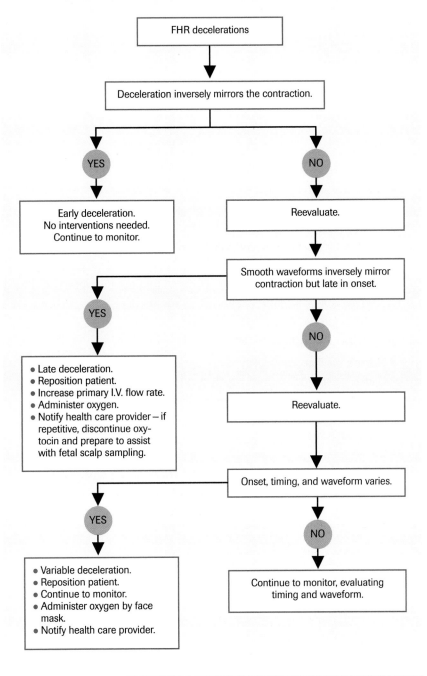

FHR decelerations

↓

Deceleration inversely mirrors the contraction.

YES → Early deceleration. No interventions needed. Continue to monitor.

NO → Reevaluate.

↓

Smooth waveforms inversely mirror contraction but late in onset.

YES →
- Late deceleration.
- Reposition patient.
- Increase primary I.V. flow rate.
- Administer oxygen.
- Notify health care provider — if repetitive, discontinue oxytocin and prepare to assist with fetal scalp sampling.

NO → Reevaluate.

↓

Onset, timing, and waveform varies.

YES →
- Variable deceleration.
- Reposition patient.
- Continue to monitor.
- Administer oxygen by face mask.
- Notify health care provider.

NO → Continue to monitor, evaluating timing and waveform.

Key facts about FHR accelerations

- Brief increases in FHR of at least 15 beats above baseline that usually last 15 to 20 seconds
- Usually above 150 beats/minute
- Caused by fetal movements or contractions
- Uniform or variable
- Indicate fetal well-being
- Require no intervention

Key facts about baseline variability

- Normal cardiac irregularity caused by interplay of the parasympathetic and sympathetic nervous systems
- Appears as slightly irregular or jittery on waveform
- *Short-term variability* refers to the beat-to-beat changes in baseline FHR; averages 6 to 10 beats/minute
- *Long-term variability* refers to rhythmic fluctuations and waves (usually three to five times per minute); ranges from 6 to 10 beats/minute occurring 3 to 10 times/minute
- Indicates adequate CNS function
- Increased by stimulation of the fetus; slowed by sleep, analgesics, and anesthetics
- Requires no treatment unless fetus shows signs of distress

– Remember that no further intervention is necessary unless fetal distress is noted
– Assess deceleration pattern for reassuring signs
  · These include a baseline rate that isn't increasing, short-term variability that isn't decreasing, decelerations that abruptly begin or end, and decelerations that last less than 50 seconds
  · If no reassuring signs are revealed, notify the health care provider
– Be aware that if rate falls below 70 beats/minute and persists for more than 60 seconds, the health care provider may choose to intervene
– Anticipate amnioinfusion for repetitive variable decelerations

Accelerations
- Caused by fetal movements or contractions
- Shape
- Uniform or variable
- Range
  – Accelerations are brief increases in the FHR of at least 15 beats above the baseline usually lasting 15 to 20 seconds
  – Accelerations are usually above 150 beats/minute
- Significance
  – Accelerations are reassuring patterns that indicate fetal well-being
  – They suggest that the fetus isn't acidotic
- Nursing interventions: none required

Baseline variability
- Normal cardiac irregularity
- Cause
  – Continuous interplay of the parasympathetic and sympathetic nervous systems
  – Short-term variability refers to the beat-to-beat changes of FHR in the baseline
  – Long-term variability refers to the rhythmic fluctuations and waves; usually occur three to five times per minute, usually over time or over a period of heart cycles
- Shape
- Slightly irregular or jittery appearance of the waveform
- Range
  – Average beat-to-beat variability is 6 to 10 beats/minute
  – Long-term variability usually ranges from 6 to 10 beats/minute occurring 3 to 10 times/minute
- Significance
  – Baseline variability indicates adequate fetal central nervous system (CNS) function

– Typically stimulation of the fetus increases baseline variability, whereas sleep slows it
- Nursing interventions
  – Keep in mind that drugs used for analgesia and anesthesia can slow baseline variability
  – Know that no treatment is required unless the fetus shows signs of distress
  – Continue to monitor FHR for changes

Increased variability

- Caused by early, mild hypoxia and fetal stimulation
- It's the earliest sign of mild fetal hypoxia
- Nursing interventions include carefully evaluating the FHR tracing for signs of fetal distress

Decreased variability

- Caused by hypoxia, acidosis, CNS depressants, and other drugs
- Significance
  – Decreased variability is benign when associated with drugs
  – It can be an ominous sign if caused by hypoxia or associated with late decelerations
- Nursing interventions
  – Reposition the patient to the left-lateral position
  – Administer I.V. fluids and oxygen as ordered
  – Assist with possible fetal blood sampling
  – Anticipate the need for insertion of internal fetal monitor as ordered

DIAGNOSTIC MEASURES

Fetal blood sampling

- Description
  – Method of monitoring fetal blood pH when indefinite or nonreassuring FHR patterns occur
  – Indicated when fetal hypoxemia is suspected
  – A blood sample is usually taken from the scalp but also may be taken from the presenting part if the fetus is in a breech presentation
  – For fetal blood sampling to occur, membranes must be ruptured, the cervix must be dilated at least 2 cm, and the presenting part must be no higher than −2 station
  – All parameters of an arterial blood gas analysis can be determined; however, pH and base excess are used primarily to evaluate the fetus's condition

Key facts about fetal blood sampling

- Method of monitoring fetal blood pH when indefinite FHR patterns occur
- Indicated when fetal hypoxemia is suspected
- Sample usually taken from the scalp (or presenting part if fetus is breech)
- Membranes must be ruptured, the cervix must be dilated at least 2 cm, and the presenting part must be no higher than –2 station
- Fetal scalp pH of 7.25 or higher is normal; value below 7.20 indicates severe acidosis and fetal distress

Key facts about fetal amnioinfusion

- Replacement of amniotic fluid volume through intrauterine infusion of an isotonic solution using a pressure catheter
- Indicated when repetitive variable decelerations aren't alleviated by maternal position change and oxygen administration
- May be performed to dilute meconium before aspiration occurs
- Helps relieve umbilical cord compression

- Nursing interventions
  - Assist the health care provider with obtaining the sample
  - Tell the patient that she should feel no pain during the procedure
  - Warn the patient that she might experience a feeling of uncomfortable pressure during the sample collection
  - Assess the patient for a period of two contractions after sample collection to ensure no further scalp bleeding
  - Keep in mind that a fetal scalp blood pH of 7.25 or higher is normal; a value below 7.20 indicates severe acidosis and fetal distress
  - Anticipate collection of another sample in 30 minutes if the pH is between 7.20 and 7.24; this level is considered preacidotic
  - Know that vacuum extraction shouldn't be used for delivery if the fetus has undergone scalp blood sampling to prevent bleeding at the puncture site

Amnioinfusion

- Description
  - Refers to the replacement of amniotic fluid volume through intrauterine infusion of an isotonic solution, such as normal saline or lactated Ringer's solution, using a pressure catheter
  - Indicated when umbilical cord compression is a factor or when repetitive variable decelerations aren't alleviated by maternal position change and oxygen administration
  - It may also be done to dilute meconium before aspiration occurs
  - Helps to relieve umbilical cord compression in such conditions as oligohydramnios associated with postmaturity, intrauterine growth retardation, and premature rupture of membranes
- Nursing interventions
  - Prepare the patient for the procedure and encourage her to lie in a lateral recumbent position
  - Assist with administration of fluid, usually a 500-ml infusion at first; anticipate adjustment in flow rate to maintain FHR pattern demonstrating no variable decelerations
  - Warm the solution for the infusion to the patient's body temperature to avoid chilling
  - Continuously monitor FHR and uterine contractions
  - Assess temperature at least every hour to detect infection
  - Monitor patient for a continuous flow of fluid via the vagina
  - Provide comfort measures, including frequent bed linen changes
  - Notify the health care provider if the fluid suddenly stops, an indication that the fetal head is engaged and fluid is collecting in the uterus; could lead to hydramnios or uterine rupture

OBSTETRIC PROCEDURES

● **Episiotomy**
- Description
  - A surgical incision of the perineum used to enlarge the vaginal outlet
  - Used to prevent the perineum from tearing, which can occur with birth
  - Helps to release the pressure on the fetal head that accompanies birth
  - The type of episiotomy done depends on the site and direction of the incision
    - Midline episiotomy
      - Involves an incision that's made in the middle of the perineum
      - Advantageous because it's associated with easier healing, decreased blood loss, and decreased postpartum discomfort
    - Mediolateral episiotomy
      - Involves an incision begun at the midline and then angled to one side away from the rectum
      - Advantageous because of the decreased risk of rectal mucosa tears
- Advantages
  - Prevents tearing (laceration) of the perineum
  - Can be repaired more easily than a tear and heals faster
  - Enlarges the vaginal outlet to facilitate manipulation or use of forceps
- Disadvantages
  - May interfere with maternal-neonatal bonding if discomfort is severe
  - Creates a potential site of infection
  - May make the patient hesitant to void or have a bowel movement

● **Amniotomy**
- Description
  - Refers to the artificial rupture of the amniotic sac
  - Performed when the membranes haven't ruptured spontaneously, as a means of augmenting or inducing labor, allowing the fetal head to contact the cervix more directly, and increasing the efficiency of the contractions
  - May be done to allow internal fetal monitoring and to access the fetus for fetal blood sampling
  - Before an amniotomy is done, the following must be present

---

Quick guide to obstetric procedures

- **Episiotomy** — surgical incision of the perineum used to enlarge the vaginal outlet; prevents tearing and relieves pressure from fetal head during birth
- **Amniotomy** — artificial rupture of amniotic sac used to augment or induce labor; allows access to the fetus for internal fetal monitoring or blood sampling
- **Forceps delivery** — use of forceps to aid delivery or relieve fetal head compression; used to shorten second stage of labor when adverse fetal or maternal conditions exist
- **Vacuum extraction** — use of plastic vacuum cup, negative pressure, and traction to facilitate descent and delivery of fetal head; alternative to forceps delivery
- **Version** — gentle pressure applied to maternal abdomen to manually turn the fetus from one presentation to another (usually breech to cephalic)

Episiotomy sites and benefits

- Midline, or middle of the perineum — easier healing, decreased blood loss, decreased postpartum discomfort
- Mediolateral, or from midline and then angled to one side away from the rectum — decreased risk of rectal mucosal tears

- The fetus must be in the vertex position with the fetal head at +2 station or lower and a Bishop score of at least 8
- The woman's cervix must be dilated at least 3 cm
– The procedure is virtually painless for the patient and the fetus because there are no nerve endings in the membranes
– After the woman is placed in a dorsal recumbent position, the membranes are torn with a hemostat or punctured with an Amniohook (a long thin instrument similar to a crochet hook) inserted into the vagina; if the tear or puncture has been performed properly, the amniotic fluid will gush out
- Advantages
  – It helps to induce or augment labor
  – It provides access to the fetus
- Disadvantages
  – There's an increased risk of umbilical cord prolapse
  – The patient is at risk for infection
  – If the patient has hydramnios, abruptio placenta may occur as a natural aftereffect of the procedure
    - As the uterus collapses due to the draining fluid, the area of placental attachment shrinks
    - The placenta no longer fits its implantation site, resulting in a decrease in surface area where fetal oxygenation occurs, possibly adversely affecting the fetus

● Forceps delivery
- Description
  – Forceps are steel instruments used to assist with delivery and to relieve fetal head compression
  – Forceps consist of two blades connected together; blades are slipped into position one at a time
  – Commonly used forceps include Kjelland's, Elliot, Piper, Tucker-McLean, and Simpson's
  – Forceps delivery may be either low-forceps or midforceps
    - A low-forceps (outlet) delivery is performed when the fetus's head reaches the perineum; typically the fetal head is at +2 station or more
    - A midforceps delivery is performed when the fetal head is engaged but is at less than +2 station; because of the increased risks of birth trauma, this type of delivery is rarely done
  – For a forceps delivery to be performed, the following must be present
    - Ruptured membranes
    - Fully dilated cervix

Basic requirements for amniotomy

- Membranes intact
- Fetus in vertex position
- Fetal head at +2 station or lower
- Bishop score of at least 8
- Cervical dilation of at least 3 cm

Basic requirements for forceps delivery

- Ruptured membranes
- Fully dilated cervix
- Empty bladder
- Absence of cephalopelvic disproportion

- Empty bladder
- Absence of cephalopelvic disproportion
- Advantage is that it shortens the second stage of labor when adverse fetal and maternal conditions exist
- Disadvantages
  - Increases perinatal morbidity and mortality (midforceps delivery)
  - Increases neonatal birth trauma and depression
  - Increases incidence of perineal lacerations, postpartum hemorrhage, and bladder injury

Vacuum extraction

- Description
  - An alternative to forceps delivery; facilitates descent of fetal head
  - A plastic vacuum cup is applied to the fetal head, negative pressure is exerted, and traction is applied to deliver the head
- Advantages
  - It's associated with a lower incidence of vaginal, cervical, and third- and fourth-degree lacerations
  - It's also associated with less maternal discomfort, because the cup doesn't occupy additional space in the birth canal
  - Little anesthesia is needed compared with that required for forceps delivery; subsequently, the neonate is born with less respiratory depression
- Disadvantages
  - Vacuum extraction is associated with a marked caput succedaneum of the neonate's head, lasting as long as 7 days after birth
  - Tentorial tears are possible from extreme pressure
  - Renewed bleeding from the scalp can occur if used for a fetus that has undergone fetal blood sampling
  - Use in preterm neonates is problematic because of the extreme softness of their skulls

Version

- Description
  - Also called external cephalic version; refers to a manual attempt to turn a fetus from one presentation to another
  - Usually used to turn a fetus in the breech presentation to a cephalic one
  - After locating the breech and vertex of the fetus, gentle pressure is applied to the abdomen to turn the fetus
  - Tocolytic agents to relax the uterus and epidural anesthesia to relieve pain may be administered
- Advantages
  - It's a noninvasive procedure

Disdvantages of version

- May cause extreme pressure
- Increases the possibility of Rh isoimmunization; thus, RhoGAM is administered to an Rh-negative women

Primary indications for cesarean birth

- Cephalopelvic disproportion
- Uterine dysfunction
- Malposition or malpresentation
- Previous uterine surgery
- Complete or partial placenta previa
- Preexisting medical condition (for example, diabetes or cardiac disease)
- Prolapsed umbilical cord
- Fetal distress

Incision types

- **Transverse** – incision made through lower portion of the uterus; most common incision; associated with decreased incidence of peritonitis and postoperative adhesions and minimal blood loss; allows for subsequent vaginal birth
- **Classic** – vertical incision made through the abdomen; used when adhesions from previous cesarean delivery exist, fetus is in transverse lie, or placenta is anteriorly implanted; limits possibility of subsequent vaginal birth

– Version may decrease the number of cesarean deliveries done as a result of breech presentation
- Disadvantages
  - The patient may feel extreme pressure during the manual turning
  - Rh isoimmunization is possible if minimal bleeding occurs, thus necessitating administration of $Rh_o(D)$ immune globulin (RhoGAM) to Rh-negative women

CESAREAN BIRTH

● Description
- Refers to the removal of the neonate from the uterus through an abdominal incision
- Indicated in specific situations
  - Cephalopelvic disproportion
  - Uterine dysfunction
  - Malposition or malpresentation
  - Previous uterine surgery
  - Complete or partial placenta previa
  - Preexisting medical condition (for example, diabetes or cardiac disease)
  - Prolapsed umbilical cord
  - Fetal distress

● Two types of incisions
- The transverse incision, also known as the "bikini" or low-segment incision, is the preferred and most common incision
  - It's associated with a decreased incidence of peritonitis and postoperative adhesions
  - Blood loss is minimal
  - Incision is made through the lower portion of the uterus that's minimally active with contractions, making the incision less likely to rupture during future labors
  - Vaginal birth after cesarean delivery is possible with this incision
- The classic, or vertical, incision is used when adhesions from previous cesarean delivery exist, when the fetus is in a transverse lie, or when the placenta is anteriorly implanted
  - The incision is made through the abdomen, high on the uterus
  - This type of incision may be used for patients with placenta previa because the incision can be made without cutting the placenta
  - The chances of vaginal birth after cesarean birth with this type of incision are low because of the incision's location in the major active contracting portion of the uterus

● **Vaginal birth after cesarean birth**
- A patient who has had a previous low-transverse cesarean delivery may attempt a vaginal birth, provided that no medical or obstetric contraindication to labor or history of prior uterine rupture exists
- The incidence of dehiscence of a former low-transverse uterine incision dehiscence during an attempted vaginal birth after cesarean birth is less than 1%

INDUCTION OF LABOR

● **Overview**
- Several conditions determine readiness
  - Fetal maturity (assessed by amniotic fluid studies and serial ultrasound examinations)
  - Fetal position (determined by ultrasound or Leopold's maneuvers)
  - Cervical dilation, effacement, consistency, and position (determined by vaginal examination and use of scoring systems such as Bishop score)
  - Trial of labor after cesarean (TOLAC) birth
    - Candidates
      - Previous one or two low-transverse incisions
      - Pelvis evaluated for adequacy
      - No other uterine scars or previous uterine ruptures
      - Health care provider readily available for intervention of urgent or immediate cesarean birth
      - Personnel and equipment for emergency resuscitation readily available
      - Anesthesia available
    - Contraindications
      - Prior classic incision
      - Contracted pelvis
      - Medical or obstetric complications that preclude vaginal delivery
      - Inability to perform an emergency cesarean birth because of staffing, anesthesia, or facility limitations
- Indications
  - Postmaturity (more than 42 weeks' gestation), which can lead to placental insufficiency or fetal compromise
  - Premature rupture of membranes, which increases the risk of intrauterine infection
  - Pregnancy-induced hypertension, which may worsen
  - Rh isoimmunization, which can produce erythroblastosis fetalis
  - Maternal diabetes, which can lead to fetal death from placental insufficiency

---

Contraindications for TOLAC

- Prior classic incision
- Contracted pelvis
- Medical or obstetric complications that preclude vaginal delivery
- Inability to perform an emergency cesarean birth because of staffing, anesthesia, or facility limitations

---

Indications for induction

- Postmaturity (more than 42 weeks' gestation)
- Premature rupture of membranes
- Pregnancy-induced hypertension
- Rh isoimmunization
- Maternal diabetes
- Chorioamnionitis
- Fetal death

Contraindications for induction

- Maternal
- Previous cesarean birth with a classic incision
- Previous hysterotomy or myomectomy
- Previous uterine rupture
- Placenta previa
- Active genital herpes infection
- Fetal
- Abnormal lie
- Distress
- Premature or low-birth-weight
- Positive oxytocin challenge test

Key facts about induction by amniotomy

- Artificial rupturing of membranes to induce labor
- Indicated for internal fetal monitoring and when oxytocin is contraindicated
- Contraindicated when presenting part is at –2 station or higher, in cases of placenta previa, when estimated date of delivery is uncertain, and when patient had active herpesvirus 2 lesions in the vagina

- Chorioamnionitis
- Fetal death
- Absolute maternal contraindications
  - Previous cesarean birth with a classic incision
  - Previous hysterotomy or myomectomy
  - Previous uterine rupture
  - Placenta previa
  - Active genital herpes infection
- Relative maternal contraindications
  - Multiparity
  - Malpresentation
  - Overdistention of the uterus
  - Cancer of the cervix
  - Structural abnormalities of the vagina, uterus, or pelvis
- Fetal contraindications
  - Abnormal lie
  - Fetal distress
  - Premature or low-birth-weight
  - Positive oxytocin challenge test
- Advantages
  - Allows the patient to prepare physically and psychologically for labor and delivery
  - Can resolve medical conditions that might endanger fetal well-being
- Disadvantages
  - Poses risks to the fetus from increased uterine activity and possible prematurity
  - Poses risks to the patient from prolonged labor, cervical laceration, and postpartum hemorrhage
  - Produces physical and psychological stress if induction fails

● **Induction by way of amniotomy**
- Description
  - Involves the artificial rupturing of membranes with a sterile instrument
  - Under favorable conditions, about 80% of patients enter labor within 24 hours
- Indications
  - When internal fetal monitoring is desired
  - When oxytocin is contraindicated
- Contraindications
  - Presenting part at −2 station or higher
  - Placenta previa
  - Abnormal presenting part

- Uncertain estimated date of delivery
- Active herpesvirus 2 lesions in the vagina
- Nursing interventions
  - Explain the purpose of the procedure to the patient
  - Wash hands and put on gloves
  - Clean the perineum with soap and water or gauze pads moistened with antiseptic agent
  - Place a linen-saver pad underneath patient's buttocks
  - Assist with insertion of device to rupture membranes; maintain sterile technique
  - Apply pressure to the uterine fundus, if ordered, as the instrument is inserted vaginally
  - Evaluate the FHR for at least 60 seconds after rupture; check for large variable decelerations, which suggest cord compression
  - Continue to frequently monitor FHR, every 5 minutes for 20 minutes and then every 30 minutes
  - Assess maternal temperature at least once every 2 hours
  - Report the presence of meconium, blood, or an unusual odor in the amniotic fluid
  - Clean and dry the perineal area
- Advantages
  - Facilitates fetal status monitoring using an internal scalp electrode, catheter, or scalp blood sampling
  - Facilitates assessment of amniotic fluid color and composition
- Disadvantages
  - Increases the risk of infection and cord prolapse
  - Increases the incidence of fetal head compression

● **Induction by way of oxytocin infusion**
- Description
  - Involves the administration of I.V. oxytocin (Pitocin) to augment or stimulate uterine contractions
  - Oxytocin is administered via an I.V. infusion pump
- Indications
  - Prolonged rupture of membranes
  - Postmaturity
  - Induction necessary because of adverse maternal or fetal conditions
- Contraindications
  - Cephalopelvic disproportion
  - Fetal distress
  - Previous uterine surgery
  - Overdistended uterus
  - Abnormal fetal presentation

Nursing interventions for induction by amniotomy

- Explain the reason for induction.
- Wash hands and put on gloves.
- Clean the perineum with soap and water or gauze pads moistened with antiseptic.
- Place linen-saver pad under patient's buttocks.
- Assist with insertion of device to rupture membranes, and apply pressure to the uterine fundus, if ordered, as instrument is inserted.
- Evaluate FHR for at least 60 seconds after rupture.
- Continue monitoring FHR every 5 minutes for 20 minutes and then every 30 minutes.
- Assess maternal temperature at least every 2 hours.
- Report meconium, blood, or unusual odor in the amniotic fluid.
- Clean and dry the perineal area.

Key facts about induction using oxytocin

- Administration of I.V. oxytocin to augment or stimulate uterine contractions
- Indicated in cases involving prolonged rupture of membranes, postmature fetus, or adverse maternal or fetal conditions
- Contraindicated in cases involving cephalopelvic disproportion, fetal distress, previous uterine surgery, overdistended uterus, or abnormal fetal presentation

Complications of oxytocin administration

Oxytocin can cause uterine hyperstimulation. This, in turn, may progress to tetanic contractions, which last longer than 2 minutes. Signs of hyperstimulation include contractions less than 2 minutes apart and lasting 90 seconds or longer, uterine pressure that doesn't return to baseline between contractions, and intra-uterine pressure that rises to more than 75 mm Hg.

WHAT ELSE TO WATCH FOR
Other potential complications include fetal distress, abruptio placentae, and uterine rupture. In addition, watch for signs of oxytocin hypersensitivity, such as elevated blood pressure. Rarely, oxytocin leads to maternal seizures or coma from water intoxication.

STOP SIGNS
Contraindications to administering oxytocin include placenta previa, diagnosed cephalopelvic disproportion, fetal distress, prior classic uterine incision or uterine surgery, and active genital herpes. Oxytocin should be administered cautiously to a patient who has an overdistended uterus or a history of cervical surgery, uterine surgery, or grand multiparity.

Signs of oxytocin administration complications

- Contractions that are less than 2 minutes apart and last 90 seconds or longer
- Uterine pressure that doesn't return to baseline between contractions
- Intrauterine pressure greater than 75 mm Hg
- Elevated blood pressure

Advantages of oxytocin administration

- Has a predictable course of action
- Doesn't directly affect the fetus
- Stimulates contractions efficiently and effectively

Disadvantages of oxytocin administration

- Increases risk of tetanic uterine contractions
- Overstimulates the uterus
- May cause fetal distress and uterine rupture

- Advantages
  - Uses a drug with a predictable action
  - Doesn't directly affect the fetus
  - Stimulates contractions efficiently and effectively
- Disadvantage
  - Increases the risk of tetanic uterine contractions
  - Also increases the risk of overstimulating the uterus, which can lead to fetal distress and uterine rupture (see *Complications of oxytocin administration*)
- Nursing interventions
  - Explain the rationale for the induction (see *What to expect in labor induction*)
  - Assess the FHR and contraction patterns by continuous electronic monitoring to ensure that they're occurring in a 20-minute span
  - Always administer oxytocin solution as a piggyback to the primary I.V. line using an infusion pump; if a problem occurs such as decelerations of the FHR or fetal distress, the piggyback infusion can be stopped immediately and the primary line resumed
  - Know that the typical recommended labor-starting dosage for administration is 0.5 to 1 mU/minute and the maximum dosage is 20 mU/minute
  - Because the onset of oxytocin action is immediate, be prepared to start monitoring uterine contractions

TIME-OUT FOR TEACHING

What to expect in labor induction

Be sure to discuss the following topics when teaching a patient who's about to have labor induced:
- rationale for induction
- type of induction being used
- possible risks and benefits to patient and fetus
- signs and symptoms to report
- necessary assessments and monitoring activities to be performed.

 – Increase the oxytocin dosage as ordered
    • Never infuse more than 2 mU/minute once every 30 to 60 minutes
    • Typically, the dosage continues at a rate that maintains activity closest to normal labor
 – Before each increase, be sure to assess contractions, maternal vital signs, fetal heart rhythm, and FHR
    • If using an external fetal monitor, the uterine activity strip or grid should show contractions occurring every 2 to 3 minutes; contractions should last for about 60 seconds and be followed by uterine relaxation
    • When using an internal fetal monitor, look for an optimal baseline value ranging from 5 to 15 mm Hg; the goal is to verify uterine relaxation between contractions
 – Assist with comfort measures, such as repositioning the patient on her other side, as needed
 – Stop the infusion immediately if fetal distress or tetanic uterine contractions occur
 – Continue assessing maternal and fetal responses to the oxytocin
    • Review the infusion rate to prevent uterine hyperstimulation
    • To manage hyperstimulation, discontinue the infusion, administer oxygen, and notify the health care provider
    • To reduce uterine irritability, try to increase uterine blood flow by changing the patient's position and increasing the infusion rate of the primary I.V. line.
    • After hyperstimulation resolves, resume the oxytocin infusion according to facility policy and the physician's order

● **Induction using prostaglandin**
 • Description
    – Induction using prostaglandin (prostaglandin E_2 such as dinoprostone [Cervidil, Prepidil or Prostin E_2]); involves the intracervical or

---

Nursing interventions during oxytocin induction

- Explain the reason for induction.
- Assess FHR and contraction patterns to ensure that they're occurring in a 20-minute span.
- Administer oxytocin solution using an infusion pump piggybacked to the primary I.V. line (recommended labor-starting dosage is 0.5 to 1 mU/minute; maximum dosage is 20 mU/minute).
- Never infuse more than 2 mU/minute once every 30 to 60 minutes.
- Be prepared to start monitoring uterine contractions.
- Before increasing the dosage, be sure to assess contractions, maternal vital signs, fetal heart rhythm, and FHR.
- Assist with comfort measures, such as repositioning.
- Stop the infusion immediately if fetal distress or tetanic uterine contractions occur.
- Monitor maternal and fetal responses.
- Review the infusion rate to prevent uterine hyperstimulation.

Key facts about induction using prostaglandin

- Intracervical or intravaginal insertion of prostaglandin gel to soften the cervix
- Initiates the breakdown of collagen
- Indicated for cases involving postmaturity; long, thick cervix at time of induction; or adverse maternal or fetal conditions
- Contraindicated in cases involving maternal temperature greater than 100° F, asthma or cardiac disorder, vaginal bleeding, contraindications to vaginal delivery, allergy to prostaglandin, or Bishop score higher than 5

How to apply prostaglandin gel

- To the interior surface of the cervix with a catheter or suppository
- To the external surface of the cervix with a diaphragm
- By vaginal insertion

intravaginal insertion of prostaglandin gel to soften (ripen) the cervix
- The drug initiates the breakdown of the collagen that keeps the cervix tightly closed
- Prostaglandin gel is applied to the interior surface of the cervix by a catheter or suppository, to the external surface of the cervix by applying it to a diaphragm and then placing the diaphragm against the cervix, or by vaginal insertion
- Additional doses may be applied every 6 hours (however, two or three doses are usually enough to cause ripening)
- The woman should remain flat after the application of the gel to prevent the medication from leaking
- Indications
  - Postmaturity
  - Long, thick cervix at the time of induction
  - Induction necessary because of adverse maternal or fetal conditions
- Contraindications
  - Maternal temperature greater than 100° F (37.8° C)
  - Asthma or cardiac disorder
  - Vaginal bleeding
  - Any contraindication for a vaginal delivery
  - Allergy to prostaglandin
  - Bishop score higher than 5
- Advantages
  - Decreases the likelihood of cesarean birth or failed induction
  - Requires lower doses of oxytocin
  - Reduces the need for analgesia or such instruments as forceps
  - Shortens labor
- Disadvantage is that it increases the risk of uterine hyperstimulation
- Nursing considerations
  - Know that additional cervical softening is unlikely to result from additional doses when the Bishop score is 7 or higher
  - Keep the patient recumbent for at least 30 to 60 minutes after gel insertion
  - Perform continuous external fetal monitoring for 4 hours after gel insertion
  - Ensure that a responsible health care provider is readily available
  - Continuously monitor FHR for at least 30 minutes after each application and up to 2 hours after vaginal insertion
  - Assess the patient for possible adverse reactions to prostaglandin, such as headache, vomiting, fever, diarrhea, and hypertension.

– Use prostaglandins cautiously in women with asthma, glaucoma, renal, or cardiac disease
– Don't use oxytocin and prostaglandin concurrently
  · Any prostaglandin cervical-ripening product should be removed from the cervix before oxytocin administration because prostaglandin potentiates oxytocin's effect
  · The prostaglandin should also be removed before amniotomy
– Don't administer more than 6 doses; once labor begins, expect to discontinue the drug
– Have appropriate personnel and equipment readily available for delivery and possible neonatal resuscitation

OBSTETRIC ANALGESIA AND ANESTHESIA

● **Pain perception theories**
  • Specificity—A specific pain system carries messages from pain receptors in the body to a pain center in the brain
  • Pattern—Particular networks of nerve impulses are produced by sensory input at the dorsal horn cells; pain results when the output of these cells exceeds a critical level
  • Gate control—Local physical stimulation can balance the pain stimuli by closing down a hypothetical gate in the spinal cord that blocks pain signals from reaching the brain

● **Sources of pain during labor**
  • Dilation and stretching of the cervix
  • Hypoxia of the uterine muscle cells during a contraction
  • Lower uterine segment stretching
  • Pressure by the presenting part on adjacent structures
  • Distention of the vagina and perineum
  • Emotional tension

● **Circumstances affecting pain perception**
  • Cultural background
    – Individuals tend to react to pain in ways that are acceptable in their culture
    – Some women react to pain by becoming silent and avoiding interaction with other individuals, as learned through previous experiences or conditioning; others scream, verbalize their feelings of distress, or become verbally abusive to others
    – Determining the level of comfort each woman desires as well as the manner in which she chooses to express her discomfort is important

Sources of pain during labor

● Dilation and stretching of cervix
● Hypoxia of uterine muscle cells during a contraction
● Lower uterine segment stretching
● Pressure by the presenting part on adjacent structures
● Distention of the vagina and perineum
● Emotional tension

Factors affecting pain perception

● Cultural background (can also affect amount and type of analgesia a woman may choose to have during labor)
● Personal significance (self-concept)
● Fatigue and sleep deprivation
● Attention and distractions (preoccupation with another activity can lessen perceived pain)

– Culture and families also play a role in pain perception and in determining the amount and type of analgesia a woman may choose to have during labor

– If childbirth is viewed as a natural process that doesn't disrupt the usual functioning of the family unit, the woman is less likely to show an outward reaction to labor pains and less likely to require pharmacologic pain relief

• Personal significance: Self-concept is closely aligned with how an individual regards pain

• Fatigue and sleep deprivation: A tired individual has less energy and can't focus on such strategies as distraction

• Attention and distractions: Preoccupation with another activity (such as breathing techniques) lessens perceived pain

PAIN RELIEF DURING LABOR AND DELIVERY

● **General information**

• Labor and the birth of a child usually produce a significant amount of discomfort and are emotionally draining for the woman who's experiencing them

• Prenatal education and planning and the presence of a support person (commonly called a birthing partner or coach) during labor and birth can alleviate the woman's anxiety and increase her self-esteem and feelings of control over the experience (empowerment), thus reducing the discomfort she feels or, more appropriately, increasing her ability to deal with it

• The end result of these measures is a decrease in the amount or total avoidance of analgesia or anesthesia necessary during the birthing process

● **Nonpharmacologic measures**

• Relaxation

– Most childbirth education classes teach relaxation techniques to their students

– Turns the woman's focus away from the pain, which reduces tension, effectively breaking the pain cycle—less tension leads to a perception of decreased pain, which leads to less tension

– Part of the relaxation process is positioning; the woman should be taught to shift her position during labor to find the one that's most comfortable for her

– Commonly, the position of the fetus and the presenting part affect the most comfortable position for the mother

• For example, a woman with a fetus in an occiput posterior position usually experiences intense back pain during labor

TOP 8

Nonpharmacologic ways to relieve pain during labor and delivery

1. Relaxation techniques — exercises to focus attention away from pain

2. Focusing — concentration on an object

3. Imagery — visualization of a person, place, or thing

4. Effleurage — light abdominal massage

5. Lamaze — patterns of controlled breathing

6. Hypnosis — alteration in state of consciousness

7. Acupuncture and acupressure — stimulation of trigger points with needles or pressure

8. Yoga — deep-breathing exercises, body-stretching postures, and meditation to promote relaxation

Understanding effleurage

Effleurage is a light fingertip massage that the woman or her partner performs on her abdomen or thighs during contractions. This illustration shows the tracing patterns used for effleurage.

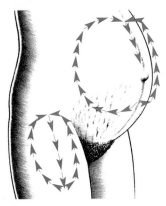

> • A change from a back- or side-lying position to one on the hands and knees with the head lower than the hips usually helps to ease this pain

- Focusing
  - Method of distraction; involves the use of a photograph or object that's important, has special meaning, or is particularly appealing to the woman
  - Patient concentrates intently on the object during contractions
  - Keeps the sensory input perceived during the contraction from reaching the pain center in the cortex of the brain
- Imagery
  - Also known as *visualization;* involves the mental concentration on a person, place, or thing
  - Sound, or what the woman hears during this process, is an important part of effective imagery that aids in maintaining her concentration on the image
  - When using imagery involving a place, the woman mentally places herself in a different environment, usually on a beach with the sound of waves crashing on shore, in a forest or meadow with the sound of rustling leaves or singing birds, or near a stream or river with the sound of the water flowing by.
  - If a person is included as part of the woman's visualization, he should be speaking softly and offering words of comfort
  - The person could also be singing or reading a favorite poem; an example of an item that could be used during visualization might be a music box playing a favorite tune
- Effleurage
  - Light abdominal massage in which the woman or her coach traces a pattern on the skin—repeating it over and over (see *Understanding effleurage*)

Spotlight on imagery

- Mental concentration on a person, place, or thing
- Also known as *visualization*
- Sound plays important part in maintaining concentration on the image
- In place imagery, the woman mentally places herself in a different environment

Three key Lamaze breathing techniques

1. Slow – inhaling through the nose and exhaling through the mouth or nose six to nine times per minute
2. Accelerated-decelerated – inhaling through the nose and exhaling through the mouth as contractions become more intense
3. Pant-blow – performing rapid, shallow breathing through the mouth only throughout contractions, particularly during the transitional phase

Spotlight on TENS

- Stimulation of large-diameter neural fibers by electric currents
- May be more effective in reducing back pain associated with labor than with pain caused by uterine contractions

Spotlight on hypnosis

- Alteration in state of consciousness that allows perception and motor control to be influenced by suggestion
- Infrequently used
- Requires meeting with hypnotherapist during pregnancy for evaluation and conditioning

- The rate of effleurage is slow and remains constant, even though the rate of breathing may change
- If the patient has external fetal monitoring, the effleurage can be performed on the thigh
- Effective for mild to moderate discomfort
- Distraction
  - Involves the diversion of attention from discomfort during early labor
  - Examples include playing games or recalling pleasant experiences
- Lamaze breathing techniques
  - These techniques involve three patterns of controlled chest breathing
    - Slow—Inhale through the nose and exhale through the mouth or nose six to nine times per minute
    - Accelerated-decelerated—Inhale through the nose and exhale through the mouth as contractions become more intense
    - Pant-blow—Perform rapid, shallow breathing through the mouth only throughout contractions, particularly during the transitional phase
  - These techniques are used primarily during the active and transitional phases of labor
- Transcutaneous electrical nerve stimulation (TENS)
  - Stimulation of large-diameter neural fibers through electric currents to alter pain perception
  - Although not documented as being significant in reducing the pain caused by uterine contractions, TENS may be effective in reducing the extreme back pain that some woman have during contractions
- Hypnosis
  - Involves an altered state of consciousness allowing perception and motor control to be influenced by suggestion
  - Though used infrequently, hypnosis can provide a satisfactory method of pain relief for the woman who follows hypnotic suggestions
  - The woman must meet with the hypnotherapist several times during her pregnancy for evaluation and conditioning
  - If it's determined that she's a good candidate for this method of pain relief, she'll be given a posthypnotic suggestion that she'll experience either reduced pain during labor or no pain at all
- Acupuncture and acupressure
  - Methods of pain relief sometimes used during labor
  - Acupuncture is the stimulation of key trigger points with needles; it's unnecessary for these points to be near the affected organ be-

cause their activation causes the release of endorphins, which reduce the perception of pain

- – Acupressure is finger pressure or massage at the same trigger points
- – Holding and squeezing the hand of a woman in labor may trigger the point most commonly used for acupuncture and acupressure during labor
- • Yoga
  - – Uses a series of deep-breathing exercises, body-stretching postures, and meditation to promote relaxation, slow the respiratory rate, lower blood pressure, improve physical fitness, reduce stress, and allay anxiety
  - – May help reduce the pain of labor by helping the body relax and possibly releasing endorphins

● **Analgesics**
- • Opioids
  - – Commonly used drugs include meperidine (Demerol), fentanyl (Sublimaze), butorphanol (Stadol), and nalbuphine (Nubain)
  - – Common maternal adverse reactions include respiratory depression, nausea and vomiting, drowsiness, and transient hypotension
  - – Common fetal-neonatal adverse reactions include neonatal respiratory depression (if medication is given within 2 hours of delivery), hypotonia, and lethargy
- • Sedatives
  - – Barbiturates, such as secobarbital (Seconal) and pentobarbital (Nembutal), are sometimes used in false labor or in the early latent phase of labor
  - – Benzodiazepines, such as midazolam (Versed), may be used by some health care providers but their use requires strict monitoring
  - – Common maternal-fetal-neonatal adverse reactions include transient decrease in variability, neonatal respiratory depression, and decreased level of alertness
- • Intrathecal opioid analgesia
  - – Involves the injection of an opioid into the spinal cord
  - – An opioid such as fentanyl is injected via a catheter inserted into the subarachnoid space
  - – Advantages
    - · Onset of pain relief is rapid without the effects of sedation
    - · No motor block occurs, so the patient can ambulate
    - · The urge to push isn't blocked, thereby allowing her to participate more fully
    - · No sympathetic nervous system block occurs, so hypotension isn't a problem

---

Primary benefits of yoga

- ● Promotes relaxation
- ● Slows the respiratory rate
- ● Lowers blood pressure
- ● Reduces stress
- ● Allays anxiety

Analgesics used during labor and delivery

- ● Opioids (meperidine, fentanyl, butorphanol, and nalbuphine)
- ● Sedatives
- – Barbiturates (secobarbital, pentobarbital)
- – Benzodiazepines (midazolam)
- ● Intrathecal opioid analgesia: injection of opioid into spinal cord

Key facts about general anesthesia

- Administered I.V. or by inhalation
- Results in unconsciousness
- Used only if regional anesthesia is contraindicated or in an emergency
- Maternal adverse reactions include vomiting, aspiration, increased uterine relaxation and, possibly, postpartum uterine atony
- Fetal-neonatal adverse reactions include respiratory depression, fetal acidosis, hypotonia, and lethargy

Quick guide to regional anesthesia

- **Local anesthesia** – administered to block pain neuropathways that pass from the uterus to the spinal cord
- **Lumbar epidural** – injection into the epidural space in lumbar region
- **Spinal anesthesia** – injection into the cerebrospinal fluid in the spinal canal; used for urgent cesarean births because of its rapid onset
- **Local infiltration** – injection of anesthesia into the perineal nerves
- **Pudendal block** – blockage of the pudendal nerve; used to ease pain during delivery
- **Paracervical block** – blockage of nerves in the peridural space at the sacral hiatus; used during first and second stages of labor as well as during delivery

- Disadvantages
  - Limited duration of action
  - Possible level of inadequate pain relief

● **Anesthetics**
- General anesthesia
  - Administered I.V. or by inhalation, resulting in unconsciousness
  - Used only if regional anesthesia is contraindicated or if an emergency situation develops suddenly
  - Inhaled anesthetics used include nitrous oxide, isoflurane (Forane), and halothane (Fluothane)
  - I.V. anesthetics (usually reserved for patients with massive blood loss) include thiopental (Pentothal) and ketamine (Ketalar)
  - Maternal adverse reactions include vomiting and aspiration, and increased uterine relaxation, possibly leading to postpartum uterine atony
  - Fetal-neonatal adverse reactions include respiratory depression, fetal acidosis, hypotonia, and lethargy
- Regional anesthesia
  - Local anesthesia administered to block pain neuropathways that pass from the uterus to the spinal cord by way of sympathetic nerves
  - Lumbar epidural anesthesia involves the injection of medication into the epidural space in the lumbar region
    - Advantages
      - Leaves the patient awake and cooperative for delivery without adverse fetal effects
      - Provides analgesia for the first and second stages of labor and anesthesia for birth
    - Disadvantages
      - Hypotension (uncommon, although incidence increases if the patient doesn't receive a proper fluid load before the procedure)
      - Decreased urge to push (uncommon because of the low concentration of local anesthetic used)
      - Risk of dural puncture, leading to postspinal headache or transient complete motor paralysis
      - Urine retention
      - Maternal fever that may be due to hyperventilation and decreased heat dissipation (that is, decreased sweating from pain relief); it may cause an increase in fetal temperature thus increasing the demand for oxygen, subsequently leading to fetal hypoxia and acidosis

- It differentiates the source of fever (that is, epidural versus infection); other changes, such as white blood count, drainage odor, and fetal tachycardia, should be assessed
– Spinal anesthesia involves the injection of medication into the cerebrospinal fluid in the spinal canal
  - Advantages
    - Low incidence of adverse effects
    - Useful for urgent cesarean births because of its rapid onset
  - Disadvantages
    - Short duration
    - Possible development of postspinal headache
    - Risk of transient complete motor paralysis
    - Increased incidence and degree of hypotension
    - Urine retention
– Local infiltration involves the injection of anesthesia into the perineal nerves
  - This method is advantageous because of its ease of administration
  - The major disadvantage is that the woman receives relief from discomfort only at delivery, not during labor
– Pudendal block is the blockage of the pudendal nerve
  - This method is used only for delivery, not for labor
  - It's advantageous because it's a simple, safe method that usually doesn't depress the fetus
  - The major disadvantage is that the woman receives no relief from discomfort of uterine contractions, only discomfort from perineal distention
– Paracervical block refers to blockage of nerves in the peridural space at the sacral hiatus
  - Advantages
    - Allows patient to be awake
    - Provides analgesia for the first and second stages of labor
    - Provides anesthesia for delivery
  - Disadvantages
    - Increased incidence of hypotension
    - Increased use of forceps
    - Increased episodes of fetal bradycardia
    - Increased risk of hematomas
    - Possible risk of injecting directly into the fetus

- **Nursing interventions**
  - Know each type of anesthesia and analgesia used, including action, possible adverse reactions, and requirements for administration and monitoring

Advantages of lumbar epidural anesthesia

- Patient awake and cooperative for delivery
- No adverse fetal effects
- Provides analgesia for the first and second stages of labor and anesthesia for birth

Disadvantages of lumbar epidural anesthesia

- Hypotension
- Decreased urge to push
- Risk of dural puncture
- Urine retention
- Maternal fever

Key nursing interventions during medication administration

- Know action, adverse reactions, and administration and monitoring requirements of each drug used.
- Answer any questions the patient has to allay fears and anxiety.
- Closely monitor the patient and fetus for complications.
- Act promptly if adverse reactions occur; notify the health care provider immediately; have emergency equipment ready.

- Allay the patient's fears and anxieties about medication, and answer her questions
- Assist with preparation and administration of medications as appropriate
- Closely monitor the patient and fetus; watch for possible maternal, fetal, or neonatal complications from administered medications
- Take swift action if adverse reactions occur; notify the health care provider immediately; have emergency equipment readily available should problems arise
- If the patient is receiving an opioid analgesic, have naloxone (Narcan) readily available

ALTERNATIVE BIRTHING EXPERIENCES

● Birthing centers
- May be found in maternity facilities located in a hospital or separate institution close to a hospital
- Provide a warm, homelike environment
- Require families to take more responsibility for the birth experience
- Not appropriate for high-risk deliveries
- Most care is provided by nurse-midwives

● Home births
- Advantageous because they allow the family unit to remain intact
- May be considered controversial because of inadequate medical backup
- The woman is responsible for ensuring that the home is adequately prepared for the birth
- Typically, the woman must be in good health, have adequate support for assistance before, during, and after labor and delivery, and be able to adjust to changing events

Alternative birthing experiences

- Birthing center
- Home birth
- Siblings present
- Side-lying, squatting, sitting, or semi-Fowler's position
- Leboyer method

● Siblings present at birth
- Prenatal education of and active participation by siblings
- Fosters the integration of the neonate into the family

● Alternative positions
- Side-lying
- Squatting
- Sitting
- Semi-Fowler's

● Leboyer method
- Controversial birthing method
- Focuses on a soothing, tender approach to handling the neonate immediately after delivery
  - Lights are dimmed
  - Noise is diminished

– Neonate is gently placed in a warm bath after the umbilical cord has been clamped

● **Water birth**

• Involves the woman sitting or reclining in a warm water bath during labor
• The neonate is born under water and then immediately brought out of the water for the first breath
• Advantages
  – The water fosters a feeling of weightlessness
  – Relaxation occurs secondary to the warm water
• Disadvantages
  – Risk of fecal contamination of the water (from bearing down)
  – May lead to uterine infection and neonatal aspiration of water during birth

ROLE OF THE COACH DURING LABOR AND DELIVERY

● **Coach**

• Of great value during labor and delivery, especially if the patient and coach have attended prenatal classes together
• May be the patient's husband or any significant other
• In some cases, the patient may also opt to have another woman present during labor and delivery for support
  – This person is called a doula and is skilled in events of labor and delivery
  – Using a doula can free the patient's partner from stress of the events and coaching
  – Some research suggests that use of a doula reduces the incidence of oxytocin augmentation, epidural anesthesia, and cesarean birth
• Benefits
  – Emotional support
  – Physical support (such as back rubs)
  – Enhanced communication between the patient and staff if necessary (for example, to overcome a language barrier)
  – Reduction in anxiety and pain perception
  – Aid in the initiation of bonding with the neonate

Spotlight on water birth

• Woman sits or reclines in warm water during labor
• Neonate is born under water (immediately brought up for first breath)
• Water fosters feeling of weightlessness and relaxation
• Places patient at risk for uterine infection
• Risk of neonatal aspiration of water

Key facts about a birthing coach

• May be patient's husband or a significant other
• May also be a doula (a woman skilled in events of labor and delivery)
• Provides emotional support
• Provides physical support
• Helps reduce anxiety and pain perception
• Aids initiation of bonding with the neonate

TOP 12

Items to study for your next test on normal labor and delivery

1. Four components of labor
2. Types of fetal presentation, lie, position, and attitude
3. Normal and abnormal contraction patterns
4. Four stages of true labor
5. Seven cardinal movements of labor
6. Maternal physiologic responses to labor
7. Maternal assessment during labor
8. Fetal evaluation during labor
9. Fetal heart rate patterns
10. Maternal and fetal diagnostic procedures during labor
11. Cesarean birth and induction of labor
12. Types of obstetric analgesia and anesthesia

NCLEX CHECKS

It's never too soon to begin your NCLEX preparation. Now that you've reviewed this chapter, carefully read each of the following questions and choose the best answer. Then compare your responses with the correct answers.

1. What's the most common type of pelvis found in women?
- ☒ **A.** Gynecoid
- ☐ **B.** Anthropoid
- ☐ **C.** Android
- ☐ **D.** Platypelloid

2. What separates the false pelvis from the true pelvis?
- ☐ **A.** Pelvic inlet
- ☐ **B.** Pelvic outlet
- ☒ **C.** Linea terminalis
- ☐ **D.** Pelvic cavity

3. Which of the following pelvic diameters would pose a problem for vaginal delivery?
- ☐ **A.** True conjugate of 4⅜″ (11 cm) or greater.
- ☒ **B.** Transverse diameter of inlet of less than 5″ (12.7 cm)
- ☐ **C.** Anteroposterior diameter of outlet of 4⅝″ (11.7 cm)
- ☐ **D.** Intertuberous diameter of 4½″ (11.5 cm)

4. Which of the following attitudes refers to the "military" position?
- ☐ **A.** Complete flexion
- ☒ **B.** Moderate flexion
- ☐ **C.** Partial extension
- ☐ **D.** Complete extension

5. Which of the following is characteristic of Braxton Hicks contractions?
- ☒ **A.** Irregular pattern
- ☐ **B.** Unaffected by activity
- ☐ **C.** Primarily felt in the back
- ☐ **D.** Moderate to strong intensity

6. Which of the following would confirm spontaneous rupture of membranes?
- ☐ **A.** Negative ferning
- ☐ **B.** Absence of fluid pooling at cervix
- ☐ **C.** Pain with fluid gushing
- ☐ **D.** Bright blue nitrazine paper

7. During the transition phase of the first stage of labor, which of the following occurs?

- ☐ **A.** Irregular short contractions
- ☒ **B.** Feeling the urge to push
- ☐ **C.** Onset of the first contractions
- ☐ **D.** Cervical dilation of 4 to 7 cm

8. Which of the following signs indicate that the placenta has separated and is ready to be delivered?

- ☐ **A.** Slowing of vaginal bleeding
- ☐ **B.** Cessation of uterine contractions
- ☒ **C.** Lengthening of the umbilical cord
- ☐ **D.** Round firm uterine shape
- ☒ **E.** Discoid uterine shape
- ☒ **F.** Sudden gush of vaginal blood

9. Which of the following maternal responses would be most common in the second stage of labor?

- ☒ **A** Active pushing
- ☐ **B.** Loss of control
- ☐ **C.** Concern about labor progress
- ☐ **D.** Excitement

10. Which of the following measurements indicates that the fetal presenting part is engaged?

- ☐ **A.** −2
- ☒ **B.** 0
- ☐ **C** +2
- ☐ **D.** +4

ANSWERS AND RATIONALES

1. CORRECT ANSWER: A

Gynecoid pelvis is the most common type of female pelvis, occurring in about 50% of females. Its round shape with adequate diameters allow easy passage of fetal skull and shoulders. Anthropoid pelvis is found in about 25% of females. It's oval and may pose difficulty in passage, except when the fetus is in the occiput posterior position. Android pelvis is the third most common type of pelvis, found in about 20% of females, and is heart-shaped. Platypelloid pelvis is found in about 5% of females. Its oval or flat shape may pose difficulty for the fetus to rotate sufficiently to match the shape of this pelvis at the appropriate diameters.

2. CORRECT ANSWER: C

The linea terminalis is an imaginary line that separates the false pelvis from the true pelvis. The pelvic inlet is the entrance to the true pelvis. The pelvic outlet is the inferior portion of the pelvis. The pelvic cavity is the curved area between the pelvic inlet and outlet.

3. CORRECT ANSWER: B

To be adequate for vaginal delivery, the transverse diameter of the inlet should measure 5⅜" (13.5 cm) or greater. A true conjugate of 4⅜" (11 cm) or greater, anteroposterior diameter of outlet of 4⅝" (11.7 cm), and an inter-tuberous diameter ranging from 3⅞" to 5⅜" (10 to 13.7 cm) are considered adequate for vaginal delivery.

4. CORRECT ANSWER: B

The military position refers to moderate flexion, which involves a sinciput (forehead) presentation through the birth canal. It's commonly known as the military position because the straightness of the head makes the fetus appear to be "at attention." With complete flexion, the neck of the fetus is completely flexed, and the head is tucked down onto the chest, with the chin touching the sternum. The fetus's arms are folded over the chest with the elbows flexed, the lower legs are crossed, and the thighs are drawn up onto the abdomen, with the calf of each leg pressed against the thigh of the opposite leg. Partial extension involves a brow presentation through the birth canal. The neck of the fetus is extended, with the head moved backward slightly so that the brow becomes the first part of the fetus to pass through the pelvis during delivery. Complete extension involves a face presentation through the birth canal. The head and neck of the fetus are hyperextended with the occiput touching the fetus's upper back; the back is usually arched, increasing the degree of hyperextension.

5. CORRECT ANSWER: A

Braxton Hicks contractions are irregular with the length of time between them and strength varying widely. Although they may gradually increase in frequency and intensity through the pregnancy, they maintain an irregular pattern. Braxton Hicks contractions can be diminished with increased activity, eating, drinking, or changing position. Braxton Hicks contractions are typically painless—especially early in pregnancy. Many women feel only a tightening of the abdomen in the first or second trimester, but if the woman does feel pain from these contractions, it's felt only in the abdomen and the groin—never in the back.

6. CORRECT ANSWER: D

The nitrazine test involves the use of litmus paper to detect the pH of the secretions; change in the paper color to bright blue indicates a change in pH from amniotic fluid with rupture of membranes. Appearance of "ferning" when a specimen of fluid is applied to a slide and viewed under a microscope indicates rupture of membranes. A vaginal examination with a speculum with pooling of fluid at the base of cervix indicates rupture of membranes. Spontaneous rupture of the membranes isn't painful because the membranes have no nerve supply.

7. CORRECT ANSWER: B

During the transition phase, the woman typically feels the urge to push. Irregular short contractions are typical of the latent phase. The onset of the first contractions signifies the beginning of the first stage of labor. Cervical dilation of 4 to 7 cm occurs during the active phase.

8. CORRECT ANSWERS: C, E, AND F

Signs that the placenta has separated and is ready to be delivered include lengthening of the umbilical cord, sudden gush of vaginal blood, and change in the shape of the uterus from round to discoid. After delivery of the neonate, uterine contractions commonly cease for several minutes. The uterus can be felt as a round mass, firm to the touch, just below the level of the umbilicus. After the brief period of rest, when the contractions resume, the uterus takes on a discoid shape and remains that way until the placenta has separated from the uterus. Separation of the placenta from the uterus occurs after the uterus resumes contractions.

9. CORRECT ANSWER: A

During the second stage of labor, maternal behavior changes from coping with contractions to actively pushing. Loss of control is more common during the transitional phase of the first stage of labor. During active phase, the patient becomes serious and concerned about the progress of labor; she may ask for pain medication or use breathing techniques. Excitement is a common response early during the first stage of labor.

10. CORRECT ANSWER: B

Engagement occurs when the fetal presenting part is at the level of the ischial spines, or station 0. A −2 station indicates that the fetal presenting part is 2 cm above the ischial spines. A +2 station indicates that the fetal presenting part is 2 cm below the ischial spines. A +4 station indicates that the fetal presenting part is at the perineum, commonly called "crowning."

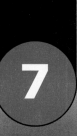

Complications and high-risk conditions of labor and delivery

LEARNING OBJECTIVES

After studying this chapter, you should be able to:

● List possible complications of labor and delivery.

● Describe management of the patient in premature labor.

● Describe immediate steps to follow when an umbilical cord prolapses.

CHAPTER OVERVIEW

During labor and delivery, conditions may develop that cause complications or place the patient at risk. Throughout this period, the nurse must be alert for these conditions to ensure early identification and prompt intervention, thereby minimizing the risk to the patient and fetus.

PREMATURE LABOR

● **Description**

• Also known as *preterm labor;* the onset of rhythmic uterine contractions that produce cervical changes after fetal viability but before fetal maturity

• Usually occurs between 20 and 37 weeks' gestation

• Fetal prognosis depends on birth weight and length of gestation

– Neonates who weigh less than 737 g and are less than 26 weeks' gestation have a survival rate of about 10%
– Those who weigh 737 to 992 g and are between 27 and 28 weeks' gestation have a survival rate of more than 50%
– Those who weigh 992 to 1,219 g and are more than 28 weeks' gestation have a 70% to 90% survival rate
• Premature labor increases the risk of neonate morbidity or mortality from excessive maturational deficiencies

Maternal causes
• Cardiovascular and renal disease
• Diabetes mellitus
• Pregnancy-induced hypertension
• Infection
• Abdominal surgery or trauma
• Incompetent cervix
• Placental abnormalities
• Premature rupture of membranes

Fetal causes
• Infection
• Hydramnios
• Multiple pregnancy

Assessment findings
• Onset of rhythmic uterine contractions
• Possible rupture of membranes, passage of the cervical mucus plug, and a bloody discharge
• Typically 20 to 37 weeks' gestation
• Cervical effacement and dilation on vaginal examination

Treatment
• Designed to suppress preterm labor when tests show immature fetal lung development, cervical dilation of less than 4 cm, and the absence of factors that contraindicate continuation of pregnancy
• Such treatment consists of bed rest and, when necessary, drug therapy with a tocolytic
• In general, tocolytics are contraindicated if:
– Gestation is less than 20 weeks
– Cervical dilation is more than 4 cm
– Cervical effacement is more than 50%
• Terbutaline (Brethine), a beta-adrenergic blocker, is the most commonly used tocolytic
– It's a $beta_2$ receptor stimulator that causes smooth-muscle relaxation

Key facts about premature labor
• Usually occurs between 20 and 37 weeks' gestation
• Fetal prognosis depends on birth weight and length of gestation
• Premature labor increases the risk of infant morbidity or mortality
• Treatment may consist of a tocolytic such as terbutaline, magnesium sulfate, indomethacin, and nifedipine

Maternal causes of premature labor
• Cardiovascular and renal disease
• Diabetes mellitus
• Pregnancy-induced hypertension
• Infection
• Abdominal surgery or trauma
• Incompetent cervix
• Placental abnormalities
• Premature rupture of membranes

Fetal causes of premature labor
• Infection
• Hydramnios
• Multiple pregnancy

Facts about terbutaline

- Beta-adrenergic agent
- Most commonly used tocolytic
- Brand name Brethine
- Maternal adverse effects include tachycardia, diarrhea, nervousness and tremors, nausea and vomiting, headache, hyperglycemia or hypoglycemia, hypokalemia, and pulmonary edema
- Fetal adverse effects include tachycardia, hypoxia, hypoglycemia, and hypocalcemia
- Antidote is propranolol

Facts about magnesium sulfate

- First drug used to halt contractions
- CNS depressant that helps relax uterus
- Contraindicated in cases of severe abdominal pain of unknown origin and oliguria
- Maternal adverse effects include drowsiness, flushing, warmth, nausea, headache, slurred speech, and blurred vision
- Fetal adverse effects include hypotonia and bradycardia
- Antidote is calcium gluconate

Facts about indomethacin

- Prostaglandin synthesis inhibitor
- Brand name Indocin
- Typically isn't used after 32 weeks' gestation
- May cause premature closure of the ductus arteriosus

– Contraindications
  - Severe pregnancy-induced hypertension
  - Cardiac disease
– Adverse effects on the mother include tachycardia, diarrhea, nervousness and tremors, nausea and vomiting, headache, hyperglycemia or hypoglycemia, hypokalemia, and pulmonary edema
– Adverse effects on the fetus include tachycardia, hypoxia, hypoglycemia, and hypocalcemia
– Antidote is propranolol (Inderal)
- Magnesium sulfate is typically the first drug used to halt contractions
  – It's a central nervous system (CNS) depressant that prevents reflux of calcium into the myometrial cells, thereby keeping the uterus relaxed
  – Contraindications include severe abdominal pain of unknown origin and oliguria
  – Adverse effects on the mother
    - Drowsiness
    - Flushing
    - Warmth
    - Nausea
    - Headache
    - Slurred speech
    - Blurred vision
  – Drug is associated with toxicity, which is manifested by CNS depression in the mother
    - Respirations less than 12 breaths/minute
    - Hyporeflexia
    - Oliguria
    - Cardiac arrhythmias
    - Cardiac arrest
  – Adverse effects on the fetus include hypotonia and bradycardia
  – Antidote is calcium gluconate
- Indomethacin (Indocin) is a prostaglandin synthesis inhibitor; typically not used after 32 weeks' gestation to avoid premature closure of the ductus arteriosus
  – Mechanism: nonsteroidal anti-inflammatory that decreases production of prostaglandins, which are lipid compounds associated with the initiation of labor
  – Contraindications
    - GI bleeding
    - Ulcers
    - Rectal bleeding
    - Severe cardiovascular, renal, or hepatic disease (use cautiously)

– Adverse effects on the mother
  · Nausea, vomiting, and dyspepsia
  · Additive CNS effects if given with magnesium sulfate
– Adverse effects on the fetus include premature closure of ductus arteriosus
– There's no antidote; discontinue drug
• Nifedipine (Procardia) is a calcium channel blocker
  – It decreases the production of calcium, a substance associated with the initiation of labor
  – Contraindications
    · Sick sinus syndrome
    · Second- or third-degree atrioventricular heart block
    · Systolic blood pressure less than 90 mm Hg
  – Adverse effects on the mother
    · Headache
    · Flushing
    · Additive CNS effects if given with magnesium sulfate
  – Adverse effects on the fetus is minimal
  – There's no antidote; discontinue drug
• For prevention in a patient with a history of premature labor, a purse-string suture (cerclage) may be inserted at 14 to 18 weeks' gestation to reinforce an incompetent cervix

● **Nursing interventions**
• Closely observe the patient in preterm labor for signs of fetal or maternal distress and provide comprehensive supportive care
• Provide guidance about the hospital stay, potential for delivery of a premature infant, and the possible need for neonatal intensive care
• During attempts to suppress preterm labor, make sure the patient maintains bed rest; provide appropriate diversionary activities
• Administer medications as ordered (see *Administering terbutaline,* page 224)
• Because sedatives and analgesics can harm the fetus, use them sparingly (minimize the need for them by providing comfort measures, such as frequent repositioning and good perineal and back care)
• Monitor blood pressure, pulse rate, respirations, fetal heart rate (FHR), and uterine contraction pattern when administering a beta-adrenergic stimulant, a sedative, or a narcotic (minimize adverse reactions by keeping the patient in a side-lying position as much as possible to ensure adequate placental perfusion)
• Monitor the status of contractions, notifying the physician if the patient experiences more than 4 contractions per hour
• If the mother's pulse rises above 120 beats/minute or her systolic blood pressure drops below 90 mm Hg, or if the fetus's heart rate

TOP 4

Interventions for premature labor

1. Observe for signs of fetal or maternal distress.
2. Administer medications as ordered.
3. Monitor the status of contractions, and notify the physician if they occur more than four times per hour.
4. Encourage the patient to lie on her side to prevent vena caval compression, supine hypotension, and fetal hypoxia.

Administering terbutaline

I.V. terbutaline may be ordered for a woman in premature labor. When administering this drug, follow these steps:

- Obtain baseline maternal vital signs, fetal heart rate (FHR), and laboratory studies, including serum glucose and electrolyte levels and hematocrit.
- Institute external monitoring of uterine contractions and FHR.
- Prepare the drug with lactated Ringer's solution instead of dextrose and water to prevent additional glucose load and possible hyperglycemia.
- Administer the drug as an I.V. piggyback infusion into a main I.V. solution so that the drug can be discontinued immediately if the patient experiences adverse reactions.
- Use microdrip tubing and infusion pump to ensure an accurate flow rate.
- Expect to adjust infusion flow rate every 10 minutes until contractions cease or adverse reactions become problematic.
- Monitor maternal vital signs every 15 minutes while infusion rate is being increased and then every 30 minutes thereafter until contractions cease; monitor FHR every 15 to 30 minutes.
- Auscultate breath sounds for evidence of crackles or changes; monitor the patient for complaints of dyspnea and chest pain.
- Be alert for maternal pulse rate greater than 120 beats/minute, blood pressure less than 90/60 mm Hg, or persistent tachycardia or tachypnea, chest pain, dyspnea, or abnormal breath sounds because these could indicate developing pulmonary edema. Notify the physician immediately.
- Watch for fetal tachycardia or late or variable decelerations in FHR pattern because these could indicate uterine bleeding or fetal distress necessitating an emergency birth.
- Monitor intake and output closely, every hour during the infusion and the every 4 hours after.
- Expect to continue the infusion for 12 to 24 hours after contractions have ceased and then switch to oral therapy.
- Administer the first dose of oral therapy 30 minutes before discontinuing the I.V. infusion.
- Instruct the patient on how to take the oral therapy, continuing therapy until 37 weeks' gestation or until fetal lung maturity has been confirmed by amniocentesis; alternatively, if the patient is prescribed subcutaneous terbutaline therapy via a continuous pump, teach the patient how to use the pump.
- Teach the patient how to measure her pulse rate before each dose of oral terbutaline, or at the recommended times with subcutaneous therapy; instruct the patient to call the physician if her pulse rate exceeds 120 beats/minute or she experiences palpitations or severe nervousness.

rises above 180 beats/minute or drops below 110 beats/minute, notify the health care provider

- Administer fluids as ordered to ensure adequate hydration
- Frequently assess deep tendon reflexes when administering magnesium sulfate
- Monitor the neonate for signs of magnesium toxicity, including neuromuscular and respiratory depression

Warning signs during premature labor

- Maternal pulse rate above 120 beats/minute
- Maternal systolic blood pressure below 90 mm Hg
- Fetal heart rate above 180 beats/minute or below 110 beats/minute

TIME-OUT FOR TEACHING

Home tocolytic therapy

Be sure to include these topics in your teaching plan for the patient who will be receiving home tocolytic therapy:
- rationale for therapy
- drug dosage, frequency, and route
- adverse effects
- signs and symptoms of true labor
- daily fetal movement counts
- contraction and pulse rate monitoring
- signs and symptoms to notify health care provider
- activity restrictions
- supportive services.

- During active premature labor, remember that a preterm neonate has a lower tolerance for the stress of labor and is much more likely to become hypoxic than a term neonate
    - If necessary, administer oxygen to the patient through a nasal cannula
    - Encourage the patient to lie on her left side or sit up during labor to prevent vena caval compression, which can cause supine hypotension and subsequent fetal hypoxia
- Observe maternal and fetal response to labor through continuous monitoring
    - Prevent maternal hyperventilation, using a rebreathing bag, as necessary
    - Continually reassure the patient throughout labor to help reduce her anxiety
- Help the patient get through labor with as little analgesic and anesthetic as possible
    - To minimize fetal CNS depression, avoid administering an analgesic when delivery seems imminent
    - Monitor fetal and maternal response to local and regional anesthetics
- If labor is suppressed, begin discharge teaching with the woman and her support person about tocolytic therapy at home; anticipate referral for home care follow-up (see *Home tocolytic therapy*)

DYSFUNCTIONAL LABOR

● Description
- Also known as *inertia;* refers to a sluggishness in the force of labor (contractions)
    - Dysfunctional labor is somewhat different from dystocia
    - Dysfunctional labor results in a prolonged labor
    - Dystocia refers to a difficult labor

Ways to prevent hypoxia during active premature labor

- If necessary, administer oxygen to the patient through a nasal cannula.
- Encourage the patient to lie on her left side or sit up during labor to prevent vena caval compression.

Key facts about dysfunctional labor

- It refers to sluggish contractions.
- It can occur at any point in labor but is generally classified as primary (occurring at the onset of labor) or secondary (occurring later in labor).
- The incidence of maternal postpartal infection and hemorrhage and infant mortality is higher in women who have prolonged labors than in those who don't.

- Dysfunctional labor can occur at any point in labor but is generally classified as primary (occurring at the onset of labor) or secondary (occurring later in labor)
- The incidence of maternal postpartal infection and hemorrhage and infant mortality is higher in women who have prolonged labors than in those who don't, which is why it's vital to recognize and prevent dysfunctional labor

● **Causes**
- Prolonged labor can result from various problems
- It may be related to problems with the passenger, passage, or power
    – Problems related to the passenger include fetal malposition or malpresentation or an unusually large fetus
    – Problems related to passage include pelvic contractures
    – Problems related to power include uterine contractions that are hypotonic, hypertonic, or uncoordinated
- Such medications as analgesics or anesthetics given too early during labor and other conditions, such as a distended bladder or bowel, can contribute to dysfunctional labor

● **Assessment findings**
- Hypotonic contractions (most common during the active phase, resulting in a protracted active phase)
    – Number of contractions is usually low or infrequent
        · May not increase beyond two or three in a 10-minute period
        · Pattern is highly irregular and typically doesn't cause pain
    – The resting tone of the uterus remains below 10 mm Hg
    – Strength of contractions doesn't rise above 25 mm Hg
- Hypertonic contractions (most common during the latent phase, resulting in a prolonged latent phase)
    – Intensity of contractions may be no stronger than with hypotonic contractions
    – Tend to occur frequently
    – Hypertonic uterine contractions are marked by an increase in resting tone to more than 15 mm Hg
    – The woman complains of pain
- Uncoordinated contractions

● **Treatment**
- Management of hypotonic contractions involves improving the strength of contractions
    – If contractions are too weak or infrequent to be effective, labor may need to be induced or augmented to make uterine contractions stronger

Evaluating cervical readiness

Bishop's scale is a tool that you can use to assess whether a woman is ready for labor. A score ranging from 0 to 3 is given for each of five factors: cervical dilation, length (effacement), station, consistency, and position. If the woman's score exceeds 8, the cervix is considered suitable for induction.

SCORING FACTOR	SCORE			
	0	**1**	**2**	**3**
Dilation (cm)	0	1 to 2	3 to 4	3 to 4
Effacement (%)	0 to 30	40 to 50	60 to 70	80
Station	–3	–2	–1 to 0	+1 to +2
Consistency	Firm	Medium	Soft	
Position	Posterior	Mild position	Anterior	

Adapted with permission from Bishop, E.H. "Pelvic Scoring for Elective Induction," *Obstetrics and Gynecology* 24:266, 1964.

– Labor may need to be induced if the cervix is deemed ready for dilation, as evidenced by a score of 8 on the cervical readiness scale (see *Evaluating cervical readiness*)

- Labor may need to be induced if the cervix is deemed ready for dilation, as evidenced by a score of 8 on the cervical readiness scale (see *Evaluating cervical readiness*)
  - Labor may need to be augmented if the fetus is in danger or if labor doesn't occur spontaneously and the fetus appears to be at term
  - Cervical ripening via stripping of membranes or application of prostaglandin gel or laminaria may be done to prepare for the induction of labor
  - Oxytocin is administered to induce or augment labor
- Management of hypertonic contractions involves promoting rest, providing analgesia with a drug such as morphine sulfate, possibly inducing sedation so the woman can rest
  - Measures to promote comfort may include changing the linen and the mother's gown, darkening room lights, and decreasing noise and stimulation
  - If the FHR decelerates, the first stage of labor is abnormally long, or progress isn't made with pushing (second stage arrest), cesarean birth may be necessary

Nursing interventions
- Explain the events to the patient and her support person; explain that the contractions are ineffective
- Provide comfort measures, including nonpharmacologic pain relief measures

Five factors evaluated by Bishop's scale
1. Cervical dilation
2. Cervical effacement
3. Station
4. Consistency
5. Position

TOP 4
Ways to manage dysfunctional labor
1. Administer oxytocin to induce or augment labor.
2. Promote rest.
3. Provide analgesia or sedate the patient so she can rest.
4. Know that cesarean birth may be necessary if the FHR decelerates, the first stage of labor is abnormally long, or progress isn't made with pushing.

Key facts about PROM

- It refers to membrane rupture 1 or more hours before the onset of labor. (*Preterm PROM* refers rupture in a preterm gestation.)
- It is a spontaneous break in the amniotic sac before onset of regular contractions.
- It results in progressive cervical dilation.
- The mother is at risk for chorioamnionitis if the time between rupture of membranes and onset of labor is longer than 24 hours.
- The risks of fetal infection, sepsis, and perinatal mortality increase with every hour of ruptured membranes and labor, and every vaginal examination or other invasive procedure.

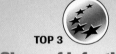

TOP 3

Signs of infection with PROM

1. Maternal fever
2. Fetal tachycardia
3. Foul-smelling vaginal discharge

- Continuously monitor uterine contractions and FHR patterns
- Offer fluids as appropriate; institute I.V. therapy to supply glucose to replace depleted stores from prolonged labor
- Assist with measures to induce or augment labor; monitor oxytocin infusion, if used
- Encourage frequent voiding to prevent bladder distention from interfering with labor contractions

PREMATURE RUPTURE OF MEMBRANES

● Description

- Premature rupture of membranes (PROM) refers to membrane rupture 1 or more hours before the onset of labor; *preterm PROM* refers to rupture of the membranes before the onset of labor in a preterm gestation
- PROM is a spontaneous break or tear in the amniotic sac before onset of regular contractions, resulting in progressive cervical dilation
- The mother is at risk for chorioamnionitis if the latent period (time between rupture of membranes and onset of labor) is longer than 24 hours
  - Signs include fetal tachycardia, maternal fever, foul-smelling amniotic fluid, and uterine tenderness
  - Development of chorioamnionitis can lead to sepsis and death
  - Risk of development increases exponentially after 18 hours of ruptured membranes without delivery
- The risks of fetal infection, sepsis, and perinatal mortality increase with PROM; risks increase with every hour of ruptured membranes, every hour of labor, and every vaginal examination or other invasive procedure

● Causes

- Unknown
- Malpresentation and a contracted pelvis commonly accompany the rupture
- Predisposing factors include poor nutrition and hygiene and lack of prenatal care, an incompetent cervix, increased intrauterine tension due to hydramnios or multiple pregnancies, defects in the amniotic membrane, and uterine, vaginal, and cervical infections (most commonly group B streptococcal, gonococcal, chlamydial, and anaerobic organisms)

● Assessment findings

- Typically, PROM causes blood-tinged amniotic fluid containing vernix caseosa particles to gush or leak from the vagina
- Maternal fever, fetal tachycardia, and foul-smelling vaginal discharge indicate infection

- Alkaline pH of fluid collected from the posterior fornix turns nitrazine paper deep blue
- A smear of fluid, placed on a slide and allowed to dry, takes on a fern-like pattern (because of the high sodium and protein content of amniotic fluid); considered a positive finding that confirms that the substance is amniotic fluid

● Treatment

- Depends on fetal age and the risk of infection
- In a term pregnancy, if spontaneous labor and vaginal delivery don't result within a relatively short time (usually within 24 hours after the membranes rupture), labor is usually induced with oxytocin; if induction fails, cesarean delivery is performed
- Management of a preterm pregnancy of less than 34 weeks is controversial
  - With a preterm pregnancy of 28 to 34 weeks, treatment includes hospitalization and observation for signs of infection (such as maternal leukocytosis or fever, and fetal tachycardia) while awaiting fetal maturation
  - If clinical status suggests infection, baseline cultures and sensitivity tests are appropriate
  - If these tests confirm infection, labor must be induced, followed by I.V. administration of an antibiotic
  - A culture of gastric aspirate or a swabbing from the neonate's ear may be done to determine the need for antibiotic therapy
  - With delivery, resuscitative equipment must be readily available to treat neonatal distress

● Nursing interventions

- Prepare the patient for a vaginal examination
- Before physically examining a patient who is suspected of having PROM, explain all diagnostic tests and clarify any misunderstandings
- During the examination, stay with the patient
  - Offer reassurance
  - Provide sterile gloves and sterile lubricating jelly
  - Don't use iodophor antiseptic solution; it discolors nitrazine paper and makes pH determination impossible
- After the examination, provide proper perineal care
- Send fluid specimens to the laboratory promptly because bacteriologic studies need immediate evaluation
- If the patient has streptococcal B infection, anticipate the need to administer a prophylactic antibiotic to reduce the risk of infecting in the neonate
- Administer I.V. fluids as ordered
- If labor starts, observe the mother's contractions and monitor her status

How to confirm the presence of amniotic fluid

- Place a smear of fluid on a slide and allow it to dry.
- Check the results. If the fluid takes on a fernlike pattern, it's amniotic fluid.

Treatment for PROM

- Depends on fetal age and the risk of infection.
- In a term pregnancy, within 24 hours of membrane rupture, labor is usually induced with oxytocin; cesarean delivery is performed if induction fails.
- In a preterm pregnancy of 28 to 34 weeks, the patient is typically hospitalized and observed for signs of infection while awaiting fetal maturation. If an infection is detected, labor is induced and an antibiotic administered.

Key nursing interventions for PROM

- Explain all diagnostic tests.
- Assist with examination and specimen collection.
- Administer I.V. fluids.
- Observe for initiation of labor (monitor vital signs frequently).
- Offer emotional support.
- Teach the patient with a history of PROM how to recognize it and to report it promptly.

TOP 3

Conditions associated with precipitate labor

1. Multiparity
2. Oxytocin induction
3. Amniotomy

Assessment findings in precipitate labor

- Strong uterine contractions with signs of premature placental separation
- Cervical dilation during active phase of more than 5 cm/hour in a nullipara and 10 cm/hour in a multipara

– Monitor vital signs every 2 hours
– Watch for signs of maternal infection, such as fever, abdominal tenderness, and changes in amniotic fluid (including purulence or foul odor) and fetal tachycardia (which may precede maternal fever); report such signs immediately

- Encourage the patient and her family to express their feelings and concerns for the infant's health and survival
- Teach the patient in the early stages of pregnancy how to recognize premature rupture of the membranes; make sure she understands that amniotic fluid doesn't always gush (it sometimes leaks slowly)
- Stress that she must immediately report premature rupture because prompt treatment may prevent dangerous infection
- Warn the patient not to engage in sexual intercourse, douche, or take tub baths after the membranes rupture

PRECIPITATE LABOR

Description

- Refers to labor that lasts 3 hours or less
- More common in multiparous patients and in women who have received oxytocin induction or amniotomy
- The mother is at risk for hemorrhage secondary to premature separation of the placenta and for lacerations due to the force and rapidity of the birth
- The fetus is at risk for hemorrhage and subdural hematoma, possibly from the rapid release of pressure on the fetal head

Cause

- Lack of maternal tissue resistance to the passage of the fetus

Assessment findings

- Strong uterine contractions with signs of premature placental separation
- Cervical dilation during the active phase of more than 5 cm/hour in a nulliparous woman and greater than 10 cm/hour in a multiparous woman

Treatment

- A tocolytic may be administered to reduce the strength and frequency of the contractions
- Plans for immediate delivery are commonly necessary
- If the woman has a history of precipitate labor, plans may be made for induction near term to control the onset and progression of labor

Nursing interventions

- Provide emotional and physical support to the woman and her support person
- Explain all procedures and treatments being initiated

- Encourage the woman to relax as much as possible
- Continuously monitor uterine contractions and FHR patterns
- Instruct the woman with a history of precipitate labor that it may occur with future pregnancies; advise the woman to plan for such an occurrence in advance

AMNIOTIC FLUID EMBOLISM °

Description
- Refers to the escape of amniotic fluid into maternal circulation
- Results from a defect in the membranes after rupture or from partial abruptio placentae
- The fetus is at risk for possible deposition of meconium, lanugo, and vernix in the pulmonary arterioles

Causes
- Believed to be an anaphylactoid type of response
- Predisposing factors include intrauterine fetal death, high parity, abruptio placentae, oxytocin augmentation, and advanced maternal age

Assessment findings
- Sudden dyspnea
- Cyanosis
- Tachypnea
- Hemorrhage
- Chest pain
- Coughing with pink frothy sputum
- Increasing restlessness and anxiety
- Shock disproportionate to blood loss

Treatment
- Administration of oxygen, blood, and heparin
- Insertion of a central venous pressure line
- Close monitoring of cardiopulmonary status
- Immediate delivery of the infant

Nursing interventions
- Know that the prognosis of the mother and fetus depends on the size of the embolism and the skill and speed of the emergency interventions
- Administer oxygen via face mask or cannula, as ordered, and assess vital signs at least every 15 minutes for changes
- Anticipate the need for endotracheal intubation to maintain pulmonary function
- Prepare to initiate cardiopulmonary resuscitation (CPR) (vital organs are deprived of oxygen supply due to the embolism; within minutes sudden cardiopulmonary arrest may occur)

Key nursing interventions for precipitate labor

- Provide emotional support.
- Explain all procedures and treatments.
- Encourage the woman to relax.
- Continuously monitor uterine contractions and FHR.

Key facts about amniotic fluid embolism

- Escape of amniotic fluid into maternal circulation
- Results from a defect in the membranes after rupture or from partial abruptio placentae
- Fetal risk for deposition of meconium, lanugo, and vernix in the pulmonary arterioles
- Predisposing factors: intrauterine fetal death, high parity, abruptio placentae, oxytocin augmentation, and advanced maternal age

Assessment findings in amniotic fluid embolism

- Sudden dyspnea
- Cyanosis
- Tachypnea
- Hemorrhage
- Chest pain
- Coughing with pink frothy sputum
- Increasing restlessness and anxiety
- Shock disproportionate to blood loss

- Arrange to transfer the patient to the intensive care unit and prepare for immediate delivery of the fetus by cesarean birth
- Assess the patient for signs and symptoms of disseminated intravascular coagulation (DIC), which may develop from the presence of particles in the bloodstream
- Administer fibrinogen as ordered to counteract DIC

PROLAPSED UMBILICAL CORD

Description
- Refers to the descent of the umbilical cord into the vagina before the presenting part (see *Umbilical cord prolapse*)
- This prolapse may occur any time after the membranes rupture, especially if the presenting part isn't fitted firmly in the cervix
- Umbilical cord prolapse is an emergency requiring prompt action to save the fetus; the cord may become compressed between the fetus and maternal cervix or pelvis, thus compromising fetoplacental perfusion

Cause
- It's most common with these conditions:
  - PROM
  - Fetal presentation other than cephalic
  - Placenta previa
  - Intrauterine tumors preventing the presenting part from engaging
  - Small fetus
  - Cephalopelvic disproportion preventing firm engagement
  - Hydramnios
  - Multiple gestation
- It may also occur if any factor interferes with fetal descent

Assessment findings
- Cord may be palpable at the perineum during vaginal examination
- An ultrasound helps confirm it
- FHR pattern shows variable decelerations

Treatment
- Focuses on relieving the pressure on the cord
  - Trendelenburg or knee-chest position to cause the fetal head to fall back from cord
  - Elevating the head up and off the cord with a sterile gloved hand inserted vaginally
- Oxygen is usually administered to promote adequate fetal oxygenation
- FHR monitoring is begun if not already in place, with frequent observations for decelerations

---

Key nursing interventions for amniotic fluid embolism

- Administer oxygen via face mask or cannula, as ordered.
- Assess vital signs every 15 minutes.
- Prepare to initiate CPR.
- Prepare for immediate delivery of the fetus by cesarean birth.
- Assess for signs and symptoms of DIC.

Key facts about umbilical cord prolapse

- The descent of the umbilical cord into the vagina before the presenting part
- May occur any time after the membranes rupture
- An emergency requiring prompt action to save the fetus (the cord may become compressed between the fetus and maternal cervix or pelvis, thus compromising fetoplacental perfusion)

Causes of umbilical cord prolapse

- PROM
- Fetal presentation other than cephalic
- Placenta previa
- Intrauterine tumors preventing the presenting part from engaging
- Small fetus
- Cephalopelvic disproportion preventing firm engagement
- Hydramnios
- Multiple gestation

Umbilical cord prolapse

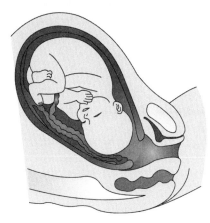
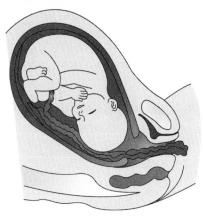

Umbilical cord prolapse with cord remaining within the uterus

Umbilical cord prolapse with cord appearing at the perineal area

- If the cord is exposed, saline-soaked sterile dressings are applied over any portion of the cord
- Vaginal delivery may be done if the woman's cervix is fully dilated; cesarean delivery is performed if cervical dilation is incomplete

● Nursing interventions

- Always auscultate fetal heart sounds immediately after rupture of the membranes occurring either spontaneously or by amniotomy
- Assist with measures to relieve cord compression
- Administer oxygen at 10 L/minute by face mask as ordered
- Anticipate the use of a tocolytic to reduce uterine activity and pressure on the fetus
- Monitor uterine contractions and FHR patterns closely; notify the physician of any variable decelerations
- Cover any exposed areas of the cord with sterile saline-soaked dressings
- Prepare the patient for delivery
  - Explain to the patient and her support person what's happening and any treatments and procedures being done
  - Offer emotional support

UTERINE INVERSION

● Description

- A rare phenomenon, occurring in about 1 in 15,000 births
- With this condition, the uterus actually turns inside out

Causes of uterine inversion

- Application of traction to the uterine fundus when the uterus isn't contracted
- Insertion of the placenta at the fundus

Assessment findings in uterine inversion

- A large, sudden gush of blood from the vagina
- Nonpalpable fundus in the abdomen
- Signs and symptoms of shock if bleeding continues
- Possible exsanguination if bleeding continues unchecked

Treatment of uterine inversion

- I.V. fluid and blood component may be given to replace fluid volume and blood loss.
- General anesthesia, nitroglycerin, or a tocolytic may be given to relax the uterus.
- The physician will try to replace the uterus.
- Oxytocin may be used to promote contraction of the replaced uterus.
- Antibiotic therapy may be given postpartally.
- As a last resort, an emergency hysterectomy may be required.

- The inverted fundus may lie within the uterine cavity of the vagina or, in total inversion, protrude from the vagina

● **Causes**
- May occur after the birth of the neonate, especially if traction is applied to the uterine fundus when the uterus isn't contracted
- May also occur when the placenta is inserted at the fundus; during birth, the passage of the fetus pulls the fundus down

● **Assessment findings**
- A large, sudden gush of blood from the vagina
- Nonpalpable fundus in the abdomen
- Signs and symptoms of shock if the loss of blood continues unchecked for more than a few minutes
    - Hypotension
    - Dizziness
    - Pallor
    - Diaphoresis
- Possible exsanguination if bleeding continues unchecked

● **Treatment**
- I.V. fluid and blood component therapy may be necessary to replace fluid volume and blood loss
- General anesthesia, nitroglycerin, or a tocolytic may be administered to relax the uterus
- After administration, the physician will attempt to manually replace the uterus
- Once replaced, oxytocin may be used to promote uterine contraction
- Due to uterine exposure, antibiotic therapy is indicated postpartally
- As a last resort, the patient may require an emergency hysterectomy

● **Nursing interventions**
- Provide emotional support to the woman and her support person; explain what's happening and any treatments and procedures being done
- Never attempt to replace the inversion because without good pelvic relaxation this may only increase bleeding
- Never attempt to remove the placenta if it's still attached because this will only create a larger bleeding area
- Keep in mind that administering an oxytocic only compounds the inversion
- Initiate I.V. fluid therapy as ordered
    - Use a large-gauge needle because blood will need to be replaced
    - If the woman has an I.V. line already in place, increase the flow rate to achieve optimal flow of fluid to try to restore fluid volume
- Administer oxygen by mask as ordered

- Monitor vital signs at least every 15 minutes
- Be prepared to perform CPR if the woman's heart fails from the sudden blood loss
- Assist with measures to relax the uterus
- Expect to administer oxytocin after manual replacement to help the uterus contract
- Anticipate administering an antibiotic, as ordered, in the postpartum period because the uterine endometrium was exposed

UTERINE RUPTURE

Description
- Occurs in about 1 in 1,500 births (rare)
- Occurs when the uterus undergoes more strain than it's capable of sustaining and then ruptures
- Impending rupture is usually preceded by a pathologic retraction ring (see *Understanding a pathologic retraction ring,* page 236)
- Rupture can be complete, going through endometrium, myometrium, and peritoneum, or incomplete, leaving the peritoneum intact
- The viability of the fetus depends on the extent of the rupture and the time that elapses between the rupture and abdominal extraction
- The woman's prognosis depends on the extent of the rupture and blood loss

Causes
- Usually occurs from a previous cesarean birth, such as when a vertical scar from a previous incision is present
- Can also occur from hysterotomy repair
- Other causes include:
  - Prolonged labor
  - Faulty presentation
  - Multiple gestation
  - Use of oxytocin
  - Obstructed labor
  - Traumatic maneuvers using forceps or traction

Assessment findings
- Indentation appearing across the abdomen over the uterus (pathologic retraction ring)
- Strong uterine contractions without any cervical dilation
- Indications of complete uterine rupture
  - Sudden, severe pain during a strong labor contraction
  - Report of a tearing sensation
  - Cessation of uterine contractions
  - Hemorrhage

Key facts about pathologic retraction rings

- Also called *Bandl's rings*
- Most common type of constriction ring responsible for dysfunctional labor
- Key sign of impending uterine rupture
- Appears as horizontal indentation across abdomen, usually during second stage of labor
- Prevents further passage of the fetus

Indications of complete uterine rupture

- Sudden, severe pain during a strong labor contraction
- A tearing sensation
- Cessation of uterine contractions
- Hemorrhage
- Signs of shock
- Change in abdominal contour with distinct swelling
- Absent fetal heart sounds

Surgeries for uterine rupture

- Laparotomy to control bleeding
- Hysterectomy to remove the damaged uterus
- Tubal ligation to prevent future conception

Understanding a pathologic retraction ring

A pathologic retraction ring, also called *Bandl's ring*, is the most common type of constriction ring responsible for dysfunctional labor. It's a key warning sign of impending uterine rupture.

A pathologic retraction ring appears as a horizontal indentation across the abdomen, usually during the second stage of labor (see arrow on illustration). The myometrium above the ring is considerably thicker than it is below the ring. When present, the ring prevents further passage of the fetus, holding the fetus in place at the point of the retraction. The placenta is also held at that point.

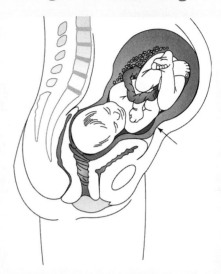

- – Signs of shock
- – Change in abdominal contour with two distinct swellings
  - · Retracted uterus
  - · Extrauterine fetus
- – Absent fetal heart sounds
- Indications of incomplete rupture less apparent
  - – Localized tenderness and persistent ache over lower uterine segment
  - – Gradual onset of absent fetal heart sounds, absent contractions, and vital sign changes

Treatment

- At the end of pregnancy the uterus is a highly vascular organ making uterine rupture an immediate emergency situation, comparable to a splenic or hepatic rupture
- Treatment focuses on the following measures:
  - – Fluid replacement
  - – I.V. oxytocin to contract the uterus and minimize bleeding
- A cesarean birth, if possible, will be done to ensure safe birth of the fetus
- Manual removal of the placenta under general anesthesia may be necessary in the event of placental-stage pathologic retraction rings
- A laparotomy may be necessary as an emergency measure to control bleeding and repair the rupture; hysterectomy (removal of the damaged uterus) or tubal ligation may be performed at the time of the laparotomy

- It's inadvisable for a woman to conceive again after uterine rupture, unless it occurred in the inactive lower segment

● **Nursing interventions**
- Administer emergency fluid replacement therapy as ordered
- Anticipate the use of I.V. oxytocin to contract the uterus and minimize bleeding
- Prepare the woman for a possible laparotomy as an emergency measure to control bleeding and repair the rupture
- Immediately provide information to the support person and inform him about the fetal outcome, the extent of the surgery, and the woman's safety
- Offer emotional support and expect them to grieve, not only for the loss of this child (if applicable) but also for the loss of having future children through pregnancies (if a hysterectomy or tubal ligation was performed)
- Allow them time to express their emotions without feeling threatened

CEPHALOPELVIC DISPROPORTION

● **Description**
- Refers to the narrowing of the birth canal
- Involves a disproportion between the size of the normal fetal head and the pelvic diameters
- Results in failure to progress in labor
- With cephalopelvic disproportion (CPD), the fetus's head doesn't engage
    - The head remains a floating entity, possibly resulting in malposition, further complicating the situation
    - If membranes rupture, the possibility of cord prolapse greatly increases

● **Causes**
- The physical size of the maternal pelvis is a major contributor
    - Inlet contraction occurs when the narrowing of the anteroposterior diameter is less than 11 cm or the maximum transverse diameter is 12 cm or less
    - This type of sizing may stem from rickets in the early life of the mother or from an inherited small pelvis
- In primigravidas, the fetal head normally engages at weeks 36 to 38 of pregnancy
    - When this event occurs before labor begins, it's assumed that the pelvic inlet is adequate

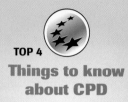

TOP 4

**Things to know
about CPD**

1. Labor fails to progress.
2. The fetus's head doesn't engage.
3. The head remains a floating entity, which may result in malposition.
4. If membranes rupture, the possibility of cord prolapse greatly increases.

– When a head engages or proves it fits into the pelvic brim, it's likely that it will also be able to pass through the midpelvis and through the outlet

• Outlet contraction can also be a contributing factor

– There's a narrowing of the transverse diameter (located at the distance between the ischial tuberosities) at the outlet to less than 11 cm

– Although this measurement is easily determined during prenatal visits and thus can be anticipated before labor begins, it can also be determined during labor

● **Assessment findings**

• Lack of fetal head engagement in a primigravida due to a fetal abnormality, such as a larger-than-usual head, or a pelvic abnormality, such as a smaller-than-usual pelvis

● **Treatment**

• If the pelvic measurements are borderline or just adequate, especially the inlet measurement, and the fetal lie and position are good, the physician may allow a trial labor to determine whether labor can progress normally

• A trial labor may be allowed to continue if descent of the presenting part and dilation of the cervix are occurring

• If labor doesn't progress or complications develop, cesarean birth is the delivery method of choice

● **Nursing interventions**

• Instruct the primiparous patient to maintain her prenatal visit schedule so that pelvic measurements are taken and recorded before week 24 of pregnancy

• Monitor progress of the trial labor—if, after 6 to 12 hours, adequate progress in labor can't be documented or if fetal distress occurs, prepare the woman for a cesarean birth

• Remember that it may be difficult for women to undertake a labor they know they may be unable to complete

– Be alert to the feelings of the patient

· Some women having a trial labor feel as if they're on trial, with feelings of self-consciousness and being judged

· If dilation doesn't occur, they may feel discouraged and inadequate, as if they're somehow at fault

– Know that sometimes it doesn't become evident until the labor progresses and the woman is in denial that it isn't going as expected (A woman may not be aware how much she wanted the trial labor to work until she's told that it isn't working)

• Allow the patient to verbalize her feelings and beliefs related to being needlessly subjected to pain

**Key nursing
interventions for CPD**

• Monitor progress of trial labor.
• Provide emotional support.
• Explain necessity of cesarean birth, if appropriate.
• Offer support to the patient's support person.

- Emphasize that it's best for the neonate to be born vaginally, if possible
- If the trial labor fails and cesarean birth is scheduled, provide an explanation about why it's necessary and is best for the neonate
- Provide support for the patient's support person; he may also be frightened and feel helpless when a problems occurs in labor and birth
- Inform the patient and support person that a cesarean birth isn't an inferior birth method
  - Remind them that it's an alternative method
  - In this instance, it's the method of choice, allowing them to achieve their goal of a healthy mother and a healthy child

PLACENTAL ANOMALIES

● **Description**
- Involve abnormalities in the size of the placenta or the blood vessels connected to it
  - The normal placenta weighs about 500 g, is 15 to 20 cm in diameter, and is 1.5 to 3.0 cm thick
  - Its weight is approximately one-sixth that of the fetus
- Several different types of placental anomalies can occur
  - The battledore placenta involves an alteration in the way the cord is attached; it's inserted marginally rather than centrally
  - With placenta succenturiata, one or more accessory lobes are connected to the main placenta by blood vessels
  - With placenta circumvallata, the membrane covering is altered (ordinarily, the chorion membrane begins at the edge of the placenta and spreads to envelop the fetus)
    - With this type of anomaly, there's no chorion totally covering the fetal side of the placenta
    - The umbilical cord enters the placenta at the usual midpoint; large vessels spread out from there but end abruptly at the point where the chorion folds back onto the surface
  - With placenta marginata, the fold of chorion reaches just to the edge of the placenta
  - With velementous insertion of the cord, the cord doesn't enter the placenta directly; instead, it separates into small vessels that reach the placenta by spreading across a fold of amnion
  - With vasa previa, the umbilical cord insertion crosses the cervical os, possibly with the cord being delivered before the fetus
  - With placenta accreta, the chorionic villi are deeply attached onto or into the myometrium, resulting in an unusually deep attachment of the placenta to the uterine myometrium; this leads to problems in which the placenta won't loosen and deliver as it normally should

---

Types of placental anomalies

- **Battledore placenta** – the cord is inserted marginally rather than centrally
- **Placenta succenturiata** – one or more accessory lobes are connected to the main placenta by blood vessels
- **Placenta circumvallata** – the fetal side of the placenta lacks chorion
- **Placenta marginata** – the fold of chorion reaches just to the edge of the placenta
- **Velementous insertion of the cord** – the cord separates into small vessels that reach the placenta by spreading across a fold of amnion
- **Vasa previa** – the umbilical cord insertion crosses the cervical os
- **Placenta accreta** – the chorionic villi are deeply attached onto or into the myometrium

Treatment of placental anomalies

- Complete visual inspection of the placenta is necessary after birth.
- With placenta succenturiata, manual removal of the placenta is indicated.
- With vasa previa, cesarean birth is the method of choice to prevent blood loss associated with tearing.
- With placenta accreta, methotrexate may be given to destroy the remaining attached tissue; alternatively, a hysterectomy may be necessary.

Nursing interventions for placental anomalies

- Make sure the placenta is inspected after delivery.
- Assist with manual removal of placenta succenturiata.
- Prepare the patient for the possibility of cesarean birth.
- Offer emotional support.
- Monitor the patient closely immediatly after delivery.

Causes
- Exact cause is unknown
- Possible contributors include:
  - A woman with diabetes may have an unusually enlarged placenta
  - With certain diseases, such as syphilis or erythroblastosis, the placenta may be so large that it weighs half as much as the fetus
  - A placenta wider in diameter may occur if the uterus has scars or a septum, possibly due to being forced to spread out to find implantation space

Assessment findings
- Typically noted during visual examination of the placenta after birth

Treatment
- Complete visual inspection of the placenta is necessary after birth
- With placenta succenturiata, manual removal of the placenta is indicated
- With vasa previa, cesarean birth is the method of choice to prevent blood loss associated with tearing
- With placenta accreta, methotrexate may be given to destroy the remaining attached tissue; alternatively a hysterectomy may be necessary

Nursing interventions
- Make sure that the placenta is inspected after delivery
- Assist with manual removal of placenta succenturiata
- Prepare the patient for the possibility of cesarean birth
- Offer emotional support and explain all treatments and procedures to the patient and her support person
- Monitor the patient closely in the immediate postpartum period

EARLY POSTPARTUM HEMORRHAGE

Description
- Refers to blood loss of 500 ml or more during the first hour after delivery
  - Normally, after vaginal delivery, a blood loss up to 500 ml is considered acceptable
  - The acceptable range for blood loss after cesarean birth is typically 1,000 to 1,200 ml
- This risk is greatest during the first hour after birth, after the placenta has detached, leaving the highly vascular yet denuded uterus widely exposed

Causes
- The primary cause of early postpartum hemorrhage is uterine atony (relaxation of the uterus)

Understanding lacerations

Lacerations are tears in the perineum, vagina, or cervix that occur from stretching of tissues during delivery. Perineal lacerations are classified as first, second, third, or fourth degree:

- A first-degree laceration involves the vaginal mucosa and the skin of the perineum to the fourchette.
- A second-degree laceration involves the vagina, perineal skin, fascia, levator ani muscle, and perineal body.
- A third-degree laceration involves the entire perineum and the external anal sphincter.
- A fourth-degree laceration involves the entire perineum, rectal sphincter, and portions of the rectal mucous membrane.

    – Hemorrhage occurs because the uterus doesn't contract properly, leaving the vessels at the placental site open

    – Any condition that interferes with the ability of the uterus to contract can lead to uterine atony and, subsequently, postpartal hemorrhage

- Lacerations of the cervix, birth canal, or perineum also can lead to postpartum hemorrhage (see *Understanding lacerations*)
  - Cervical lacerations may result in profuse bleeding if the uterine artery is torn
  - This usually occurs immediately after the placenta is delivered
- Retained placental fragments are another cause of postpartum hemorrhage; if the fragment is large, bleeding will be apparent in the early postpartum period
- DIC may cause postpartum hemorrhage; more common in women with abruptio placenta, missed abortion, or intrauterine fetal death

● **Assessment findings**

- Bleeding that occurs suddenly in large amounts or gradually, over time, as seeping or oozing of blood
- Signs and symptoms of hypovolemic shock if blood loss is sufficient
  - Decreased sensorium
  - Rapid, shallow respirations and rapid, thready peripheral pulses
  - Decreased urine output to possibly less than 25 ml/hour
  - Cold, clammy skin
  - Mean arterial pressure below 60 mm Hg and a narrowing pulse pressure
- Perineal pads being saturated frequently
- Soft, relaxed uterus
- Oozing of blood continuously from the site of a laceration
- Soft, noncontracting uterus if due to retained placental fragments
- Pallor

Facts about postpartum hemorhage

- Refers to blood loss of 500 ml or more during the first hour after delivery
- Normally, after vaginal delivery, a blood loss of up to 500 ml is considered acceptable
- Acceptable range for blood loss after cesarean birth is 1,000 to 1,200 ml

Causes of early postpartum hemorrhage

- Any condition that interferes with the ability of the uterus to contract
- Lacerations of the cervix, birth canal, or perineum
- Retained placental fragments
- DIC

Assessment findings in early postpartum hemorrhage

- Sudden bleeding
- Signs and symptoms of hypovolemic shock
- Soft, relaxed uterus
- Oozing of blood from laceration site
- Soft, noncontracting uterus
- Pallor

Treatment of postpartum hemorrhage

- Prompt blood and fluid replacement is given to restore intravascular volume and to raise blood pressure above 60 mm Hg.
- Uterine massage is initiated for the patient with uterine atony.
- If massage is inadequate, oxytocin may be ordered.
- The physician may opt to perform a bimanual massage.
- I.M. administration of prostaglandins may be ordered.
- A hysterectomy may be done as a last resort.
- Lacerations, if present, are surgically repaired.
- Retained placental fragments typically are removed via D&C.

● **Treatment**
- Focuses on correcting the underlying cause of the hemorrhage and instituting measures to control blood loss and minimize the extent of hypovolemic shock
- Emergency treatment relies on prompt, adequate blood and fluid replacement to restore intravascular volume and to raise blood pressure and maintain it above 60 mm Hg
- Rapid infusion of normal saline or lactated Ringer's solution and, possibly, albumin or other plasma expanders may be needed to expand volume adequately until whole blood can be matched
- Uterine massage is initiated for the patient with uterine atony
  - If massage is ineffective or fails to maintain the uterus in a contracted state, oxytocin may be ordered to help with uterine contraction
  - If these measures are ineffective, the physician may opt to perform a bimanual massage
- I.M. administration of prostaglandins may be ordered to promote strong, sustained uterine contractions
- If all attempts to halt bleeding are ineffective, a hysterectomy may be done; considered only as a last resort
- Lacerations, if present, are surgically repaired
- Retained placental fragments typically are removed via a dilatation and curettage (D&C)

● **Nursing interventions**
- Frequently assess the patient's fundus and lochia
  - Initially at least every 15 minutes to detect changes
  - Notify the health care provider if the fundus doesn't remain contracted or if lochia increases
- Perform fundal massage as indicated to assist with uterine involution
  - Remain with the client, frequently reassessing the fundus to ensure that it remains firm and contracted
  - Keep in mind that the uterus may relax quickly once massage is completed, placing the patient at risk for continued hemorrhage
- Weigh perineal pads to determine the extent of blood loss
- Turn the patient to the side and inspect under the buttocks for pooling of blood; if necessary, weigh disposable bed linen pads and add this to the weight of the perineal pads to estimate blood loss
- Inspect perineal area closely for oozing from possible lacerations
- Monitor vital signs frequently for changes, noting any trends, such as a continuously rising pulse rate; immediately report any changes
- Assess intake and output
  - Report urine output less than 30 ml/hour

– Encourage the woman to void frequently to prevent bladder distention from interfering with uterine involution
– If the patient is unable to void, anticipate the need to insert an indwelling urinary catheter
• Inform the patient which danger signs and symptoms suggest hemorrhage and should be reported
• If the patient develops signs and symptoms of hypovolemic shock:
– Begin an I.V. infusion with normal saline solution or lactated Ringer's solution delivered through a large-bore (14G to 18G) catheter; assist with the insertion of a central venous line and pulmonary artery catheter for hemodynamic monitoring
– Record blood pressure, pulse and respiratory rates, and peripheral pulse rates every 15 minutes until stable
– Continuously monitor cardiac rhythm
– Monitor the patient's central venous pressure, right atrial pressure, pulmonary artery pressure, pulmonary artery wedge pressure, and cardiac output at least hourly or as ordered
– During therapy, assess skin color and temperature and note any changes; cold, clammy skin may signal continuing peripheral vascular constriction, indicating progressive shock
– Watch for signs of impending coagulopathy (such as petechiae, bruising, bleeding, or oozing from gums or venipuncture sites)
– Anticipate the need for fluid replacement and blood component therapy as ordered
– Measure arterial blood gas (ABG) levels
  · Administer oxygen by nasal cannula, face mask, or airway to ensure adequate tissue oxygenation
  · Adjust the oxygen flow rate as ABG measurements indicate
– Obtain venous blood specimens, as ordered, for a complete blood count, electrolyte measurements, type and crossmatching, and coagulation studies
– If the patient has received oxytocin I.V. for treatment of uterine atony, continue to assess the fundus closely because oxytocin's action, although immediate, is short in duration; the client may experience a recurrence of atony
– If the health care provider orders intramuscular administration of prostaglandin, be alert for possible adverse reactions, such as nausea, diarrhea, tachycardia, and hypertension
– Provide emotional support to the patient; explain all events to help alleviate fear and anxiety
– Prepare the patient for possible treatments such as bimanual massage, surgical repair of lacerations, or D&C as indicated

Nursing interventions for postpartum hemorrhage

• Frequently assess the patient's fundus and lochia and notify the primary care provider of changes.
• Perform fundal massage as indicated.
• Weigh perineal pads and bed linen pads to determine the extent of blood loss.
• Inspect perineal area for oozing.
• Monitor vital signs frequently and report changes.
• Assess intake and output.
• Encourage the woman to void frequently to prevent bladder distention from interfering with uterine involution.
• Watch for signs and symptoms of hypovolemic shock.
• Administer oxygen.

Key nursing interventions for hypovolemic shock

• Administer I.V. fluids.
• Monitor vital signs and cardiac rhythm frequently.
• Administer oxygen.
• Give medications as necessary.
• Provide emotional support.

FETAL DISTRESS

● Description

- Refers to fetal compromise that results in a stressful and potentially lethal condition
- Normally during labor, the fetus is able to respond appropriately as indicated by the following:
  - FHR ranging between 120 to 160 beats/minute
  - Reassuring FHR pattern
    - Baseline variability within acceptable parameters (short-term variability of 6 to 10 beats/minute; long-term variability of 3 to 5 cycles/minute)
    - Accelerations in FHR with movement or activity
    - Early decelerations (indicative of fetal head compression during contraction) or mild variable decelerations (indicative of cord compression relieved with maternal position changes)

● Causes

- Prematurity
- Uteroplacental insufficiency
- Congenital malformation
- ABO or Rh incompatibility
- Maternal complications, such as diabetes, heart disease, or pregnancy-induced hypertension
- Prolonged labor
- Postmaturity
- Oxytocin infusion
- Vaginal bleeding

● Assessment findings

- Nonreassuring or ominous FHR pattern
- Fetal acidosis
- Meconium-stained amniotic fluid
- Decrease in or cessation of fetal movement; increased with meconium

● Treatment

- Dependent on underlying cause

● Nursing interventions

- Monitor FHR, fetal activity, fetal heart variability
- Immediately notify the physician
- Prepare for possible placement of internal monitor and fetal scalp pH sampling
- Position the patient on her left side to enhance uteroplacental blood flow
- Administer oxygen via face mask as ordered (typically 6 to 8 L/minute)
- Expect to discontinue oxytocin infusion if in use
- Prepare the patient for delivery as indicated

What happens in fetal distress

- Ominous FHR pattern
- Fetal acidosis
- Meconium-stained amniotic fluid
- Decrease in or cessation of fetal movement

Key nursing interventions for fetal distress

- Monitor FHR, fetal activity, fetal heart variability.
- Immediately notify the physician.
- Prepare for possible placement of internal monitor and fetal scalp pH sampling.
- Position the patient on her left side to enhance uteroplacental blood flow.
- Administer oxygen via face mask as ordered (typically 6 to 8 L/minute).
- Expect to discontinue oxytocin infusion if in use.

NCLEX CHECKS

It's never too soon to begin your NCLEX preparation. Now that you've reviewed this chapter, carefully read each of the following questions and choose the best answer. Then compare your responses to the correct answers.

1. Which of the following would the nurse administer as the antidote for terbutaline?

☐ **A.** Calcium gluconate
☑ **B.** Propranolol
☐ **C.** Vitamin K
☐ **D.** Protamine sulfate

2. Hypotonic contractions are most likely to occur:

☑ **A.** during the active phase of labor.
☐ **B.** as a component of PROM.
☐ **C.** during the latent phase of labor.
☐ **D.** as an indication of premature labor.

3. Which of the following is a priority after rupture of membranes to determine possible umbilical cord prolapse?

☑ **A.** Auscultating fetal heart sounds
☐ **B.** Turning the patient onto her left side
☐ **C.** Administering oxygen via face mask
☐ **D.** Administering a tocolytic

4. With which of the following placental anomalies is the placenta deeply attached to the uterus?

☐ **A.** Battledore placenta
☐ **B.** Placenta succenturiata
☑ **C.** Placenta accreta
☐ **D.** Placenta circumvallata

5. Which of the following are considered causes of early postpartum hemorrhage? Select all that apply.

☑ **A.** Uterine atony
☐ **B.** PROM
☑ **C.** Perineal laceration
☐ **D.** Small size for gestational age
☑ **E.** Retained placental fragments
☑ **F.** DIC

6. Which of the following signs would likely indicate fetal distress?

☐ **A.** FHR of 140 beats/minute
☐ **B.** Short-term variability of 7 beats/minute
☐ **C.** Early decelerations
☑ **D.** Severe variable decelerations

TOP 10

Items to study for your next test on complications and high-risk conditions of labor and delivery

1. Signs and symptoms of premature labor
2. Medical treatment and nursing interventions for dysfunctional labor
3. Assessment findings in premature rupture of membranes
4. Medical treatment and nursing interventions for prolapsed umbilical cord
5. Signs and symptoms of uterine inversion
6. Treatment of uterine rupture
7. Nursing interventions for cephalopelvic disproportion
8. Types of placental anomalies
9. Nursing interventions for early postpartum hemorrhage
10. Signs and symptoms of fetal distress

ANSWERS AND RATIONALES

1. CORRECT ANSWER: B
Propranolol is the antidote for terbutaline. Calcium gluconate is the antidote for magnesium sulfate, vitamin K is the antidote for warfarin, and protamine sulfate is the antidote for heparin.

2. CORRECT ANSWER: A
Hypotonic contractions are most likely to occur during the active phase of labor. They aren't associated with PROM or premature labor. Hypertonic contractions typically occur during the latent phase of labor.

3. CORRECT ANSWER: A
With rupture of membranes, either spontaneously or via amniotomy, fetal heart sounds should be auscultated to determine whether umbilical cord prolapse has occurred. Turning the patient to the left side enhances utero-placental blood flow but does not help determine whether umbilical cord prolapse has occurred. Additionally, the patient needs to be placed in the Trendelenburg or knee-chest position to alleviate cord compression if pro-lapse has occurred. Administering oxygen via face mask may be used to pro-mote fetal oxygenation with cord prolapse but does not help determine whether prolapse has occurred. Tocolytics are used to treat premature labor. They may be used after prolapse has occurred to reduce uterine activity and pressure on the fetus.

4. CORRECT ANSWER: C
With placenta accreta, the chorionic villi are deeply attached onto or into the myometrium resulting in an unusually deep attachment of the placenta to the uterine myometrium. The battledore placenta involves an alteration in the way the cord is attached and inserted marginally rather than centrally. With placenta succenturiata, one or more accessory lobes are connected to the main placenta by blood vessels. With placenta circumvallata, the mem-brane covering is altered (ordinarily, the chorion membrane begins at the edge of the placenta and spreads to envelop the fetus).

5. CORRECT ANSWERS: A, C, E, AND F
Causes of postpartal hemorrhage include uterine atony, perineal laceration, retained placental fragments, and DIC. PROM and a neonate who is small for gestational age aren't considered causes of early postpartum hemor-rhage.

6. CORRECT ANSWER: D
Severe variable decelerations are an ominous sign indicating continued cord compression, which subsequently interferes with fetal oxygenation. An FHR of 140 beats/minute is within normal parameters. Short-term variability in the range of 6 to 10 beats/minute and early decelerations, which indicate fe-tal head compression during a contraction, are reassuring FHR patterns.

8

The normal neonate

LEARNING OBJECTIVES

After studying this chapter, you should be able to:

- Describe the normal physical and neurologic characteristics of the neonate.
- Explain how to perform neonatal care.
- Name the conditions included in a gestational age assessment.
- State the advantages and disadvantages of breast-feeding and bottle-feeding.

CHAPTER OVERVIEW

A neonate experiences many changes while adapting to extrauterine existence. Knowledge of these changes and of the normal physical and neurologic characteristics of the neonate provides the basis for normal neonate care.

ADAPTATION TO EXTRAUTERINE LIFE

● **Cardiovascular system**
- The first breath expands the neonate's lungs, decreasing pulmonary vascular resistance
- Clamping the cord increases systemic vascular resistance and left atrial pressure

Changes in the neonate's cardiovascular system

- Atrial pressures change and functionally close the foramen ovale.
- Po_2 increases and constricts the ductus arteriosus.
- Fibrosis of umbilical vein, arteries, and ductus venosus occurs within 3 to 7 days.

What happens in the neonate's respiratory system

- Amniotic fluid is drained from the lungs.
- Lung fluid crosses the alveolar membrane into the capillaries.
- Surfactant lowers surface tension in the alveolus.

Facts about the neonatal GI system

- Bacteria aren't normally present.
- Bowel sounds can be heard 1 hour after birth.
- The neonate has a limited ability to digest fats.
- The lower intestine contains meconium at birth.

- Major changes occur as the neonate adapts to extrauterine life
  - Changing atrial pressures functionally close the foramen ovale almost immediately after birth (fibrosis may take from several weeks to a year)
  - Increasing partial pressure of oxygen (Po_2) constricts the ductus arteriosus
    - Functional closure occurs within 15 minutes to 12 hours after birth; fibrosis within 3 weeks
    - The ductus arteriosus eventually occludes and becomes a ligament
  - Clamping and severing of the umbilical cord immediately closes the umbilical vein, arteries, and ductus venosus (fibrosis occurs within 3 to 7 days, and the structures eventually convert into ligaments)

● **Respiratory system**
- The initial breath is a reflex triggered in response to chilling, noise, light, or pressure changes
- Air replaces the fluid that filled the lungs before birth
  - Between 7 and 42 ml of amniotic fluid is squeezed or drained from the lungs during vaginal delivery; other lung fluid crosses the alveolar membrane into the capillaries
  - Fluid retention greatly impedes normal respiratory adjustment
- Surfactant maintains respiratory stability by lowering surface tension in the alveolus at the end of expiration, thus preventing collapse

● **Renal system**
- Because renal function doesn't fully mature until after the first year of life, the neonate has a minimal range of chemical balance and safety
- Low ability to excrete drugs and excessive fluid loss can rapidly lead to acidosis and fluid imbalances

● **GI system**
- Neonates born beyond 32 to 34 weeks' gestation have adequate sucking and swallowing coordination
- Bacteria aren't normally present in the neonate's GI tract
- Bowel sounds can be heard 1 hour after birth
- Uncoordinated peristaltic activity in the esophagus exists for the first few days of life
- The neonate has a limited ability to digest fats because amylase and lipase are absent at birth
- The lower intestine contains meconium at birth; the first meconium (sterile, greenish black, and viscous) usually passes within 24 hours

– Failure to pass meconium in the first 24 to 48 hours suggests possible meconium ileus, imperforate anus, or bowel obstruction

Thermogenesis

- Temperature regulation is immature in the neonate because of a large body surface to body mass and the inability to generate heat from shivering
  - It's difficult for the neonate to conserve body heat because he has only a thin layer of subcutaneous fat
  - Other reasons the neonate has trouble maintaining body temperature
    - Blood vessels are closer to the surface of the skin
    - Vasomotor control is less developed
    - Sweat glands have little thermogenic function until the fourth week or later of life
- Normal neonates can produce sufficient heat in an optimal thermal environment
  - Full-term neonates maintain a flexed body posture, which decreases the exposure of body surface area
  - Neonates maintain temperature through nonshivering thermogenesis
  - The principle sources of thermogenesis are the heart, liver, and brain
  - Brown fat, or brown adipose tissue, is an additional source of thermogenesis unique to the neonate
    - Brown fat is metabolized leading to lipolysis and fatty acid oxidation
    - These events produce heat, which is released to the perfusing blood
- Rapid heat loss may occur in a suboptimal thermal environment by way of conduction, convection, radiation, or evaporation
  - Conduction involves heat loss to cold surfaces with which the neonate is in contact
  - Convection involves heat loss to the air that's cooler than the neonate's temperature
  - Radiation involves heat loss to solid objects that are near the neonate but not contacting the neonate
  - Evaporation involves heat loss through vaporization of liquid on the neonate's skin

Immune system

- The neonatal immune system depends largely on three immunoglobulins — IgG, IgM, and IgA

Conditions that affect thermogenesis

- Large body surface to body mass
- Inability to generate heat from shivering
- Thin layer of subcutaneous fat
- Difficulty conserving body heat

Ways that rapid heat loss occurs

- Conduction   Cold surface
- Convection   air
- Radiation   solid objects
- Evaporation   vaporate

Neonatal immunoglobulins and their functions

- IgG provides the neonate with antibodies to bacterial and viral agents.
- IgM in high levels indicates a nonspecific infection.
- IgA limits bacterial growth in the GI tract.

- IgG, a placentally transferred immunoglobin, provides the neonate with antibodies to bacterial and viral agents
  - IgG can be detected in the fetus at the third month of gestation
  - The infant first synthesizes its own IgG during the first 3 months of life, thus compensating for concurrent catabolism of maternal antibodies
- The fetus synthesizes IgM by the 20th week of gestation
  - IgM doesn't cross the placenta
  - High levels of IgM in the neonate indicate a nonspecific intrauterine infection
- IgA is not detectable at birth; it doesn't cross the placenta
  - Secretory IgA is found in colostrum and breast milk
  - IgA limits bacterial growth in the GI tract
- The neonate has fragile defenses against infection
  - The neonate's skin is fragile, thin, and easily broken allowing for easy entry of microorganisms
  - The neonate's immune response is limited to localized infections, thus spread of microorganisms is rapid

● **Hematopoietic system**

- The blood volume of the full-term neonate is 80 to 110 ml/kg of body weight, averaging about 300 ml
- The amount of blood bound to hemoglobin is less in a neonate than in a fetus
- The partial pressure of oxygen in the blood is less in a neonate than in a fetus
- Neonates are born with high erythrocyte counts secondary to the effects of fetal circulation and the need to ensure adequate oxygenation
- Levels of vitamin K in the neonate are lower than normal leading to an increase in coagulation time

● **Neurologic system**

- General neurologic function is evident by the neonate's movements
- These movements are uncoordinated and poorly controlled indicating the immaturity of the neurologic system
- The neonate demonstrates primitive reflexes, which disappear during the infancy period, being replaced by purposeful activity (see discussion later in this chapter on reflexes)
- The full-term neonate's neurologic system should produce equal strength and symmetry in responses and reflexes
- Diminished or absent reflexes may indicate a serious neurologic problem, and asymmetrical responses may indicate trauma during birth, including nerve damage, paralysis, and fracture
- Neurologic development follows a cephalocaudal, proximodistal pattern

Characteristics of the neonatal hematopoietic system

- Blood volume is 80 to 110 ml/kg of body weight.
- Levels of vitamin K are lower than normal.
- Coagulation time is increased.

Characteristics of the neonatal neurologic system

- Primitive reflexes
- Cephalocaudal, proximodistal pattern of development

● Hepatic system

- The liver continues to play a role in blood formation
- Jaundice is a major concern in the neonatal hepatic system because of increased serum levels of unconjugated bilirubin from increased red blood cell (RBC) lysis, altered bilirubin conjugation, or increased bilirubin reabsorption from the GI tract
- Physiologic jaundice (icterus neonatorum) develops in about 50% of full-term neonates and 80% of premature neonates
    - The icteric (yellow) color reflects increased serum levels of unconjugated bilirubin
    - The icteric color isn't apparent until the bilirubin levels are between 4 and 6 mg/dl
    - Unconjugated bilirubin levels seldom exceed 12 mg/dl; peak levels occur by 3 to 5 days after delivery (full-term) and 5 to 6 days (preterm)
    - Physiologic jaundice appears after the first 24 hours of extrauterine life; pathologic jaundice is evident at birth or within the first 24 hours of extrauterine life
- Breast milk jaundice appears after the first week of extrauterine life when physiologic jaundice is declining
    - Peak level is 15 to 25 mg/dl
    - Between 1% and 2% of breast-feeding neonates are affected
    - The exact cause is unknown; current theories revolve around increased intestinal absorption of bilirubin from beta-glucuronidase
- Breast-feeding-associated jaundice appears 2 to 3 days after birth in about 10% of breast-fed neonates
    - Peak level is 9 to 19 mg/dl
    - Poor caloric intake leads to decreased hepatic transport and bilirubin clearance
- Management of jaundice includes monitoring serum bilirubin levels, maintaining hydration, using bilirubin lights as needed, and providing emotional support to the parents

NEONATAL ASSESSMENT

● Initial assessment

- Ensure a proper airway via suctioning; administer oxygen as needed
- Dry the neonate under the warmer; keep the head lower than the trunk to promote drainage of secretions
- Help determine the Apgar score (see *Obtaining an Apgar score,* page 252)
    - The Apgar score quantifies neonatal heart rate, respiratory effort, muscle tone, reflexes, and color

Primary types and incidence of neonatal jaundice

- Physiologic jaundice — 50% of full-term neonates and 80% of premature neonates
- Breast milk jaundice — 1% to 2% of breast-feeding infants
- Breast-feeding-associated jaundice — 10% of breast-feeding infants

Management of jaundice

- Monitor serum bilirubin levels.
- Maintain hydration.
- Use bilirubin lights as needed.
- Provide emotional support to parents.

Apgar assessment areas

- Heart rate
- Respiratory effort
- Muscle tone
- Reflex irritability
- Skin color

What to do in the initial neonatal assessment

- Ensure a proper airway via suctioning.
- Dry the neonate.
- Help determine the initial Apgar score.
- Apply a cord clamp and monitor the neonate for abnormal bleeding.
- Observe the neonate for voiding and meconium.
- Assess for abnormalities.
- Continue to assess using the Apgar score criteria.
- Obtain clear footprints and fingerprints.
- Apply identification bands.
- Promote bonding.
- Review maternal prenatal and intrapartal data.

Obtaining an Apgar score

Follow these steps to determine a neonate's Apgar score at 1-minute and 5-minute intervals after birth:

- Assess the neonate's *heart rate.* Using a stethoscope, listen to the heartbeat for 60 seconds and then record the rate.
- Assess *respiratory effort* by noting the volume and vigor of the neonate's cry. Then, using a stethoscope, assess the depth and rate of respirations. Begin neonatal resuscitation if you detect abnormal respirations.
- Determine *muscle tone* by evaluating the degree of flexion and resistance to extension in the extremities (extend the limbs and observe their rapid return to flexion).
- Assess *reflex irritability* by observing the neonate's response to nasal suctioning or to flicking the sole.
- Observe skin *color,* especially at the extremities (if the neonate is dark skinned, inspect the oral mucosa, conjunctivae, lips, palms, and soles).

For each category listed, assign a score of 0 to 2, as shown below. A total score of 7 to 10 indicates that the neonate is in good condition; 4 to 6, in fair condition; 0 to 3, in danger (the neonate needs immediate resuscitation).

SIGN	APGAR SCORE		
	0	1	2
Heart rate	Absent	Less than 100 beats/minute	More than 100 beats/minute
Respiratory effort	Absent	Slow, irregular	Good cry
Muscle tone	Flaccid	Some flexion and resistance to extension of extremities	Active motion
Reflex irritability	No response	Grimace or weak cry	Vigorous cry
Color	Pallor, cyanosis	Pink body, blue extremities	Completely pink

- Each category is assessed at 1 minute after birth and again 5 minutes later
- Scores in each category range from 0 to 2
- The maximum score is 10
- Evaluation at 1 minute indicates the neonate's initial adaptation to extrauterine life
- Evaluation at 5 minutes gives a clearer picture of the neonate's overall status
- Apply a cord clamp and monitor the neonate for abnormal bleeding from the cord
  - Analyze the umbilical cord
  - Two arteries and one vein should be apparent
- Observe the neonate for voiding and meconium
- Assess the neonate for gross abnormalities and signs of suspected abnormalities

Taking an axillary temperature in a neonate

To take an axillary temperature in a neonate, follow these steps:
- Dry the axillary skin.
- Place the thermometer in the axilla and hold it along the outer aspect of the neonate's chest between the axillary line and the arm.
- Hold the thermometer in place until the temperature registers.

- Reassess axillary temperature in 15 to 30 minutes if it registers outside the normal range; if the temperature remains abnormal, notify the health care provider.
- Document the temperature reading.

- Continue to assess the neonate by using the Apgar score criteria, even after the 5-minute score is received
- Obtain clear footprints and fingerprints (the neonate's footprints are kept on a record that includes the mother's fingerprint)
- Apply identification bands with matching numbers to the mother (one band) and neonate (two bands) before they leave the delivery room
- Promote bonding between the mother and neonate
- Review maternal prenatal and intrapartal data to determine factors that might impact neonatal well-being

● **Ongoing physical assessments**
- Assess the neonate's vital signs
  - Count respirations with a stethoscope for 60 seconds
    - The normal respiratory rate ranges from 30 to 60 breaths/minute
    - Respiratory rate should be determined first, before the neonate becomes active or agitated
  - Take the apical pulse for 60 seconds
    - Place the stethoscope over the apical impulse on the fourth or fifth intercostal space at the left midclavicular line over the cardiac apex, listening and counting for 1 full minute
    - The normal apical pulse ranges from 120 to 160 beats/minute
    - The rate may be decreased to 110 beats/minute with neonatal sleeping
  - Take the first temperature rectally to check for rectal patency
    - Continued use of the rectal site isn't recommended because of possible rectal mucosa damage; use the axillary site instead (see *Taking an axillary temperature in a neonate*)
    - A delay in adjusting to extrauterine existence may cause temperature at birth to be 96.8° F (36° C), but this should stabilize within 8 to 12 hours at about 98.2° F (36.8° C)
    - A normal axillary temperature is 97.5° to 99° F (36.4° to 37.2° C)
- Measure and record blood pressure
  - The normal neonatal blood pressure reading ranges from 60 to 80 mm Hg systolic and 40 to 50 mm Hg

Key ongoing assessments

- Assess the neonate's vital signs: respirations, apical pulse, temperature (rectally first and axillary after that).
- Meaure and record blood pressure.
- Measure and record initial vital statistics: weight, length, head and chest circumferences.
- Complete a gestational age assessment.

Categorizing gestational age

- Preterm neonate – less than 37 weeks' gestation
- Term neonate – 37 to 42 weeks' gestation
- Postterm neonate – 42 or more weeks' gestation

– Use of a properly fitting blood pressure cuff is crucial; cuff width should be about one-half the circumference of the neonate's arm
- Measure and record the neonate's initial vital statistics (see *Obtaining size and weight measurements*)
  – Average weight is 5 lb, 8 oz to 8 lb, 13 oz (2,500 to 4,000 g)
  – Average length is 18″ to 21″ (46 to 53 cm)
  – Average head circumference is 13″ to 14″ (33 to 35 cm)
  – Average chest circumference is 12″ to 13″ (30 to 33 cm); usually 2 to 3 cm less than head circumference
- Complete a gestational age assessment, if indicated (see *Ballard gestational-age assessment tool,* pages 256 to 258)
  – Perinatal mortality and morbidity are related to gestational age and birth weight
  – The clinical assessment of gestational age is used to determine if an infant should be categorized as preterm, term, or postterm
    • Preterm — less than 37 weeks' gestation
    • Term — 37 to 42 weeks' gestation
    • Postterm — greater than or equal to 42 weeks' gestation
  – The Ballard scoring system uses physical and neurologic findings to estimate gestational age
    • This system enables estimates of gestational age to within 1 week, even in extremely premature neonates
    • This evaluation can be done anytime between birth and 42 hours of age, but the greatest reliability is at 30 and 42 hours

Administer prescribed medications
- Vitamin K (AquaMEPHYTON), 0.5 to 1 mg I.M. is administered prophylactically to prevent a transient deficiency of coagulation factors II, VII, IX, and X
  – The neonate's GI system is sterile at birth
  – This absence of intestinal flora predisposes the neonate to a deficiency of vitamin K
- Antibiotic ointment is necessary for prophylactic eye treatment of *Neisseria gonorrhoeae* and *Chlamydia*
  – Treatment is legally required in all 50 states
  – A 1 to 2 cm ribbon of ointment is used (see *Administering prophylactic eye treatment,* page 259)
  – Erythromycin ointment 0.5% is typically the drug of choice

Perform laboratory tests
- Neonates born to mothers who are Rh negative or of blood type O should have blood specimens obtained for these tests:
  – Blood type
  – Bilirubin level
  – Direct Coombs' test

Medications to administer to a neonate

- Vitamin K (AquaMEPHYTON), 0.5 to 1 mg I.M. to prevent a transient deficiency of coagulation factors II, VII, IX, and X
- Antibiotic ointment (typically erythromycin 0.5%) for prophylactic eye treatment of *Neisseria gonorrhoeae* and *Chlamydia* organisms

Obtaining size and weight measurements

Size and weight measurements establish the baseline for monitoring normal growth. When obtaining these measurements, place the neonate in a supine position in the crib or on the examination table and remove all clothing. Then follow these steps.

MEASURING HEAD CIRCUMFERENCE

- Slide a tape measure under the neonate's head at the occiput and draw the tape around snugly, just above the eyebrows. Record the measurement.

MEASURING HEAD-TO-HEEL LENGTH

- Fully extend the neonate's legs with the toes pointing up.
- Measure the distance from the heel to the top of the head using a tape measure or length board.

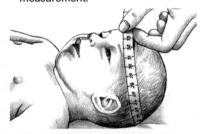
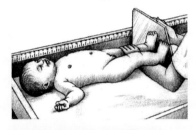

MEASURING CHEST CIRCUMFERENCE

- Place a tape measure under the back and wrap it snugly around the chest at the nipple, keeping the back and front of the tape level.
- Take the measurement after the neonate inspires and before he begins to exhale.

WEIGHING THE NEONATE

- Before a feeding, remove the neonate's diaper and place the neonate in the middle of a scale tray.
- Obtain the measurement while maintaining one hand poised over the neonate at all times.

MEASURING ABDOMINAL GIRTH

- Place a tape under the back and wrap it snugly around the abdomen just above the umbilicus.

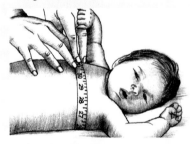

- Reticulocyte count
- Hematocrit
- Knowledge of neonatal blood type assists in determining whether an Rh or ABO incompatibility exits
- An abnormal direct Coombs' test result indicates presence of maternal antibodies in the neonate's blood, suggesting blood incompatibility
- Increased reticulocyte count indicates the body's response to RBC destruction
- Decreased hematocrit suggests anemia

Tests for neonatal blood incompatibility

- Blood type
- Bilirubin level
- Direct Coombs' test
- Reticulocyte count
- Hematocrit

Ballard gestational-age assessment tool

To use this tool, evaluate and score the neuromuscular and physical maturity criteria, total the score, and then plot the sum in the maturity rating box to determine the neonate's corresponding gestational age.

POSTURE

With the neonate supine and quiet, score as follows:
- Arms and legs extended = 0
- Slight or moderate flexion of hips and knees = 1
- Moderate to strong flexion of hips and knees = 2
- Legs flexed and abducted, arms slightly flexed = 3
- Full flexion of arms and legs = 4

SQUARE WINDOW

Flex the hand at the wrist. Measure the angle between the base of the thumb and the forearm. Score as follows:
- > 90 degrees = -1
- 90 degrees = 0
- 60 degrees = 1
- 45 degrees = 2
- 30 degrees = 3
- 0 degrees = 4

ARM RECOIL

With the neonate supine, fully flex the forearm for 5 seconds, then fully extend by pulling the hands and releasing. Observe and score the reaction according to this criteria:
- Remains extended 180 degrees or random movements = 0
- Minimal flexion (140 to 180 degrees) = 1
- Small amount of flexion (110 to 140 degrees) = 2
- Moderate flexion (90 to 110 degrees) = 3
- Brisk return to full flexion (< 90 degrees) = 4

POPLITEAL ANGLE

With the neonate supine and the pelvis flat on the examining surface, use one hand to flex the leg and then the thigh. Then use the other hand to extend the leg. Score the angle attained.
- 180 degrees = -1
- 160 degrees = 0
- 140 degrees = 1
- 120 degrees = 2
- 100 degrees = 3
- 90 degrees = 4
- < 90 degrees = 5

SCARF SIGN

With the neonate supine, take his hand and draw it across his neck and as far across the opposite shoulder as possible. You may assist the elbow by lifting it across the body. Score according to the location of the elbow:
- Elbow reaches or nears level of opposite shoulder = -1
- Elbow crosses opposite anterior axillary line = 0
- Elbow reaches opposite anterior axillary line = 1
- Elbow at midline = 2
- Elbow does not reach midline = 3
- Elbow does not cross proximate axillary line = 4

HEEL TO EAR

With the neonate supine, hold his foot with one hand and move it as near to the head as possible without forcing it. Keep the pelvis flat on the examining surface. Score as shown in the chart.

Facts about glucose

- Neonates weighing less than 2,500 g or more than 4,000 g should undergo blood glucose screening within 30 minutes of birth.
- Glucose levels less than 40 mg/dl indicate hypoglycemia.

- Neonates weighing less than 2,500 g or more than 4,000 g should undergo blood glucose screening within 30 minutes of birth to determine glucose stability
  - Glucose levels less than 40 mg/dl indicate hypoglycemia and require treatment

Ballard gestational-age assessment tool *(continued)*

NEUROMUSCULAR MATURITY

Neuromus-cular Maturity Sign	Score							Record score here
	-1	0	1	2	3	4	5	
Posture	–						–	
Square window (wrist)	>90°	90°	60°	45°	30°	0°	–	
Arm recoil	–	180°	140° to 180°	110° to 140°	90° to 100°	<90°	–	
Popliteal angle	180°	160°	140°	120°	100°	90°	<90°	
Scarf sign							–	
Heel to ear							–	
						TOTAL Neuromuscular Maturity Score		

PHYSICAL MATURITY

Physical Maturity Sign	Score							Record score here
	-1	0	1	2	3	4	5	
Skin	Sticky, friable, transparent	Gelatinous, red, translucent	Smooth, pink; visible vessels	Superficial peeling or rash; few visible vessels	Cracking; pale areas; rare visible vessels	Parchment-like; deep cracking; no visible vessels	Leathery, cracked, wrinkled	
Lanugo	None	Sparse	Abundant	Thinning	Bald areas	Mostly bald	–	
Plantar surface	Heel-to-toe 40 to 50 mm: -1; <40 mm: -2	>50 mm; no crease	Faint red marks	Anterior transverse crease only	Creases over anterior two-thirds	Creases over entire sole	–	
Breast	Impercep-tible	Barely perceptible	Flat areola; no bud	Stippled areola; 1- to 2-mm bud	Raised areola; 3- to 4-mm bud	Full areola; 5- to 10-mm bud	–	
Eye and ear	Lids fused, loosely: -1; tightly: -2	Lids open; pinna flat, stays folded	Slightly curved pinna; soft, slow recoil	Well-curved pinna; soft but ready recoil	Formed and firm; instant recoil	Thick cartilage; ear stiff	–	
Genitalia (Male)	Scrotum flat, smooth	Scrotum empty; faint rugae	Testes in upper canal; rare rugae	Testes descending; few rugae	Testes down; good rugae	Testes pendulous; deep rugae	–	
Genitalia (Female)	Clitoris prominent; labia flat	Prominent clitoris; small labia minora	Prominent clitoris; enlarging minora	Majora and minora equally prominent	Majora large; minora small	Majora cover clitoris and minora	–	
						TOTAL Physical Maturity Score		

(continued)

Ballard gestational-age assessment tool *(continued)*

MATURITY RATING

Physical Maturity Score	-10	-5	0	5	10	15	20	25	30	35	40	45	50
Gestational Age (weeks)	20	22	24	26	28	30	32	34	36	38	40	42	44

SCORE		GESTATIONAL AGE (weeks)	
Neuromuscular	_____	By dates	_____
Physical	_____	By ultrasound	_____
Total	_____	By score	_____

Adapted with permission from Ballard, J.L., et al. "New Ballad Score, expanded to include extremely premature infants," *Journal of Pediatrics* 119(3):417-23, 1991. Used with permission from Mosby–Year Book, Inc.

· The neonate should receive 10 ml/kg of body weight of formula
· Blood glucose level is checked 1 hour after feeding
· If the glucose level is higher than 45 mg/dl, another glucose level is obtained before the next feeding
– The neonate is assessed for signs of hypoglycemia, including jitteriness, irritability, seizures, hypothermia, lethargy, poor feeding, apnea, cyanosis, pallor, and a high pitched cry

NEONATAL PHYSICAL EXAMINATION

● **Head**
 • The neonate's head is about one-fourth of body size, appearing disproportionate to the rest of the neonate's body
    – The forehead is large and highly prominent
    – The chin appears somewhat receding
 • The neonate's head may appear misshapen and asymmetrical
    – Molding refers to asymmetry of the skull from overriding of cranial sutures during labor and delivery
       · This occurs as the presenting part of the fetal head, usually the vertex, adjusts to fit the shape of the birth canal
       · Normal shape usually is restored in several days
    – Cephalhematoma is the collection of blood between a skull bone and the periosteum that doesn't cross suture lines
       · This usually occurs about 24 hours after birth
       · Area appears egg shaped
       · It may take several weeks to resolve
    – Caput succedaneum is localized swelling over the presenting part that can cross suture lines; usually resolves in about 3 days (see

Charactistics of the normal neonatal head

● The head is about one-fourth of body size, appearing disproportionate to the rest of the neonate's body.
● The forehead is large and highly prominent.
● The chin appears somewhat receding.

Types of head asymmetry

● Molding: asymmetry of the skull from overriding of cranial sutures during labor and delivery.
● Cephalhematoma: collection of blood between a skull bone and the periosteum. Doesn't cross suture lines.
● Caput succedaneum: localized swelling over the presenting part. Crosses suture lines.

Administering prophylactic eye treatment

In neonates, prophylactic antibiotic ointment application is legally required to prevent damage and blindness from conjunctivitis. Follow these guidelines to administer this important treatment.

- Use a single dose ointment tube to prevent contamination and spread of infection
- Explain the procedure to the parents if present, informing them that the neonate will probably cry and that eye irritation may occur.
- Put on gloves.
- Wipe the neonate's face with a dry gauze.

- Shield the neonate's eyes from direct light and tilt his head slightly to the side of the intended treatment.
- Open one eye by applying pressure on the lower and upper lids.
- Instill a 1- to 2-cm ribbon of ointment along the lower conjunctival sac, from the inner canthus to the outer canthus.
- Close the neonate's eye to allow the ointment to be distributed across the conjunctiva.
- Repeat these steps with the other eye.

Distinguishing between caput succedaneum and cephalhematoma, page 260)

● **Fontanels**
- The diamond-shaped anterior fontanel is located at the juncture of the frontal and parietal bones
  - It measures $1\frac{1}{8}''$ to $1\frac{5}{8}''$ (3 to 4 cm) long and $\frac{3}{4}''$ to $1\frac{1}{8}''$ (2 to 3 cm) wide
  - It closes in about 18 months
- The triangular-shaped posterior fontanel is located at the juncture of the occipital and parietal bones
  - It measures about 0.5 to 1 cm across
  - It closes in about 8 to 12 weeks
- The fontanels should be flat and feel soft to the touch
  - A depressed fontanel indicates dehydration
  - Bulging fontanel requires immediate attention because it may indicate increased intracranial pressure

● **Eyes**
- The neonate's eyes are usually blue or gray because of scleral thinness
- Permanent eye color is established in 3 to 12 months
- Lacrimal glands are immature at birth, resulting in tearless crying for up to 2 months
- The neonate may demonstrate transient strabismus
- Doll's eye phenomenon may persist for about 10 days
- Subconjunctival hemorrhages may appear from vascular tension changes during birth

The shape and feel of neonatal fontanels

- They should be flat and feel soft to the touch.
- A depressed fontanel indicates dehydration.
- A bulging fontanel requires immediate attention because it may indicate increased intracranial pressure.

Facts about neonatal eyes

- Color is usually blue or gray.
- Permanent color appears in 3 to 12 months.
- Lacrimal glands are immature.
- Transient strabismus may be present.
- Doll's eye phenomenon may persist for about 10 days.
- Subconjunctival hemorrhages may appear.
- The red reflex is present.
- The neonate may follow objects to the midline.

Distinguishing between caput succedaneum and cephalhematoma

Caput succedaneum — swelling occurs below the scalp and can extend past the suture line

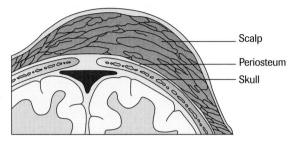

- Scalp
- Periosteum
- Skull

Cephalhematoma — swelling occurs due to blood collecting under the periosteum of the skull bone and doesn't cross the suture line

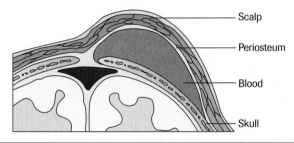

- Scalp
- Periosteum
- Blood
- Skull

TOP 7

Neonatal assessment observations

1. Collection of blood between a skull bone and the periosteum
2. Localized swelling over the presenting part
3. Strabismus
4. Persistence of doll's eye phenomenon
5. Breast engorgement
6. Scaphoid appearance of abdomen
7. Cyanosis of the hands and feet

- The red reflex is present
- The neonate may fix on objects and follow to the midline

● **Nose**
- Infants are nose breathers for the first few months of life
- Nasal passages must be kept clear to ensure adequate respirations
- Neonates instinctively sneeze to remove obstruction

● **Mouth**
- Epstein's pearls may be found on the gums or hard palate
- The neonate usually has scant saliva and pink lips
- Precocious teeth may appear
- An intact palate with a midline uvula is normal
- The neonate's tongue appears large and is prominent
  – The frenulum of the tongue in neonates should appear normal
  – In some neonates, the frenulum is attached near the tip of the tongue
- Sucking, rooting, and gag reflexes are present

● **Ears**
- The neonate's ears are characterized by incurving of the pinna and cartilage deposition

– The pinna of the external ear bends easily due to incomplete formation

– Recoil of the pinna after bending is characteristic in term neonates

- The top of the ear should be above or parallel to an imaginary line from the inner to outer canthus of the eye
- Low-set ears are associated with several syndromes, including chromosomal abnormalities such as trisomy 18 and trisomy 13
- The neonate typically responds to loud noises with the startle reflex
- Examination of the tympanic membrane is avoided due to difficulty in visualizing the eardrum and landmarks from accumulated amniotic fluid and vernix

Neck

- The neonate's neck is typically short and weak
  - The neonate's neck can't support his head
  - The head should be able to rotate freely
  - Some lifting of the head is possible when in the prone position
  - When pulled to a sitting position, head lag is noticeable
- It has deep skin folds without any webbing
- Stork beak marks or telangiectatic nevi may be noted on the back of the neck
- Neonates typically demonstrate tonic neck reflex at about 1 week of age

Chest

- Cylindrical thorax and flexible ribs are characteristic at birth
- Measurement of diameter of front to back is equal to that for side to side
- Breast engorgement may occur from maternal hormones
- Extra nipples (supernumerary) may be located below and medially to the true nipples
- Bilateral clear breath sounds typically are present
- The apex of the heart or point of maximal impulse is located at the third or fourth intercostal space
- Xiphoid process may appear prominent

Abdomen

- The abdomen is usually cylindrical with some protrusion
- A scaphoid appearance indicates diaphragmatic hernia
- Bowel sounds are present about 1 hour after birth
- The liver border is located 1 to 3 cm below the right costal margin
- Kidneys are palpable 1 to 2 cm above and on both sides of the umbilicus

Umbilical cord

- The cord is white and gelatinous with two arteries and one vein
- It begins to dry within 1 to 2 hours after delivery

Appearance of male genitals

- Rugae appear on the scrotum.
- Testes are descended into the scrotum.
- Urinary meatus is located at the penile tip (normal), on the dorsal surface (epispadias), or on the ventral surface (hypospadias).
- Foreskin is adhered to the glans.
- Penis is about 2 cm long.
- Cremasteric reflex is present.

Appearance of female genitals

- Labia majora cover the labia minora and clitoris.
- Vulva may appear edematous (from maternal hormones).
- Mucuslike, possibly blood-tinged vaginal discharge may be noted. This is called *pseudomenstruation* and results from maternal hormones.
- Hymenal tag is present.
- Urinary meatus is located below the clitoris.

- Bleeding at the cord site should be absent
- Base of the cord appears dry

● Genitals
- In males, rugae appear on the scrotum
  - Testes are descended into the scrotum
  - Urinary meatus is located at the penile tip (normal), on the dorsal surface (epispadias), or on the ventral surface (hypospadias)
  - Foreskin is adhered to the glans
  - Penis is about 2 cm long
  - Cremasteric reflex is present
- In females, labia majora cover the labia minora and clitoris
  - Vulva may appear edematous (from maternal hormones)
  - Mucuslike, possibly blood-tinged vaginal discharge may be noted
    · This is called *pseudomenstruation*
    · It results from maternal hormones
  - Hymenal tag is present
  - Urinary meatus is located below the clitoris

● Extremities
- All neonates are bowlegged and have flat feet
- Sole creases cover the anterior two-thirds of the foot
- The neonate may have abnormal extremities
  - Polydactyl—more than five digits on an extremity
  - Syndactyl—fusing together of two or more digits
- Extremities should move symmetrically with full range of motion
- Peripheral pulses are present and equal
- Nail beds are pink with a capillary refill time of less than 3 seconds
- Acrocyanosis may be present during the first 12 to 24 hours after birth
- Hip abduction should be smooth without clicks, with legs abducting to the point that they are almost flat against the surface on which the neonate is lying (see *Assessing hip abduction*)
  - Gluteal and thigh folds should be even
  - Ortolani's and Barlow's signs are negative

● Back
- The spine should be straight and flat
- Nevus pilosus at the base of the spine is commonly associated with spina bifida
- A pilonidal dimple may be present at the base of the spine; if present, further evaluation is needed to determine the presence of a sinus and its depth

● Anus
- Normally patent
- Absence of fissures

Assessing hip abduction

Assessing hip abduction helps identify whether the neonate's hip joint, including the acetabulum, is properly formed. Follow these steps:

- Place the neonate in the supine position on a bed or examination table.
- Flex the neonate's knees to 90 degrees at the hip.

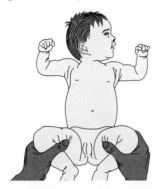

- Apply upward pressure over the greater trochanter area while abducting the hips; typically the hips should abduct to about 180 degrees, almost touching the surface of the bed or examination table.
- Listen for any sounds; normally this motion should produce no sound; evidence of a clicking or clunking sound denotes the femoral head hitting the acetabulum as it slips back into it; this sound is considered a positive Ortolani's sign suggesting hip subluxation.
- Then flex the neonate's knees and hips to 90 degrees.
- Apply pressure down and laterally while adducting the hips.
- Feel for any slipping of the femoral head out of the hip socket; evidence of slipping denotes a positive Barlow's sign suggesting hip instability and possible developmental dysplasia of the hip.

Skin

- The neonate may exhibit acrocyanosis (cyanosis of the hands and feet resulting from adjustments to extrauterine circulation)
  - The neonate's skin is pink for the first 24 to 48 hours
  - Jaundice or yellowing of the skin typically occurs at 48 to 72 hours in a full-term neonate
- Milia are clogged sebaceous glands, usually on the nose or chin
- Lanugo is fine, downy hair found after 20 weeks' gestation on the entire body except the palms and soles
- Vernix caseosa is a white cheesy protective coating composed of desquamated epithelial cells and sebum
- Erythema neonatorum toxicum is a transient, maculopapular rash
- Telangiectasia (flat, reddened vascular areas) may appear on the neck, upper eyelid, or upper lip
- Port-wine stain (nevus flammeus), a capillary angioma located below the dermis and commonly found on the face, is a flat, sharply demarcated purple-red birthmark
- Strawberry mark (nevus vasculosus), a capillary angioma located in the dermal and subdermal skin layers, is a rough, raised, sharply demarcated birthmark

Quick guide to skin spots and marks

- **Acrocyanosis:** cyanosis of the hands and feet
- **Milia:** clogged sebaceous glands
- **Lanugo:** fine, downy hair found on the entire body after 20 weeks' gestation
- **Vernix caseosa:** a white, cheesy, protective coating
- **Erythema neonatorum toxicum:** a transient, maculopapular rash
- **Telangiectasia:** flat, reddened vascular areas
- **Port-wine stain (nevus flammeus):** flat, sharply demarcated purple-red birthmark
- **Strawberry mark (nevus vasculosus):** rough, raised, sharply demarcated birthmark
- **Mongolian spots:** bluish black marks resembling bruises on the sacrum and other areas
- **Bruises, petechiae, small puncture mark, forceps marks:** marks from labor and delivery

- Mongolian spots are bluish black marks resembling bruises that appear on the sacrum, buttocks, back, and other areas
  - They're most common in neonates with dark skin
  - They usually disappear after the first few years of life
- Marks from labor and delivery may be noted
  - Bruises may possibly occur from the use of a vacuum extractor
  - Petechiae may develop due to pressure during the birth process
  - Small puncture mark may be seen due to use of internal fetal scalp electrode
  - Forceps marks over the cheeks and ears may occur from the use of forceps

● Reflexes

- Sucking—sucking motion begins when a nipple is placed in the neonate's mouth
- Swallowing—fluid is placed on the back of the tongue and the neonate swallows; it should be coordinated with the sucking reflex
- Moro's reflex—when the neonate is lifted above the crib and then suddenly lowered, the arms and legs symmetrically extend, then abduct; the fingers spread, forming a C
- Rooting—stroking the cheek makes the neonate turn his head in the direction of the stroke
- Tonic neck (fencing position)—when the neonate is in a supine position and his head is turned to one side, extremities on the same side straighten, whereas those on the opposite side flex
- Babinski's reflex—stroking the lateral sole on the side of the small toe toward and across the ball of the foot makes the toes fan upward
- Palmar grasp—placing a finger in each hand makes the neonate grasp the fingers tightly enough to be pulled to a sitting position
- Stepping—holding the neonate upright with the feet touching a flat surface elicits dancing or stepping movements
- Startle—a loud noise, such as a hand clap, elicits arm abduction and elbow flexion; the hands stay clenched
- Trunk incurvature—when a finger is run down the neonate's back, laterally to the spine, the trunk flexes and the pelvis swings toward the stimulated side
- Plantar grasp—examiner's finger touching an area below the toes causes the toes to curl over the examiner's finger (similar to palmar grasp)

Primary neonatal reflexes

- Sucking
- Swallowing
- Moro's
- Rooting
- Tonic neck
- Babinski's
- Palmar grasp
- Stepping
- Startle
- Trunk incurvature
- Plantar grasp

SENSORY ASSESSMENT

● Tactile behaviors

- Sensations of pressure, pain, and touch are present at birth or soon after

- Lips are hypersensitive
- Skin on thighs, forearms, and trunk is hyposensitive
- The neonate is especially sensitive to being cuddled and touched

● **Olfactory behaviors**
- The neonate can differentiate pleasant from unpleasant odors after mucus and amniotic fluid have been cleared from nasal passages
- The neonate can distinguish the mother's wet breast pad from those of other mothers at age 1 week

● **Vision behaviors**
- The neonate can see 7″ to 12″ (17.5 to 30.5 cm) at birth
- Eyes have immature muscle control and coordination
- Eyes are sensitive to light
- The neonate prefers complex patterns in black and white because retinal cones aren't fully developed at birth

● **Auditory behaviors**
- The neonate can detect sounds at birth
- The neonate will turn his head to familiar voices

● **Taste behaviors**
- Taste buds develop before birth
- The neonate prefers sweet tastes to bitter or sour ones
- Ability to distinguish between different tastes is present by 3 days of age

BEHAVIORAL ASSESSMENT

- Period of reactivity
  - It lasts about 30 minutes after birth
  - The neonate is awake and active
  - The neonate may demonstrate searching activities and sucking reflex
  - Respiratory rate and heart rate increase
  - Excessive respiratory secretions may be present
  - Acrocyanosis is present
  - The neonate vigorously responds to stimulation
  - It's an ideal time to initiate parental-infant bonding and breast-feeding
- Resting period
  - It lasts from several minutes to 2 to 4 hours
  - Pulse rate and respiratory rate slow, returning to baseline
  - Color appears to be stabilizing
  - The neonate may sleep for approximately 1½ hours and be difficult to arouse

---

Key neonatal sensory behaviors

- Feels sensations of pressure, pain, and touch at birth
- Is especially sensitive to being cuddled and touched
- Can differentiate pleasant from unpleasant odors
- Can see 7″ to 12″ at birth
- Can detect sounds at birth
- Can distinguish between different tastes by 3 days of age.

Key neonatal behavioral assessments

- First period of reactivity — lasts 30 minutes after birth
- Resting period — lasts several minutes to 2 to 4 hours
- Second period of reactivity — lasts 4 to 6 hours

Patterns of weight gain in neonates

- The neonate loses about 10% of his birth weight in the first few days of extrauterine life but usually regains it within 10 days.
- Infants typically gain 1 oz (28 g)/day in the first 6 months and ½ oz (14 g)/day in the second 6 months.
- Most infants double their birth weight by age 6 months and triple it by age 1 year.

Fluid facts

- Neonates need 150 to 180 ml/kg.
- They need adequate fluid because of their high metabolic rate.
- Fluid intake is essential because the neonate's body surface area promotes water loss through evaporation.

- Second period of reactivity
    - It lasts 4 to 6 hours
    - Pulse rate and respiratory rate increase again
    - Color changes occur quickly when crying or moving around
    - Mouth typically filled with mucus, causing gagging
    - Meconium stool may be passed

NUTRITION

● General information
- Proper nutrition is essential, especially in the early months, to fulfill the physiologic needs because the neonate is growing at such a high rate
    - Rapid brain growth is occurring
    - Providing nutrition also fills psychologic needs, helping to establish the parent-neonate relationship
- The neonate loses about 10% of his birth weight in the first few days of extrauterine life but usually regains it within 10 days
- Infants typically gain 1 oz (28 g)/day in the first 6 months and ½ oz (14 g)/day in the second 6 months
- Most infants double their birth weight by age 6 months and triple it by age 1 year
- Breast milk is considered the ideal nutrition for neonates
    - If breast-feeding is contraindicated, commercial formulas that are similar to breast milk are available
    - The American Academy of Pediatrics recommends that formula-fed infants be given an iron supplement for the first year

● Daily nutritional requirements
- Calories—100 to 200 kcal/kg for a term infant
- Fluid—150 to 180 ml/kg
    - Neonates need adequate fluid because of their high metabolic rate
    - Fluid intake is also essential because the body surface area of the neonate promotes water loss through evaporation
- Protein—2.2 g/kg for the first 6 months; 1.6 g/kg for the second 6 months
- Fat—30% to 60% of daily calories
- Vitamin requirements vary
    - Vitamin A—375 mcg for the first year
    - Vitamin D—7.5 mcg (retinol equivalents) for the first 6 months; 10 mcg (retinol equivalents) for the second 6 months
    - Vitamin E—3 mg (tocopherol equivalents) for the first 6 months; 4 mg (tocopherol equivalents) for the second 6 months
    - Vitamin C—30 mg for the first 6 months; 35 mg for the second 6 months

– Folacin—25 mcg for the first 6 months; 35 mcg for the second 6 months
– Niacin—5 mg (niacin equivalents) for the first 6 months; 6 mg (niacin equivalents) for the second 6 months
– Riboflavin—0.4 mg in the first 6 months; 0.5 mg in the second 6 months
– Thiamin—0.3 mg in the first 6 months; 0.4 mg in the second 6 months
– Vitamin B_6—0.3 mg in the first 6 months; 0.6 mg in the second 6 months
– Vitamin B_{12}—0.3 mg in the first 6 months; 0.5 mg in the second 6 months
• Certain minerals are also important
– Calcium—400 mg in the first 6 months; 600 mg in the second 6 months
– Phosphorus—300 mg in the first 6 months; 500 mg in the second 6 months
– Iodine—40 mcg in the first 6 months; 50 mcg in the second 6 months
– Magnesium—40 mcg in the first 6 months; 60 mcg in the second 6 months
– Zinc—5 mg in the first year
– Iron—6 mg in the first 6 months; 10 mg in the second 6 months
• If fluoridated water is unavailable, fluoride supplementation is initiated at age 6 months

● Breast-feeding
• Considered the ideal food source for the first 12 months of life
• Advantageous to the mother and the neonate
– Is economical
– Is readily available
– Promotes development of facial muscles, jaw, and teeth
– Aids in uterine involution
– Promotes transfer of maternal antibodies and possibly reduces risk of infections
• Breast milk contains secretory IgA which interferes with GI absorption of viruses and bacteria
• Lactoferrin, component of breast milk, is an iron-binding protein that interferes with bacterial growth
• Lysozyme, an enzyme found in breast milk, actively destroys bacteria
• Leukocytes, white blood cells also found in breast milk, provide protection for the neonate from common respiratory tract infections

Key nutrient requirements

• Protein
• Fluid
• Vitamins
• Minerals
• Fats

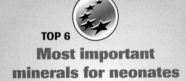

TOP 6

Most important minerals for neonates

1. Calcium
2. Phosphorus
3. Iodine
4. Magnesium
5. Zinc
6. Iron

Key benefits of breast-feeding

• Provides secretory IgA, which interferes with GI absorption of viruses and bacteria
• Provides *Lactobacillus bifidus*, which prevents growth of pathogens in the GI tract
• Enhances maternl-neonatal bonding
• Is nutritionally superior to other options

- Macrophages, cells that produce interferon, offer protection from viral invasion
- *Lactobacillus bifidus,* a bacteria found in breast milk, aids in preventing episodes of diarrhea through its interference with growth of pathogenic bacteria in the GI tract
  - Enhances maternal-neonatal bonding
  - Is nutritionally superior to all other options
    - Breast milk is more easily digested because of the greater abundance of lactalbumin, the higher percentage of amino acids, and softer curd formation
    - It has a higher calcium-phosphorus ratio, reducing the risk of tetany in the neonate
  - Reduces incidence of allergies, colic, and spitting up
  - Reduces incidence of maternal breast cancer
  - Reduces dental-arch malformations secondary to the sucking mechanism used when breast-feeding
  - Provides adequate electrolyte and mineral composition for the neonate's needs without overloading his renal system
- Breast-feeding is also associated with some disadvantages
  - Prevents others from feeding the infant unless milk is expressed or pumped
  - Limits the paternal role in infant feeding
  - Compels the mother to monitor her diet carefully
  - May be difficult for a working mother to maintain
  - Digests more quickly necessitating more frequent feedings
- Determination of whether the infant is getting enough breast milk is based on the infant's behavior; adequate nutrition is evidenced by the following:
  - Neonate or infant is content between feedings
  - Neonate or infant wets 6 to 8 diapers per day
  - Neonate or infant is gaining weight

Bottle-feeding

- Commercial formulas typically provide 20 calories per ounce when diluted properly
- These formulas are classified as milk based, soy based, or elemental
  - Milk-based formulas—for example, Enfamil and Similac—are those usually prescribed for the average infant; some may be "lactose-free"—that is, they're used for infants with galactosemia or lactose intolerance
  - Soy-based formulas, such as Isomil and Nursoy, are used for infants allergic to cow's milk protein
  - Elemental formulas are commonly prescribed for infants who have protein allergies or fat malnutrition

Evidence of adequate nutrition in breast-feeding

- Neonate or infant is content between feedings.
- Neonate or infant wets 6 to 8 diapers per day.
- Neonate or infant is gaining weight.

Classifications of commerical formulas

- Milk-based — prescribed for the average infant; some may be "lactose-free" for infants with galactosemia or lactose intolerance
- Soy-based formulas — used for infants allergic to cow's milk protein
- Elemental formulas — prescribed for infants who have protein allergies or fat malnutrition

- Commercially prepared formulas are similar in content to breast milk
- Formulas are available in several forms
  - Powder, which is combined with water (least expensive)
  - Condensed liquid that must be diluted
  - Ready to feed
  - Individually prepackaged prepared bottles (most expensive, but easiest to use)
- Formula feeding has several advantages
  - Permits the father and other family members to feed the infant
  - Poses fewer restrictions on the mother than breast-feeding
  - Allows more accurate measurement of intake
  - Enables the mother to take medications without risk to the infant
  - Requires fewer feedings than breast-feeding
  - Enables the mother to feed the infant in public without embarrassment
- Formula feeding has disadvantages
  - Costs more than breast-feeding
  - Requires greater preparation time and effort
  - Requires cleanliness of hands, water, and equipment
  - Requires adequate refrigeration and storage
  - Doesn't promote transfer of maternal antibodies
  - Doesn't benefit the mother physiologically

GENERAL INFANT CARE

Body temperature
- Maintain normal body temperature (97.7° to 98.6° F [36.5° to 37° C])
- Use a thermoregulator, such as a radiant warmer, or a temperature-controlled incubator to control environmental temperature until the neonate's temperature stabilizes (see *Understanding thermoregulators,* page 270)
  - Make sure the warmer is set to the desired temperature
  - Warm blankets, washcloths, or towels under a heat source
  - Keep the neonate under the radiant warmer until his temperature remains stable
  - When an incubator is used, keep it away from cold walls or objects, and perform all required procedures quickly, closing the portholes in the hood after completion
- Take an axillary temperature every 15 to 30 minutes until it stabilizes and then every 4 hours to ensure stability
- Apply a cap to the neonate's head to prevent heat loss
- Single- or double-wrap the infant snugly

Understanding thermoregulators

Thermoregulators preserve neonatal body warmth in various ways. A radiant warmer maintains the neonate's temperature by radiation. An incubator maintains the neonate's temperature by conduction and convection.

TEMPERATURE SETTINGS

Radiant warmers and incubators have two operating modes: nonservo and servo. The nurse manually sets temperature on nonservo equipment; a probe on the neonate's skin controls temperature settings on servo models.

OTHER FEATURES

Most thermoregulators come with alarms. Incubators have the added advantage of providing a stable, enclosed environment, which protects the neonate from evaporative heat loss.

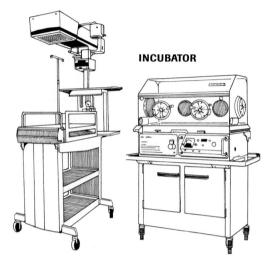

RADIANT WARMER

INCUBATOR

- Avoid exposing the infant to drafts, wetness, and direct or indirect contact with cold surfaces

● Vital signs
- Check the neonate's pulse and respiratory rates frequently until they stabilize
- Take an apical pulse and monitor respirations every 4 hours and then once every shift

● Proper cleaning and bathing techniques
- Give the first bath when vital signs have stabilized
- Wear gloves when giving the first bath
- Give the neonate a sponge bath until the umbilical cord falls off, usually within 10 to 14 days
- Use a mild, hexachlorophene-free soap
- Don't use soap on the infant's face
- Wash, rinse, and dry each portion of the body separately to minimize heat loss
  - Begin the bath with the eyes and face first, proceeding from the cleanest to the least cleanest areas
  - Clean the diaper area last

Proper techniques for bathing a neonate

- Wear gloves.
- Give a sponge bath until the umbilical cord falls off.
- Use a mild soap.
- Don't use soap on neonate's face.
- Wash, rinse, and dry each portion of the body separately, cleaning the diaper area last.
- Bathe the neonate before feedings.
- Apply alcohol if ordered to the base of the umbilical cord.

- Bathe before feedings instead of afterward to prevent vomiting
- Apply alcohol, if ordered, to the base of the umbilical cord with each diaper change and bath

Positioning the neonate
- Position the infant on his back for sleeping. This position has been linked to a decrease in the incidence of sudden infant death syndrome.
- Teach the mother the football hold, which provides adequate support for the infant while freeing a hand (for more teaching tips, see *Parental care of the normal neonate*)

Diaper changing
- Change the neonate's diaper before and immediately after feeding
- Place the diaper below the umbilical cord to prevent contamination
- Gently clean an uncircumcised penis; don't attempt to retract the foreskin
- Wipe the vulva of a female infant from front to back to avoid rectal contamination of the urethra or vagina

Suctioning
- Suction the nose and mouth as needed
- Have a bulb syringe available to promptly remove excessive mucus or milk from air passages

Circumcision care
- Observe and record the first voidance after circumcision
- Apply a thin layer of petroleum gauze to the site to control bleeding and prevent the diaper from adhering to the penis
- Wash the penis gently with water and apply fresh petroleum gauze to the glans with each diaper change
- Apply gentle pressure with a sterile 4" × 4" gauze pad if bleeding occurs; notify the physician if bleeding continues

Changing the neonate's diaper
- Change the diaper before and after feeding.
- Place the diaper below the umbilical cord.
- Gently clean an uncircumcised penis; don't retract the foreskin.
- Wipe the vulva of a female from front to back.

Care after circumcision
- Observe and record the first voidance.
- Apply a thin layer of petroleum gauze to the site.
- Wash the penis with water and apply fresh petroleum gauze with each diaper change.
- Apply gentle pressure with a sterile gauze pad if bleeding occurs; notify the physician if bleeding continues.

- Teach parents to keep the area clean and covered with petroleum gauze if appropriate for about 3 days and to report any redness or tenderness

● Prevention of infection

- Adhere to infection-control guidelines in the nursery and the maternity unit to reduce the neonate's risk for infection due to his limited ability to respond to infection
- Perform a scrub at the beginning of each work period
- Wash hands for 10 to 15 seconds after caring for one neonate and beginning to care for another
- Assist parents in washing their hands before handling the neonate
- Prevent individuals with colds and other infections from coming in contact with the neonate
- Keep the neonate's equipment and supplies separate from those used for other neonates
- Assess the mother for possible infection
- Continually assess the neonate for signs of possible infection, which may be subtle or represent other disease processes

● Prevention of neonate abduction

- Teach parents how to recognize birth facility personnel, including the use of photo identification badges with specific markings
- Instruct parents never to give their neonate to anyone who doesn't have proper identification
- Apply an electronic device, if used by the facility, to the neonate's ankle or wrist, so that if the neonate is removed from the unit, an alarm will sound
- Ensure that entrances to the unit are monitored and have limited access
  - Some units are kept locked
  - Some units require the person entering to knock on the door, press a buzzer, or use a code or card-key
- Be alert for people displaying typical characteristics for abducting a neonate
  - The person is usually a woman who knows the facility
  - The woman may have had a previous pregnancy loss or not be able to have children of her own

NCLEX CHECKS

It's never too soon to begin your NCLEX preparation. Now that you've reviewed this chapter, carefully read each of the following questions and choose the best answer. Then compare your responses to the correct answers.

1. When the neonate takes his first breath, which of the following occurs?

☐ **A.** Systemic vascular resistance increases
☐ **B.** Left atrial pressure increases
☒ **C.** Pulmonary vascular resistance decreases
☐ **D.** Foramen ovale closes

2. When inspecting the umbilical cord, the nurse would identify the presence of which of the following as normal?

☐ **A.** One artery and one vein
☐ **B.** One artery and one ligament
☐ **C.** One artery and two veins
☒ **D.** Two arteries and one vein

3. When determining the Apgar score, the nurse flicks the sole of the neonate's foot to assess which of the following?

☐ **A.** Muscle tone
☒ **B.** Reflex irritability
☐ **C.** Color
☐ **D.** Heart rate

4. Which of the following would the nurse document when assessment reveals a localized area of swelling on the neonate's head that crosses the suture lines?

☒ **A.** Caput succedaneum
☐ **B.** Molding
☐ **C.** Cephalhematoma
☐ **D.** Acrocyanosis

5. When palpating a neonate's anterior fontanel, which of the following would the nurse consider a normal finding?

☐ **A.** Complete closure
☐ **B.** Bulging
☐ **C.** Depression
☒ **D.** Softness

6. One minute after birth, a neonate is crying vigorously, has a heart rate of 98 beats/minute, is active with normal reflexes, and has a pink body and blue extremities. What Apgar score should this neonate receive?

TOP 7
Items to study for your next test on the normal neonate

1. The ways in which each body system adapts to extrauterine life
2. The steps in determing the Apgar score
3. Which medications to administer after birth and their purpose
4. The key neonatal assessment observations
5. The key neonatal behavioral assessment findings
6. The nutritional requirements of neonates
7. The points to include in a teaching plan for the parents of a normal neonate

ANSWERS AND RATIONALES

1. CORRECT ANSWER: C

The first breath expands the lungs, thereby decreasing pulmonary vascular resistance. Increased systemic vascular resistance and left atrial pressure result from clamping of the umbilical cord. Closure of the foramen ovale results from the changing atrial pressure.

2. CORRECT ANSWER: D

The umbilical cord should consist of two arteries and one vein. Any other combination is abnormal.

3. CORRECT ANSWER: B

Flicking the sole of the neonate's foot is used to assess reflex irritability. Nasal suctioning can also be used. Flexing and resistance to extension are used to assess muscle tone. Observing the neonate's skin, especially the extremities, is done to assess color. Auscultating the heartbeat with a stethoscope is used to assess heart rate.

4. CORRECT ANSWER: A

Caput succedaneum is localized swelling over the presenting part that can cross suture line. Molding refers to asymmetry of the skull from overriding of cranial sutures during labor and delivery as the presenting part of the fetal head, usually the vertex, adjusts to fit the shape of the birth canal. Cephalhematoma is the collection of blood between a skull bone and the periosteum that doesn't cross suture lines and appears egg shaped. Acrocyanosis refers to the cyanosis of the hands and feet resulting from adjustments to extrauterine circulation

5. CORRECT ANSWER: D

The anterior fontanel should feel soft and flat to the touch. It typically doesn't close until age 18 months. Bulging suggests increased intracranial pressure. Depression suggests dehydration.

6. CORRECT ANSWER: 8

According to Apgar scoring, this neonate should receive two points for muscle tone, two points for reflex irritability, and two points for respiratory effort. He lost one point out of a possible two points for a slower than normal heart rate and one point out of two points for acrocyanosis (as evidenced by a pink body with blue extremities). Therefore, this neonate's total Apgar score is 8.

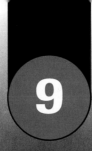

The high-risk neonate

LEARNING OBJECTIVES

After studying this chapter, you should be able to:

- Identify potential complications in high-risk neonates.
- State the signs of respiratory distress syndrome in a neonate.
- Identify clinical manifestations of drug addiction in a neonate.
- Discuss the effect of maternal infectious diseases on a fetus or neonate.
- Describe the physical characteristics of premature, postmature, small-for-gestational age, and large-for-gestational age neonates.

CHAPTER OVERVIEW

Some neonates experience conditions that complicate the neonatal period or place them at high risk for present and future problems. Knowledge of the pathophysiology and contributing factors of these conditions allows for early identification and prompt management, which is vital in preventing or minimizing long-term effects.

RESPIRATORY DISTRESS SYNDROME

- ### Description
  - A disease related to immaturity of lung tissue

Risk factors for RDS

- Prematurity
- Maternal diabetes mellitus
- Stress during delivery that produces acidosis in the neonate

Pathophysiology of RDS

- Lack of surfactant in lungs
- Leads to atelectasis as well as labored breathing, respiratory acidosis, and hypoxemia
- Blood flow to lungs decreases
- Alveoli become necrotic
- Capillaries are damaged
- Hyaline membrane forms

Initial assessment findings for RDS

- Increased respiratory rate
- Retractions
- Satisfactory color
- Good air movement on auscultation

- May also be called *hyaline membrane disease*
- A complex disorder manifested by signs of respiratory distress
- Risk factors for respiratory distress syndrome (RDS) include prematurity, maternal diabetes mellitus, and stress during delivery that produces acidosis in the neonate
  - RDS is seen almost exclusively in premature neonates
  - RDS is associated with a high risk of long-term respiratory and neurologic complications
- Prenatal diagnosis can evaluate lung maturity while the fetus is in utero
  - Evaluation of lecithin/sphingomyelin ratio of the amniotic fluid is performed
  - Lecithin and sphingomyelin are two surfactant phospholipids
  - Evaluation of fetal lung maturity gives insight into how the fetus will fare after birth and may precipitate treatment to delay labor or to mature the neonate's lungs before delivery

● Pathophysiology

- RDS is characterized by poor gas exchange and ventilatory failure due to a lack of surfactant in the lungs
  - Surfactant is a phospholipid secreted by the alveolar epithelium
  - It coats the alveoli, keeping them open so gas exchange can occur
  - In premature neonates, the lungs may not be fully developed and therefore may not have sufficient surfactant available
  - The result is the inability to maintain alveolar stability
- The lack of surfactant leads to atelectasis, labored breathing, respiratory acidosis, and hypoxemia
- With worsening atelectasis, pulmonary vascular resistance increases, which decreases blood flow to the lungs
- Right-to-left shunting of blood perpetuates fetal circulation by keeping the foramen ovale and ductus arteriosus patent
- The alveoli can become necrotic and the capillaries are damaged
- Ischemia allows fluid to leak into the interstitial and alveolar spaces, and a hyaline membrane forms
- This membrane greatly hinders respiratory function by decreasing the compliance of the lungs

● Assessment findings

- RDS can produce respiratory distress acutely after birth or within a few hours of birth
- Initial assessment may reveal various findings
  - Increased respiratory rate
  - Retractions
  - Satisfactory color
  - Good air movement on auscultation

- As respiratory distress becomes more obvious, other findings may be noted
  - Further increased respiratory rate
  - Labored breathing
  - More pronounced substernal retractions
  - Fine crackles on auscultation
  - Cyanosis
  - Nasal flaring
  - Expiratory grunting (see *Silverman-Anderson index,* page 278)
- Signs and symptoms—such as hypoxemia, hypercapnia, and acidosis—are nonspecific to RDS
  - Specific laboratory tests must be carried out to evaluate the neonate for complications
  - These tests may include blood, urine, and cerebrospinal fluid (CSF) cultures and blood glucose, serum calcium, and arterial blood gas (ABG) levels
- Radiographic evaluation reveals various findings
  - Alveolar atelectasis shown by a diffuse granular pattern that resembles ground glass over all lung fields
  - Dilated bronchioles shown by dark streaks within granular pattern

Treatment
- Thermoregulation
- Oxygen administration
- Mechanical ventilation, if needed
- Prevention of hypotension
- Prevention of hypovolemia
- Correction of respiratory acidosis by ventilatory support
- Correction of metabolic acidosis by sodium bicarbonate administration
- Administration of surfactant and such other drugs as an antibiotic, a sedative, a paralyzant, and a diuretic
- Protection from infection
- Administration of parenteral feedings

Nursing interventions
- Provide continuous monitoring and close observation
- Obtain necessary specimens for laboratory testing
- Continuously monitor pulse oximetry or transcutaneous oxygen levels
  - Administer oxygen as ordered
  - Anticipate the need for ventilatory support, including mechanical ventilation, continuous positive airway pressure, or positive end-expiratory pressure
- Suction the neonate as indicated
- Institute measures to maintain thermoregulation

Assessment areas on Silverman-Anderson index

- Upper chest
- Lower chest
- Xiphoid retractions
- Nares dilation
- Expiratory grunt

Silverman-Anderson index

The Silverman-Anderson index can be used to evaluate five areas of a neonate's respiratory status: upper chest, lower chest, xiphoid retractions, nares dilation, and expiratory grunt. Each area is graded 0 (no respiratory difficulty), 1 (moderate difficulty), or 2 (maximum difficulty), with a total score ranging from 0 (no respiratory difficulty) to 10 (maximum respiratory difficulty).

	GRADE 0	GRADE 1	GRADE 2
Upper chest	Synchronized	Lag on inspiration	Seesaw
Lower chest	No retractions	Just visible	Marked
Xiphoid retractions	None	Just visible	Marked
Nares dilation	None	Minimal	Marked
Expiratory grunt	None	Audible with stethoscope	Audible to naked ear

Reproduced with permission from *Pediatrics,* vol. 17, pages 1-10. Copyright 1956.

- Provide parenteral nutrition and avoid gavage and oral feedings during the acute stage of the disease because these situations increase respiratory rate and oxygen consumption
- Cluster nursing activities to provide the neonate with rest periods; disturb the neonate with RDS as little as possible to decrease oxygen consumption
- Administer drugs as ordered
- Provide meticulous skin and mouth care
- Educate the parents about the disease, treatments, and procedures as well as what to expect
- Orient the parents to the intensive care unit
- Provide emotional support, especially during the acute stage
- Assist with referrals to social services, the chaplain, and other supportive resources as necessary

TRANSIENT TACHYPNEA OF THE NEONATE

● Description
- Also known as *type II respiratory distress syndrome* or *wet lung*
- A mild respiratory problem in neonates, typically beginning after birth and generally lasting about 2 days
- Results from delayed absorption of fetal lung fluid after birth
  - Transient tachypnea of the neonate (TNN) is commonly observed in neonates born by cesarean delivery
  - These neonates don't receive the thoracic compression that helps to expel fluid during vaginal delivery
- Additional risk factors
  - Neonates of mothers who smoked during pregnancy
  - Neonates of diabetic mothers
  - Neonates who are small for gestational age
  - Neonates who are small or premature, or who were born rapidly by vaginal delivery (may not have received effective squeezing of the thorax to remove fetal lung fluid)
- Resolution of symptoms generally occurs within 48 hours
  - Once TTN goes away, the neonate usually recovers completely
  - The neonate has no increased risk of further respiratory problems

● Pathophysiology
- Before birth, the fetal lungs are filled with fluid
  - All of the fetus's nutrients and oxygen come from the mother through the placenta
  - The fetus doesn't use his lungs to breathe
  - During the birth process, some of the neonate's lung fluid is squeezed out as he passes through the birth canal

Facts about neonatal transient tachypnea

- It's also know as *type II respiratory distress syndrome* or *wet lung.*
- It's a mild problem that lasts about 2 days.
- It results from delayed absorption of fetal lung fluid after birth.

Who's at risk for transient tachypnea

- Neonates born by cesarean delivery
- Neonates of mothers who smoked during pregnancy
- Neonates of diabetic mothers
- Neonates who are small for gestational age
- Neonates who are small, were born prematurely, or were born rapidly by vaginal delivery (haven't received effective squeezing of the thorax to remove fetal lung fluid)

Assessment findings for TTN

- Respiratory rate > 60 breaths/minute
- Expiratory grunting
- Nasal flaring
- Slight cyanosis
- Retractions
- Tachypnea
- Hypoxemia
- Decreased carbon dioxide levels

TOP 6

Steps for treating TTN

1. Administer oxygen.
2. Maintain acid-base balance.
3. Institute thermoregulation.
4. Provide adequate nutrition via gavage feedings or I.V. fluids.
5. Institute transcutaneous oxygen monitoring.
6. Protect the patient from infection.

- After birth, the remaining fluid is pushed out of the lungs as the lungs fill with air
- Any fluid that remains is later coughed out or reabsorbed into the bloodstream
- TTN results from aspiration of amniotic or tracheal fluid compounded either by delayed clearing of the airway or by excess fluid entering the lungs
- TNN spontaneously fades as lung fluid is absorbed, usually by 48 hours of life, as respiratory activity becomes effective

Assessment findings

- Increased respiratory rate (greater than 60 breaths/minute)
- Expiratory grunting
- Nasal flaring
- Slight cyanosis
- Retractions
- Tachypnea
- ABG levels may reveal hypoxemia and decreased carbon dioxide levels
- Increased carbon dioxide levels may be a sign of fatigue and impending respiratory failure
- Chest X-ray, the diagnostic standard for TTN, reveals streaking (correlates with lymphatic engorgement of retained fetal lung fluid)

Treatment

- Oxygen administration
- Ventilatory assistance (rarely needed)
- Maintenance of acid-base balance
- Thermoregulation
- Adequate nutrition via gavage feedings or I.V. fluids
    - Difficulty with oral feedings because of increased respiratory rate and increased work of breathing; coordination of neonatal mechanisms of sucking, swallowing, and breathing
    - High risk of aspiration due to rapid respiratory rate
- Transcutaneous oxygen monitoring
- Protection from infection

Nursing interventions

- Closely monitor the neonate's heart rate, respiratory rate, and oxygenation status
- Provide respiratory support, including mechanical ventilation, if necessary
- Institute measures to maintain a neutral thermal environment
- Minimize stimulation by decreasing lights and noise levels
- Provide nutritional support via gavage feedings or parenteral nutrition
- Educate the parents about the condition and its usually quick resolution
- Provide emotional support to the parents and family

MECONIUM ASPIRATION SYNDROME

● **Description**
  - Involves aspiration of meconium into the lungs
    – Meconium is the neonate's first feces
    – It may be seen in the amniotic fluid after 34 weeks' gestation and is thick, sticky, and greenish black
  - Meconium aspiration syndrome (MAS) results when the neonate inhales the meconium mixed with amniotic fluid; typically occurs with the first breath or while the neonate is in utero
  -    Risk factors for MAS
    – Maternal diabetes
    – Maternal hypertension
    – Difficult delivery
    – Fetal distress
    – Intrauterine hypoxia
    – Advanced gestational age (greater than 40 weeks)
    – Poor intrauterine growth

● **Pathophysiology**
  - Asphyxia in utero leads to increased fetal peristalsis, relaxation of the anal sphincter, passage of meconium into the amniotic fluid, and reflex gasping of amniotic fluid into the lungs
    – Neonates with MAS increase respiratory efforts to create greater negative intrathoracic pressures and improve air flow to the lungs
    – Hyperinflation, hypoxemia, and acidemia cause increased peripheral vascular resistance
    – Right-to-left shunting commonly follows
  - Meconium creates a ball-valve effect, trapping air in the alveolus and preventing adequate gas exchange
  - Chemical pneumonitis results, causing the alveolar walls and interstitial tissues to thicken, again preventing adequate gas exchange
  - Cardiac efficiency can be compromised from pulmonary hypertension

● **Assessment findings**
  - Fetal hypoxia as indicated by altered fetal activity and heart rate
  - Dark greenish staining or streaking of the amniotic fluid noted on rupture of membranes
  - Obvious presence of meconium in the amniotic fluid
  - Greenish staining of neonate's skin (if the meconium was passed long before delivery)
  - Signs of distress at delivery, such as neonate appearing limp, Apgar scores below 6, pallor, cyanosis, and respiratory distress
  - Coarse crackles when auscultating neonate's lungs

Risk factors for MAS

● Maternal diabetes or hypertension
● Difficult delivery
● Fetal distress
● Intrauterine hypoxia
● Advanced gestational age
● Poor intrauterine growth

Assessment findings for MAS

● Fetal hypoxia
● Dark greenish staining or streaking of the amniotic fluid
● Meconium in the amniotic fluid
● Greenish staining of neonate's skin
● Signs of distress at delivery
● Coarse crackles

TOP 4

Steps for treating MAS

1. Immediately provide endotracheal suctioning at delivery.
2. Offer respiratory assistance via mechanical ventilation.
3. Maintain a neutral thermal environment.
4. Administer surfactant and an antibiotic.

Assessment findings for sepsis

- Subtle, nonspecific behavioral changes
- Temperature instability
- Feeding pattern changes
- Apnea
- Hyperbilirubinemia
- Abdominal distention
- Skin color changes
- Positive blood cultures

- Chest X-ray may show patches or streaks of meconium in the lungs, air trapping, or hyperinflation

● **Treatment**
- Respiratory assistance via mechanical ventilation
- Maintenance of a neutral thermal environment
- Administration of surfactant and an antibiotic
- Extracorporeal membrane oxygenation (ECMO) in severe cases

● **Nursing interventions**
- During labor, continuously monitor the fetus for signs and symptoms of distress
- Immediately inspect any fluid passed with rupture of membranes
- Assist with immediate endotracheal suctioning during delivery as indicated
- Monitor lung status closely, including breath sounds and respiratory rate and character
- Frequently assess the neonate's vital signs
- Administer treatment modalities, such as oxygen and respiratory support, as ordered
- Institute measures to maintain a neutral thermal environment
- Teach the parents about the condition, treatments, and procedures as well as what to expect
- Provide the parents and family with emotional support and guidance

SEPSIS

● **Description**
- Occurs when pathogenic microorganisms or their toxins occur in the blood or tissues
- Can occur before, during, or after delivery
- Most common causative organisms are the gram-negative *Escherichia coli, Aerobacter,* and *Klebsiella* and the gram-positive beta-hemolytic streptococci
- Prolonged rupture of membranes increases the neonate's risk of sepsis

● **Assessment findings**
- Subtle, nonspecific behavioral changes, such as lethargy and hypotonia
- Temperature instability
- Feeding pattern changes, such as poor sucking and decreased intake
- Apnea
- Hyperbilirubinemia
- Abdominal distention
- Skin color changes, including mottling, pallor, and cyanosis
- Positive blood cultures

Treatment
- Lumbar puncture to rule out meningitis
- Urine, skin, blood, and nasopharyngeal cultures
- Gastric aspiration
- Antibiotic administration

Nursing interventions
- Collect specimens to identify the causative organism
- Assess the neonate's vital signs at least once per hour or more frequently as indicated
- Expect to administer a broad-spectrum antibiotic before culture results are received and to switch to specific antibiotic therapy after results are received
- Provide supportive care, including maintenance of a neutral thermal environment
- Administer nutritional support
- Assist with respiratory support measures, including oxygen therapy as ordered
- Monitor fluid and electrolyte balance; administer I.V. fluid therapy as ordered
- Institute measures to provide cardiovascular support

HYPERBILIRUBINEMIA

Description
- Also called *pathologic jaundice*
- Characterized by a bilirubin level that exceeds 6 mg/dl within the first 24 hours after delivery and remains elevated beyond 7 days in a full-term neonate and beyond 10 days in a premature neonate
  - A bilirubin level that rises by more than 5 mg/day
  - A level that's greater than 12 mg/dl in premature or term neonates
  - Conjugated (direct) bilirubin level that exceeds 1.5 to 2 mg/dl
- The prognosis for hyperbilirubinemia varies, depending on the cause

Pathophysiology
- Hyperbilirubinemia can develop several ways
  - Certain drugs (such as aspirin, tranquilizers, and sulfonamides) and conditions (such as hypothermia, anoxia, hypoglycemia, and hypoalbuminemia) can disrupt conjugation and usurp albumin-binding sites
  - Decreased hepatic function can result in reduced bilirubin conjugation
  - Increased erythrocyte production or breakdown can accompany a hemolytic disorder or Rh or ABO incompatibility

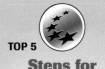

TOP 5

Steps for treating sepsis

1. Assess the neonate's vital signs frequently.
2. Administer an antibiotic as ordered.
3. Administer nutritional support.
4. Monitor fluid and electrolyte balance, and administer I.V. fluid as indicated.
5. Institute measures to provide cardiovascular support.

Characteristics of hyperbilirubinemia

- A bilirubin level that exceeds 6 mg/dl within the first 24 hours after delivery and remains elevated beyond 7 days in a full-term neonate and beyond 10 days in a premature neonate
- A bilirubin level that rises by more than 5 mg/day
- A level that's greater than 12 mg/dl in premature or term neonates
- A conjugated (direct) bilirubin level that exceeds 1.5 to 2 mg/dl

– Biliary obstruction or hepatitis may block normal bile flow
– Maternal enzymes present in breast milk can inhibit the neonate's glucuronosyltransferase-conjugating activity
- As erythrocytes break down at the end of their neonatal life cycle, hemoglobin separates into globin (protein) and heme (iron) fragments
- Heme fragments form unconjugated (indirect) bilirubin, which binds with albumin for transport to liver cells to conjugate with glucuronide, forming direct bilirubin
- Unconjugated bilirubin is fat-soluble and can't be excreted in the urine or bile; it may escape to extravascular tissue, especially fatty tissue and the brain, resulting in hyperbilirubinemia
- Unconjugated bilirubin can infiltrate the nuclei of the cerebral cortex and thalamus, leading to kernicterus (an encephalopathy)
    – Although exact level is unknown, kernicterus may occur with serum bilirubin levels at or above 20 mg/dl (full-term) and at lower levels (about 14 mg/dl) in premature neonates
    – Signs and symptoms of kernicterus include lethargy, decreased reflexes, seizures, opisthotonos, and high-pitched cry
- Possible causes include hemolytic disease of the neonate, sepsis, impaired hepatic functioning, polycythemia, enclosed hemorrhage, hypothermia, hypoglycemia, and asphyxia neonatorum

● **Assessment findings**
- Jaundice appearing anytime after the first day of life and persisting beyond 7 days
- Elevated serum bilirubin levels—levels greater than 12 mg/100 ml in a term neonate, levels greater than 15 mg/100 ml in a preterm neonate, or levels that increase more than 5 mg/100 ml in 24 hours
- Hepatosplenomegaly

● **Treatment**
- Exchange transfusion to replace the neonate's blood with fresh blood (less than 48 hours old), removing some of the unconjugated bilirubin in serum
- Phototherapy
    – Considered the treatment of choice for hyperbilirubinemia due to hemolytic disease of the neonate (after the initial exchange transfusion)
    – Uses fluorescent light to decompose bilirubin in the skin by oxidation
    – Usually discontinued after bilirubin levels fall below 10 mg/100 ml and continue to decrease for 24 hours
- Albumin administration (1 g/kg of 25% salt-poor albumin) to provide additional albumin for binding unconjugated bilirubin; done 1 to 2

Assessment findings for hyperbilirubinemia

- Jaundice that appears after the first day of life and persists longer than 7 days
- Serum bilirubin levels > 12 mg/100 ml in a term neonate, > 15 mg/100 ml in a preterm neonate, or increasing more than 5 mg/100 ml in 24 hours
- Hepatosplenomegaly

TOP 3

Steps for treating hyperbilirubinemia

1. Provide an exchange transfusion.
2. Offer phototherapy.
3. Administer albumin.

Performing phototherapy

- Set up the phototherapy unit about 18″ (45.7 cm) above the neonate's crib, and verify placement of the lightbulb shield.
- If the neonate is in an incubator, place the phototherapy unit at least 3″ (7.6 cm) above the incubator, and turn on the lights.
- Place a photometer probe in the middle of the crib to measure the energy emitted by the lights. The average range is 6 to 8 $\mu w/cm^2/$ nanometer.
- Explain the procedure to the parents.
- Record the neonate's initial bilirubin level and his axillary temperature.
- Place the opaque eye mask over the neonate's closed eyes, and fasten securely.
- Undress the neonate, and place a diaper under him. Cover male genitalia with a surgical mask or small diaper to catch urine and prevent possible testicular damage from the heat and light waves.
- Take the neonate's axillary temperature every 2 hours, and provide additional warmth by adjusting the warming unit's thermostat.

- Monitor elimination, and weigh the neonate twice daily. Watch for signs of dehydration (dry skin, poor turgor, depressed fontanels), and check urine specific gravity with a urinometer to gauge hydration status.
- Take the neonate out of the crib, turn off the phototherapy lights, and unmask his eyes at least every 3 to 4 hours (with feedings). Assess his eyes for inflammation or injury.
- Reposition the neonate every 2 hours to expose all body surfaces to the light and to prevent head molding and skin breakdown from pressure.
- Check the bilirubin level at least once every 24 hours—more often if levels rise significantly. Turn off the phototherapy unit before drawing venous blood for testing because the lights may degrade bilirubin in the blood. Notify the health care provider if the bilirubin level nears 20 mg/dl if the neonate was born at full term or 15 mg/dl if the neonate was born prematurely.

---

hours before exchange or as a substitute for a portion of the plasma in the transfused blood
- Treatment of anemia caused by hemolytic disease

● **Nursing interventions**
- Assess and record the neonate's jaundice, and note the time it began; immediately report the jaundice and serum bilirubin levels
- To prevent hyperbilirubinemia, maintain oral intake; don't skip feedings because fasting stimulates the conversion of heme to bilirubin
- Institute phototherapy as ordered (see *Performing phototherapy*)
  - Clean the neonate's eyes periodically to remove drainage
  - Offer extra water to promote bilirubin excretion
  - Explain that the neonate's stool contains some bile and may be greenish
- Assist with an exchange transfusion if indicated
- Administer $Rh_o(D)$ immune globulin (human), as ordered, to an Rh-negative mother after amniocentesis or to an Rh-negative mother

Nursing interventions during phototherapy

- Clean the neonate's eyes periodically to remove drainage.
- Offer the neonate extra water to promote bilirubin excretion.
- Tell the parents that the neonate's stool contains some bile and may be greenish.

during the third trimester (for the purpose of preventing hemolytic disease once the neonate is born), after the birth of an Rh-positive neonate, or after spontaneous or elective abortion
- Reassure parents that most neonates experience some degree of jaundice
- Explain hyperbilirubinemia, its causes, diagnostic tests, and treatment

HEMOLYTIC DISEASE

● **Description**
- Formerly called *erythroblastosis fetalis*
- Involves a breakdown of red blood cells (RBCs)
- The majority of neonates affected are female

● **Pathophysiology**
- During pregnancy, maternal antibodies are passed via the placenta to the fetus, causing RBC breakdown
- This disorder is usually caused by ABO incompatibility but may also be caused by Rh incompatibility
  - ABO incompatibility can occur when fetal blood type differs from maternal blood type
    · The most common incompatibility occurs when a type O mother carries a type A or type B fetus; type O blood contains anti-A and anti-B antibodies that travel transplacentally to the fetus, causing jaundice and hepatosplenomegaly
    · ABO incompatibility can occur with the first pregnancy and is usually milder and of shorter duration than Rh incompatibility
  - Rh incompatibility occurs when an Rh-negative mother carries an Rh-positive fetus
    · Leakage of fetal Rh antigens commonly occurs during delivery, at the time of placental separation
    · Maternal antibodies are produced in response; in a subsequent pregnancy with an Rh-positive fetus, maternal antibodies enter the fetal circulation transplacentally, causing erythroblastosis

● **Assessment findings**
- Hemolytic anemia
- Hyperbilirubinemia within the first 24 hours after birth
- Jaundice
- Hepatosplenomegaly

● **Treatment**
- Drug therapy, such as erythropoietin to stimulate RBC formation
- Initiation of early feeding (breast- or bottle-feeding)
- Family support

Key facts about hemolytic disease

- It involves a breakdown of RBCs.
- The majority of neonates affected are female.
- It's caused by ABO or Rh incompatibility.

Assessment findings for hemolytic disease

- Hemolytic anemia
- Hyperbilirubinemia within 24 hours after birth
- Jaundice
- Hepatosplenomegaly

- Phototherapy
- Exchange transfusion
- Monitoring of bilirubin levels

● **Nursing interventions**
- During pregnancy, institute preventive measures
  - Prevention involves administration of Rh immune globulin (RhoGAM) within 72 hours of delivery to prevent antibody formation
  - RhoGAM is ineffective when the woman is already sensitized
  - RhoGAM should be administered to an Rh-negative, D_u-negative woman who has had an abortion or whose neonate is Rh positive or D_u positive
  - RhoGAM can be administered at 28 weeks' gestation to decrease the incidence of maternal isoimmunizations
- Keep in mind that Rh sensitization can occur during pregnancy if the cellular layer separating maternal and fetal circulation is disrupted
- Encourage the woman to feed the neonate, if appropriate
- Prepare the neonate and parents for treatment procedures, such as phototherapy or exchange transfusion
- Monitor the neonate's vital signs closely during and after an exchange transfusion
- Provide explanations and emotional support to the parents and family

FETAL ALCOHOL SYNDROME

● **Description**
- Defined as a cluster of birth defects resulting from in utero exposure to alcohol
- Includes at least one abnormality in each of the following categories: growth retardation, central nervous system (CNS) abnormalities, and facial malformations
- Commonly found in neonates of women who ingested varying amounts of alcohol during pregnancy
- Birth defects associated with prenatal alcohol exposure can develop in the first 3 to 8 weeks of pregnancy, before a woman even knows she's pregnant
- The risk of teratogenic effects increases proportionally with increased daily alcohol intake
- No safe level of alcohol intake during pregnancy has been established
- Fetal alcohol syndrome (FAS) has been detected in neonates of moderate drinkers (1 to 2 oz [30 to 59 ml] of alcohol daily)

TOP 5

Steps for treating hemolytic disease

1. Administer drug therapy such as erythropoietin.
2. Initiate early feeding.
3. Provide phototherapy.
4. Provide an exchange transfusion.
5. Monitor bilirubin levels.

Key facts about pregnancy and alcohol

- FAS is a cluster of birth defects (growth retardation, CNS abnormalities, and facial malformations) resulting from in utero exposure to alcohol.
- Defects can develop in the first 3 to 8 weeks of pregnancy.
- The risk increases proportionally with increased daily alcohol intake.
- No safe level of alcohol intake during pregnancy has been established.
- Alcohol interferes with passage of amino acids across the placental barrier.
- Variables that affect the extent of fetal damage include the amount of alcohol consumed, timing of consumption, and pattern of use.

Assessment findings for FAS

- Growth retardation
- Difficulty establishing respirations
- Irritability
- Lethargy
- Seizure activity
- Tremulousness
- Opisthotonos
- Poor sucking reflex
- Abdominal distention
- Facial anomalies
- CNS dysfunction

Treatment for FAS

- Prevention through education
- Careful prenatal history and education
- Identification of women at risk and referrals for treatment
- Prompt identification of neonates with FAS

Pathophysiology

- Alcohol is a teratogenic substance that's particularly dangerous during critical periods of organogenesis
- Alcohol interferes with the passage of amino acids across the placental barrier
- When a pregnant woman ingests alcohol, so does her unborn child
- Alcohol crosses through the placenta and enters the blood supply of the fetus
- Alcohol interferes with healthy development of the fetus
- Variables that affect the extent of damage caused to the fetus by alcohol include the amount of alcohol consumed, timing of consumption, and pattern of alcohol use

Assessment findings

- Prenatal and postnatal growth retardation
- Characteristic findings within the first 24 hours of life
  - Difficulty establishing respirations
  - Irritability
  - Lethargy
  - Seizure activity
  - Tremulousness
  - Opisthotonos
  - Poor sucking reflex
  - Abdominal distention
- Facial anomalies, such as microcephaly, micro-ophthalmia, maxillary hypoplasia, and short palpebral fissures (see *Common facial characteristics of infants with FAS*)
- CNS dysfunction, including decreased IQ, developmental delays, neurologic abnormalities such as decreased muscle tone, poor coordination, and small brain

Treatment

- Prevention through public education
- Careful prenatal history and education
- Identification of women at risk, with referral to alcohol treatment centers if necessary
- Prompt identification of neonates with FAS to ensure early intervention and appropriate referrals

Nursing interventions

- Institute measures for prevention
  - Increase public awareness about the dangers of alcohol consumption during pregnancy
  - Ensure increased access to prenatal care
  - Provide educational programs

Common facial characteristics of infants with FAS

Eyes	• Short palpebral fissures • Strabismus • Ptosis • Myopia
Nose	• Short • Upturned • Flat or absent groove above upper lip
Mouth	• Thin upper lip • Receding jaw

- – Assist with screening women of reproductive age for alcohol problems
- – Use appropriate resources and strategies for decreasing alcohol use
- Closely assess any neonate born to a mother who has used alcohol
- Prevent and treat respiratory distress, including assessing breath sounds frequently, being alert for signs of distress, and suctioning as needed
- Encourage successful feeding; assist with developing measures to enhance neonate's intake
- Monitor weight and measure intake and output
- Promote parent-neonate attachment
  - – Encourage frequent visiting and rooming in if possible
  - – Encourage physical contact between the parents and the neonate
  - – Educate parents about neonate's complications
- Provide emotional support

DRUG ADDICTION

● Description
- Results from maternal drug use during pregnancy
- Pregnant women who use drugs are at higher risk for abruptio placentae, spontaneous abortion, preterm labor, and precipitous labor
- Neonates who are born drug addicted are at risk for urogenital malformations, cerebrovascular complications, low birth weight, decreased head circumference, respiratory problems, drug withdrawal, and death

● Pathophysiology
- Neonatal drug addiction results from intrauterine exposure
- The drug acts as a teratogen, causing abnormalities in embryonic or fetal development

TOP 3

Ways to promote parent-neonate attachment

1. Encourage frequent visiting and rooming in if possible.
2. Encourage physical contact between parents and neonate.
3. Educate parents about neonate's complications.

Key facts about neonatal drug addiction

- Results from maternal drug use during pregnancy
- Increases risk of abruptio placentae, spontaneous abortion, preterm labor, and precipitous labor
- Increases neonatal risk of urogenital malformations, cerebrovascular complications, low birth weight, decreased head circumference, respiratory problems, drug withdrawal, and death

● **Assessment findings**
- High-pitched cry
- Jitteriness
- Tremors
- Irritability
- Poor feeding habits
- Hyperactive Moro's reflex
- Increased tendon reflexes
- Frequent sneezing and yawning
- Poor sleeping pattern
- Diarrhea
- Vigorous sucking on hands
- Low birth weight or small for gestational age
- Signs and symptoms of withdrawal (dependent on the length of maternal addiction, the drug ingested, and the time of last ingestion before delivery); usually within 24 to 48 hours of delivery (see *Signs and symptoms of opiate withdrawal*)

● **Treatment**
- Tight swaddling for comfort
- A quiet, dark environment to decrease environmental stimuli
- A pacifier to meet sucking needs (heroin withdrawal)
- Gavage feeding for poor sucking reflex (methadone withdrawal)
- Maintenance of fluid and electrolyte balance
- Avoidance of breast-feeding
- Assessment for jaundice (methadone withdrawal)
- Medication to treat withdrawal manifestations (paregoric, phenobarbital, chlorpromazine, and diazepam)
- Promotion of maternal-infant bonding
- Evaluation for referral to child protective services, if warranted

● **Nursing interventions**
- Provide supportive care
- Maintain a patent airway; have resuscitative equipment readily available
- Elevate the neonate's head during feeding; offer pacifier if neonate demonstrates vigorous sucking (common in neonates of heroin-addicted mothers)
  - Provide small, frequent feedings
  - Position nipple correctly so sucking is effective
  - Monitor weight
- Maintain fluid and electrolyte balance
  - Monitor intake and output
  - Give supplemental fluids as ordered
  - Evaluate serum electrolyte levels as ordered

Signs and symptoms of opiate withdrawal

CNS SIGNS AND SYMPTOMS	GI SIGNS AND SYMPTOMS	AUTONOMIC SIGNS AND SYMPTOMS
• Seizures	• Poor feeding	• Increased sweating
• Tremors	• Uncoordinated and constant sucking	• Nasal stuffiness
• Irritability	• Vomiting	• Fever
• Increased wakefulness	• Diarrhea	• Mottling
• High-pitched cry	• Dehydration	• Temperature instability
• Increased muscle tone	• Poor weight gain	• Increased respiratory rate
• Increased deep tendon reflexes		• Increased heart rate
• Increased Moro's reflex		
• Increased yawning		
• Increased sneezing		
• Rapid changes in mood		
• Hypersensitivity to noise and external stimuli		

- Assess the neonate for signs and symptoms of respiratory distress and report them immediately if present
- Assess breath sounds frequently for changes
- Administer supplemental oxygen, as ordered, and assist with ventilatory support
- Monitor ABG and transcutaneous oxygen levels
- Cluster care to prevent overstimulation, and allow for adequate rest
- Firmly swaddle the neonate to promote comfort
- Protect the neonate from injury during seizures
- Maintain skin integrity
  - Provide meticulous skin care
  - Frequently change the neonate's position

CONGENITAL SYPHILIS

● Description
- Results from infection by the spirochete *Treponema pallidum*
- Occurs when the spirochete crosses the placenta from a pregnant infected woman to her fetus
- Diagnosed with serologic tests at 3 to 6 months
- The development of antibodies is necessary to make a diagnosis

● Assessment findings
- Vesicular lesions on the soles and palms
- Irritability
- Small size for gestational age
- Failure to thrive
- Rhinitis

Key signs and symptoms of opiate withdrawal

- Seizures
- Irritability
- High-pitched cry
- Increased Moro's reflex
- Hypersensitivity to noise and external stimuli
- Vomiting
- Diarrhea
- Increased sweating
- Mottling
- Increased respiratory rate
- Increased heart rate

Assessment findings for congenital syphilis

- Vesicular lesions on the soles and palms
- Irritability
- Small size for gestational age
- Failure to thrive
- Rhinitis
- Red rash around mouth and anus
- Copper rash on face, soles, and palms

TOP 2

Steps for treating congenital syphilis

1. Provide penicillin therapy.
2. Take precautions to control infection.

Assessment findings for ophthalmia neonatorum

- Fiery red conjunctivae
- Thick purulent discharge from the eyes
- Eyelid edema
- Corneal ulceration and destruction, if untreated

TOP 3

Steps for treating ophthalmia neonatorum

1. Administer I.V. antibiotic therapy.
2. Follow standard and contact infection-control precautions.
3. Irrigate the eyes with sterile saline solution.

- Red rash around mouth and anus
- Copper rash on face, soles, and palms

● **Treatment**
- Penicillin therapy
- Infection-control precautions
- Covering of neonatal hands to minimize skin trauma from scratching

● **Nursing interventions**
- Make sure all pregnant women are screened for syphilis at the first prenatal visit
- Assist with laboratory testing (Venereal Disease Research Laboratory or Rapid plasma reagin) on neonatal cord blood to check for intrauterine exposure
- Administer drugs as ordered

OPHTHALMIA NEONATORUM

● **Description**
- A severe eye infection that occurs in neonates at birth or during the first few months
- Results from exposure to the causative organism during vaginal delivery
- Most commonly caused by *Neisseria gonorrhoeae* or *Chlamydia trachomatis*
- Prophylactic administration of antibiotic ointment at birth to all neonates is a primary preventive strategy

● **Assessment findings**
- Fiery red conjunctivae
- Thick purulent discharge from the eyes
- Eyelid edema
- Corneal ulceration and destruction, if untreated
- Culture of exudate reveals causative organism

● **Treatment**
- I.V. antibiotic therapy
- Standard and contact infection-control precautions
- Sterile saline solution eye irrigation
- Treatment of mother for infection

● **Nursing interventions**
- Administer prophylactic antibiotic eye ointment to all neonates after delivery
- Monitor the appearance of the eyes for redness and drainage
- Institute standard and contact precautions
- Perform eye irrigation as ordered; wear goggles if splashing is likely

- Advise the mother to receive treatment for her infection; also suggest treatment for the mother's sexual partners

HYDROCEPHALUS

● Description
- An excessive accumulation of CSF within the ventricular spaces of the brain
- This accumulation leads to dilation of the ventricles, which causes potentially harmful pressure on the brain tissue
- Compression of brain tissue and cerebral blood vessels may lead to ischemia and, eventually, cell death
- May be communicating or noncommunicating
  - Communicating hydrocephalus results from faulty absorption of CSF
  - Noncommunicating hydrocephalus occurs as a result of obstruction of CSF flow
- Causes of hydrocephalus aren't well understood; possible causes include:
  - Genetic inheritance
  - Neural tube defects, such as spina bifida and enancephalocele
  - Complications of premature birth such as intraventricular hemorrhage
  - Meningitis
  - Tumors
  - Traumatic head injury
  - Subarachnoid hemorrhage
  - Prenatal maternal infections

● Pathophysiology
- With hydrocephalus, CSF production is increased, flow is obstructed, or reabsorption is altered
- As a result, intracranial pressure (ICP) increases causing brain displacement or motor and mental damage

● Assessment findings
- Increased head circumference
- Bulging fontanels
- "Sunset eyes"
- Widened sutures
- Forehead prominence
- Thin, shiny, fragile-looking scalp skin
- Irritability
- Weakness
- Seizures

Key facts about hydrocephalus

- Excessive accumulation of CSF in ventricular spaces of brain that leads to dilation of the ventricles
- Compression of brain tissue and cerebral blood vessels may lead to ischemia and, eventually, cell death
- May be communicating or noncommunicating

Possible causes of hydrocephalus

- Genetic inheritance
- Neural tube defects
- Complications of premature birth
- Meningitis
- Tumors
- Traumatic head injury
- Subarachnoid hemorrhage
- Prenatal maternal infections

Key assessment findings for hydrocephalus

- Increased head circumference
- Bulging fontanels
- "Sunset eyes"
- Widened sutures
- Forehead prominence
- Thin, shiny, fragile-looking scalp skin
- High-pitched, shrill cry
- Projectile vomiting

- Sluggish pupils with unequal response to light
- High-pitched, shrill cry
- Projectile vomiting
- Feeding problems

● **Treatment**
- Skin care to prevent breakdown and infection
- Careful head support during handling
- Measurement of head circumference
- Emotional support and education for the parents
- Assessment of neurologic status and progression of symptoms
- Shunt insertion to eliminate excess CSF
- Management of shunt and prevention of infection at the surgical site

● **Nursing interventions**
- Assess closely for signs and symptoms of increasing ICP
- Frequently measure head circumference, reporting any changes
- Maintain adequate nutrition
    - Provide a flexible feeding schedule to accommodate procedures
    - Offer small, frequent feedings, allowing extra time for feedings as necessary
- Provide meticulous skin care, repositioning the neonate's head often to reduce the risk of skin breakdown
- Teach the parents about the condition, treatments, and procedures
- Provide the parents and family with emotional support
- Prepare the neonate for shunt insertion as indicated; complete all preoperative procedures and teaching
- Perform postoperative care, including positioning the neonate on the unaffected side, monitoring the surgical site closely, and obtaining head circumference

PHENYLKETONURIA

● **Description**
- A rare hereditary condition
    - Phenylketonuria (PKU) is a disease of protein metabolism characterized by the inability of the body to metabolize the essential amino acid phenylalanine
    - It's considered an inborn metabolic error
    - It's inherited as an autosomal recessive trait; both parents must pass the gene on for the child to be affected
- Persons with PKU have almost no activity of phenylalanine hydroxylase, an enzyme that helps convert phenylalanine to tyrosine
- As a result, phenylalanine accumulates in the blood and urine and tyrosine levels are low

TOP 4

Steps for treating hydrocephalus

1. Provide skin care to prevent breakdown and infection.
2. Carefully support the head during handling.
3. Manage shunt and prevent infection at the surgical site.
4. Monitor for signs and symptoms of increasing ICP.

Key facts about PKU

- It's a rare hereditary condition that affects protein metabolism.
- It's considered an inborn metabolic error.
- It's inherited as an autosomal recessive trait (both parents must pass on the gene).
- It causes accumulation of phenylalanine that affects the development of the brain and CNS.
- It's treated with a special diet that limits phenylalanine intake.

● **Pathophysiology**
  - Accumulation of phenylalanine and its abnormal metabolites in the brain
  - This accumulation affects the normal development of the brain and CNS
  - Tyrosine is needed to form the pigment melanin and the hormones epinephrine and thyroxine
  - Decreased melanin production results in the similar fair appearance of children with PKU
  - CNS damage can be minimized if treatment is initiated before age 3 months; mental retardation can occur if the condition is untreated

● **Assessment findings**
  - Failure to thrive
  - Vomiting
  - Rashes and eczematous skin lesions
  - Decreased pigmentation
  - Seizures and tremors
  - Microcephaly
  - Hyperactivity and irritability
  - Purposeless, repetitive motions
  - Musty odor from skin and urinary excretion of phenylacetic acid
  - Positive Guthrie test result
    – This heelstick blood test is required by most states
    – It should be performed at least 24 hours after initiation of feedings

● **Treatment**
  - Low-phenylalanine formula (such as Lofenalac)
  - Continued special diet that limits phenylalanine intake

● **Nursing interventions**
  - Provide low phenylalanine formula for neonate
  - Inform the parents about the neonate's need for limited phenylalanine intake
  - Provide the parents with a list of foods to allow in the neonate's diet as well as those to avoid
  - Offer emotional support to the parents (because the disorder is genetic, the parents may feel responsible)

TORCH SYNDROME

● **Description**
  - Refers to a group of maternal infectious diseases (*To*xoplasmosis, *R*ubella, *C*ytomegalovirus, *H*erpesvirus type II)
  - Can lead to serious complications in the embryo, fetus, or neonate

Assessment findings for PKU

● Failure to thrive
● Vomiting
● Rashes; eczematous skin lesions
● Decreased pigmentation
● Seizures, tremors
● Microcephaly
● Hyperactivity, irritability
● Purposeless, repetitive motions
● Musty odor from skin and urinary excretion of phenylacetic acid
● Positive Guthrie test result

Four infections of TORCH syndrome

1. TOxoplasmosis
2. Rubella
3. Cytomegalovirus
4. Herpesvirus type II

Key facts about toxoplasmosis

- Primarily transmitted to fetus via mother's contact with contaminated cat box filler
- Abortion is recommended before 20 weeks' gestation
- Causes stillbirths, neonatal death, severe congenital anomalies, deafness, retinochoroiditis, seizures, and coma

Key facts about rubella

- Poses greatest risk during first trimester
- Causes congenital heart disease, intrauterine growth retardation, cataracts, mental retardation, and hearing impairment
- Abortion is recommended during first trimester

Key facts about CMV

- Most common cause of viral infections in fetuses
- Common cause of mental retardation
- Causes auditory difficulties, small size for gestational age, and blueberry muffin syndrome
- Antivirals are ineffective

Key facts about herpesvirus type II

- Affected neonates may be asymptomatic for 2 to 12 days
- Causes jaundice, increased temperature, and vesicular lesions
- Cesarean delivery can protect the fetus from infection

TORCH infections and their implications

INFECTION	DESCRIPTION AND IMPLICATIONS
Toxoplasmosis	• Toxoplasmosis is transmitted to the fetus primarily via the mother's contact with contaminated cat box filler. • A therapeutic abortion is recommended if the diagnosis is made before the 20th week of gestation. • Effects include increased frequency of stillbirths, neonatal deaths, severe congenital anomalies, deafness, retinochoroiditis, seizures, and coma. • Maternal treatment involves anti-infective therapy—for example, with a sulfa or clindamycin.
Rubella	• Rubella is a chronic viral infection. • The greatest risk occurs within the first trimester. • Effects include congenital heart disease, intrauterine growth retardation, cataracts, mental retardation, and hearing impairment. • Management includes therapeutic abortion if the disease occurs during the first trimester, and emotional support for parents. • Women of childbearing age should be tested for immunity and vaccinated if necessary. • The neonate may persistently shed the virus for up to 1 year.
Cytomegalovirus (CMV)	• CMV is a herpesvirus that can be transmitted from an asymptomatic mother transplacentally to the fetus or via the cervix to the neonate at delivery. • It's the most common cause of viral infections in fetuses. • CMV is a common cause of mental retardation. • Principal sites of damage are the brain, liver, and blood. • Other effects include auditory difficulties and a birth weight that's small for gestational age. • The neonate may also demonstrate a characteristic pattern of petechiae called *blueberry muffin syndrome*. • Antiviral drugs can't prevent CMV or treat the neonate.
Herpesvirus type II	• The fetus can be exposed to the herpesvirus through indirect contact with infected genitals or via direct contact with those tissues during delivery. • Affected neonates may be asymptomatic for 2 to 12 days but then may develop jaundice, seizures, increased temperature, and characteristic vesicular lesions. • A cesarean delivery can protect the fetus from infection. • Pharmacologic treatment may include acyclovir and vidarabine I.V. after exposure.

● Pathophysiology
- Infection results when the organisms cross the placenta or travel up through the birth canal
- Once present, the organisms can cause severe problems with fetal growth and development (see *TORCH infections and their implications*)

RETINOPATHY OF PREMATURITY

● Description
- Refers to an alteration in vision leading to partial or total blindness

- Typically results from prolonged exposure to high concentrations of oxygen or fluctuations in oxygen administration levels

- **Pathophysiology**
  - High oxygen concentrations lead to vasoconstriction of immature retinal blood vessels
  - Fluctuating oxygen administration levels lead to rapid vasodilation and vasoconstriction of immature, fragile retinal blood vessels
  - Subsequent rupture of vessels occurs with partial or complete retinal detachment

- **Assessment findings**
  - Include retinal changes, which are evident upon ophthalmologic examination

- **Treatment**
  - Monitoring of oxygen concentration
  - Monitoring of ABG levels
  - Monitoring of transcutaneous oxygen levels and pulse oximetry
  - Ophthalmologic examinations at regular intervals during and after hospitalization
  - Administration of vitamin E (reduces incidence of retinopathy of prematurity by modifying tissues' response to effects of oxygen)
  - Cryosurgery or laser surgery

- **Nursing interventions**
  - Closely monitor oxygen concentration levels being administered; obtain transcutaneous oxygen and ABG levels and pulse oximetry readings as ordered
  - Administer oxygen carefully, ensuring that the lowest concentration necessary is being used
  - Explain the condition and its treatments to the parents
  - Instruct the parents in the need for follow-up eye examinations
  - Provide preoperative and postoperative care as indicated

TRACHEOESOPHAGEAL FISTULA

- **Description**
  - Refers to a congenital anomaly resulting from exposure to some teratogen that doesn't allow the esophagus and trachea to separate normally
  - There's an abnormal connection between the trachea and esophagus

- **Pathophysiology**
  - Abnormal development of the trachea and esophagus occurs during the embryonic period

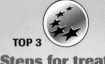

Assessment findings for tracheoesophageal fistula

- Signs of respiratory distress
- Excessive frothy oral mucus
- Difficulty feeding

TOP 4

Steps for treating tracheoesophageal fistula

1. Maintain a patent airway.
2. Withhold food and fluids.
3. Position the patient in high Fowler's position.
4. Provide a pacifier to meet sucking needs.

- Typically, the esophagus ends in blind pouch with trachea communicating by a fistula with lower esophagus and stomach

● **Assessment findings**
- Signs of respiratory distress
- Excessive frothy oral mucus
- Difficulty inserting a nasogastric tube
- Difficulty feeding (results in choking or aspiration)

● **Treatment**
- Maintenance of patent airway
- Withholding of food and fluids (nothing by mouth) until repaired
- Surgical correction
- Positioning of patient in high Fowler's position to prevent aspiration of gastric contents
- Laryngoscope and endotracheal tube at bedside in case of extreme edema causing obstruction
- Frequent shallow suctioning
- Pacifier to meet sucking needs
- Possible gastrostomy tube feedings postoperatively

● **Nursing interventions**
- Keep the neonate on nothing-by-mouth status
- Administer I.V. fluids to maintain hydration and provide nutrition; offer a pacifier to meet the neonate's sucking needs
- Assess airway for patency
- Frequently monitor vital signs and respiratory status; watch for signs and symptoms of aspiration
- Position the neonate upright or on his right side to minimize the risk of gastric secretions entering the lungs
- Maintain a neutral thermal environment
- Provide comfort measures, and institute measures to reduce the risk of the neonate's crying; the risk for vomiting and aspiration increases with crying because air entering the stomach from the fistula leads to distention
- Prepare the parents and neonate for surgical correction
- Provide postoperative care as appropriate
- Offer emotional support to the parents and family

DEVELOPMENTAL DYSPLASIA OF THE HIP

● **Description**
- Refers to the improper formation and function of the hip socket
- Commonly called *congenital hip dysplasia*
- Causes the femur head to ride out of or dislocate from the acetabulum

- **Pathophysiology**
  - Exact cause is unknown
  - The acetabulum is flattened or too shallow
  - As a result, the head of the femur dislocates upward and backward

- **Assessment findings**
  - Positive Ortolani's sign
  - Positive Barlow's sign
  - Shortened femur on affected side
  - Asymmetrical gluteal folds

- **Treatment**
  - Positioning and maintaining the head of the femur in the acetabulum with triple diapers, a Frejka pillow splint, or a Pavlik harness
  - Hip-spica cast and braces if other means prove ineffective
  - Possible surgical correction
  - Parent education about use of device for maintaining position

- **Nursing interventions**
  - Maintain the affected hip in a flexed, abducted position
  - Instruct the parents in measures to position and maintain the head of the femur
    - Teach the parents how to apply triple diapers, a splint, or a harness
    - Show parents how to properly care for the skin, especially areas under the device
  - Offer emotional support and guidance to parents
  - Encourage parents to interact with the neonate and hold the neonate, even with a device in place
  - Inform parents about the possibility of the need for surgical correction later on when the neonate is older

APNEA

- **Description**
  - Refers to the cessation of breathing for more than 15 seconds
  - Commonly seen in preterm neonates and neonates with secondary stress, such as those with infection, hyperbilirubinemia, hypoglycemia, or hypothermia

- **Pathophysiology**
  - The respiratory control centers located in the brain are immature
  - Additionally, the amount of surfactant may be insufficient
  - Other possible causes include acidosis, anemia, hypoglycemia or hyperglycemia, hypothermia or hyperthermia, upper airway obstruction, hypocalcemia, and sepsis

Assessment findings for developmental dysplasia of the hip

- Positive Ortolani's sign
- Positive Barlow's sign
- Shortened femur on affected side
- Asymmetrical gluteal folds

Nursing interventions for developmental dysplasia of the hip

- Maintain the affected hip in a flexed, abducted position.
- Teach parents how to maintain the hip in the correct position.
- Show parents how to properly care for the skin, especially areas under the device.

Kay facts about apnea

- Cessation of breathing for more than 15 seconds
- Commonly seen in preterm neonates and neonates with secondary stress
- May be caused by immaturity of the respiratory control centers in the brain, insufficient amount of surfactant, acidosis, anemia, hypoglycemia or hyperglycemia, hypothermia or hyperthermia, upper airway obstruction, hypocalcemia, and sepsis

Assessment findings for apnea

- Breathing stops for more than 20 seconds
- Bradycardia
- Early cyanosis

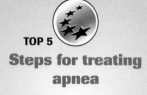

TOP 5

Steps for treating apnea

1. Provide respiratory support.
2. Provide tactile stimulation.
3. Evaluate ABG levels.
4. Provide suctioning.
5. Initiate home apnea monitoring.

> ### TIME-OUT FOR TEACHING
> # Home apnea monitoring
>
> Be sure to include these topics in your teaching plan for the parents of a neonate receiving home apnea monitoring:
> - rationale for use
> - signs and symptoms of apnea
> - equipment and procedure for use
>
> - frequency and duration of use
> - signs and symptoms requiring notification of the health care provider
> - measures to stimulate respirations
> - cardiopulmonary resuscitation technique
> - follow-up care.

Assessment findings
- Breathing stops for more than 20 seconds
- Bradycardia
- Early cyanosis

Treatment
- Respiratory support
- Tactile stimulation
- Correction of underlying cause
- Gentle handling
- Evaluation of ABG levels
- Suctioning
- Home apnea monitoring (for teaching tips, see *Home apnea monitoring*)
- Caffeine or medications such as theophylline

Nursing interventions
- Assess respiratory status closely and frequently, including after feeding because a full stomach may increase pressure on the diaphragm
- Use an apnea monitor to aid in detecting episodes; have emergency resuscitation equipment readily available
- If apnea is noted, gently flick the neonate's sole or shake the neonate
- Anticipate the need for ventilatory support if the neonate experiences frequent apneic episodes or the episodes are difficult to correct
- Maintain a neutral thermal environment to reduce added stress
- Handle the neonate gently to avoid excessive fatigue
- Avoid measuring the neonate's temperature rectally, which causes vagal stimulation and, subsequently, bradycardia and apnea

PREMATURITY

Description

- Refers to delivery of a neonate before the end of the 37th week of gestation
- Associated with numerous problems
  - All body systems are immature
  - The extent of immaturity depends on gestational age and level of development at delivery
- Premature neonates between 28 and 37 weeks' gestation have the best chance of survival

Pathophysiology

- Preterm delivery may occur because of maternal disease that necessitates delivery of the neonate for the health of the mother — for example, preeclampsia
- Preterm delivery may also be a direct result of preterm labor

Assessment findings

- Inspection findings
  - Low birth weight
  - Minimal subcutaneous fat deposits
  - Proportionally large head in relation to body
  - Prominent sucking pads in the cheeks
  - Wrinkled features
  - Thin, smooth, shiny skin that's almost translucent
  - Veins clearly visible under the thin, transparent epidermis
  - Lanugo hair over the body
  - Sparse, fine, fuzzy hair on the head
  - Soft, pliable ear cartilage; the ear may fold easily
  - Minimal creases in the soles and palms
  - Prominent eyes, possibly closed
  - Few scrotal rugae (males)
  - Undescended testes (males)
  - Prominent labia and clitoris (females)
- Neurologic examination findings
  - Inactivity (although may be unusually active immediately after birth)
  - Extension of extremities
  - Absence of suck reflex
  - Weak swallow, gag, and cough reflexes
  - Weak grasp reflex
  - Ability to bring the neonate's elbow across the chest when eliciting the scarf sign
  - Ability to easily bring the neonate's heel to his ear

- Additional findings
  - Inability to maintain body temperature
  - Limited ability to excrete solutes in the urine
  - Increased susceptibility to infection, hyperbilirubinemia, and hypoglycemia
  - Periodic breathing, hypoventilation, and periods of apnea

● **Treatment**
- Cardiac and respiratory assessment and assistance
- Resuscitation if necessary
- Maintenance of fluid and electrolyte balance
- Nutritional support
- Prevention of infection
- Assessment of neurologic status
- Maintenance of body temperature and neutral thermal environment
- Monitoring of renal function
- Emotional support to parents
- Assessment of glucose and bilirubin levels

● **Nursing interventions**
- Closely assess all body systems
- Anticipate the need for endotracheal intubation and mechanical ventilation
  - Administer oxygen as ordered, avoiding concentrations that are too high
  - Monitor transcutaneous oxygen levels or pulse oximetry readings
  - Have emergency resuscitation equipment readily available
- Administer medications to support cardiac and respiratory function
- Institute measures to maintain a neutral thermal environment; anticipate need for incubator or radiant warmer
- Avoid vigorous stroking and rubbing; use firm but gentle touch when handling neonate
- Support the head and maintain extremities close to the body during position changes
- Monitor fluid and electrolyte balance, assess intake and output, and administer I.V. fluid therapy as ordered
- Administer nutritional therapy as ordered
  - Keep in mind that neonates born before 34 weeks' gestation have uncoordinated sucking and swallowing reflexes, so gavage or I.V. feeding may be necessary
  - Provide nonnutritive sucking via a pacifier as appropriate
- Provide education, support, and guidance to the parents and family
- Explain all procedures and treatments to the parents; allow parents to verbalize their concerns; correct any misconceptions or erroneous information
- Assist with referrals for supportive services

Key nursing interventions for prematurity

- Closely assess all body systems.
- Administer oxygen as ordered.
- Administer medications.
- Maintain a neutral thermal environment.
- Monitor fluid and electrolyte balance; assess intake and output.
- Administer nutritional therapy as ordered.
- Provide education, support, and guidance to the parents and family members.

SMALL FOR GESTATIONAL AGE

● **Description**
- Birth weight at or below the 10th percentile on intrauterine growth chart
- May also be referred to as *small for date* and *intrauterine growth retardation*
- The neonate may be premature, term, or postmature
- Being small for gestational age (SGA) places the neonate at risk for certain problems
  - Perinatal asphyxia
  - Hypoglycemia
  - Hypocalcemia
  - Aspiration syndromes
  - Increased heat loss
  - Feeding difficulties
  - Polycythemia

● **Pathophysiology**
- The underlying problem is intrauterine growth retardation
- Conditions in the mother may contribute to the birth of a SGA neonate
  - Poor nutrition
  - Advanced diabetes
  - Pregnancy-induced hypertension
  - Smoking
  - Age older than 35
  - Drug use
- Partial placental separation and malfunction may also be a cause
- Conditions in the fetus may also contribute to the birth of a SGA neonate
  - Intrauterine infection
  - Chromosomal abnormalities and malformations

● **Assessment findings**
- Wide-eyed look
- Sunken abdomen
- Loose, dry skin
- Decreased chest and abdomen circumferences
- Decreased subcutaneous fat
- Thin, dry umbilical cord
- Sparse scalp hair

● **Treatment**
- Supportive care
- Nutritional support

Neonatal risks associated with SGA

- Perinatal asphyxia
- Hypoglycemia
- Hypocalcemia
- Aspiration syndromes
- Increased heat loss
- Feeding difficulties
- Polycythemia

Maternal conditions that contribute to SGA

- Poor nutrition
- Advanced diabetes
- Pregnancy-induced hypertension
- Smoking
- Age older than 35
- Drug use

Key findings associated with SGA neonates

- Wide-eyed look
- Sunken abdomen
- Loose, dry skin
- Decreased chest and abdomen circumferences
- Decreased subcutaneous fat

Nutrition facts about SGA neonates

- SGA neonates have high caloric needs and benefit from frequent feedings.
- Hypoglycemia is common because of reduced glycogen stores.
- I.V. glucose may be needed if blood glucose levels are less than 40 mg/dl.

Key facts about LGA neonates

- Have birth weights at or above the 90th percentile on intrauterine growth chart
- Were subjected to an overproduction of growth hormone in utero

Neonatal risks associated with LGA

- Increased incidence of cesarean deliveries, birth trauma, and injury
- Hypoglycemia
- Polycythemia

● **Nursing interventions**
- Support respiratory efforts; monitor respiratory status closely for changes; institute respiratory care measures, as indicated by the neonate's condition
- Institute measures to provide a neutral thermal environment
- Protect the neonate from infection
- Provide appropriate nutrition
  - Keep in mind that SGA neonates have higher caloric needs and benefit from frequent feedings
  - Monitor blood glucose levels as ordered
    · Hypoglycemia is common due to reduced glycogen stores
    · I.V. glucose may be needed if blood glucose levels are less than 40 mg/dl
- Maintain adequate hydration, monitor intake and output, administer I.V. fluid therapy as ordered
- Cluster nursing care activities to minimize the neonate's energy expenditures
- Provide meticulous skin care
- Facilitate growth and development; encourage parental interaction with neonate to promote bonding
- Keep parents informed, and provide support to the entire family

LARGE FOR GESTATIONAL AGE

● **Description**
- Birth weight at or above the 90th percentile on the intrauterine growth chart
- Also called *macrosomia*
- Large for gestational age (LGA) neonates are subjected to an overproduction of growth hormone in utero
- LGA places the neonate at risk for certain problems
  - Increased incidence of cesarean deliveries, birth trauma, and injury
  - Hypoglycemia
  - Polycythemia

● **Pathophysiology**
- LGA may result from a genetic factor
  - Male neonates tend to be larger than females
  - Neonates of large parents tend to be large
  - Neonates of multiparous women tend to be larger
- Neonates of diabetic mothers also tend to be LGA
  - High maternal blood glucose levels provide a stimulus for continued insulin production by the fetus
  - This constant state of hyperglycemia leads to excessive growth and fat deposition

● **Assessment findings**
- Weight generally more than 4,000 g (8 lb 13 oz)
- Plump and full faced
- Fractures or intracranial hemorrhage due to exposure to trauma during vaginal delivery
- Immature reflexes
- Possible asymmetry of chest secondary to diaphragmatic paralysis occurring from edema of phrenic nerve

● **Treatment**
- Close observation
- Supportive care (although large in size, the neonate is immature, requiring care similar to that for a premature neonate)

● **Nursing interventions** (see Nursing interventions for "Prematurity," page 302)

POSTMATURITY

● **Description**
- Refers to a neonate born after 42 weeks' gestation
- The placenta has the growth potential of only 40 to 42 weeks
- After that time, calcium deposits collect, making the placenta unable to function, possibly resulting in lack of oxygen, fluids, and nutrients
- The postmature neonate is at risk for problems
  - Meconium aspiration
  - Placental insufficiency
  - Hypoxia
  - Hypoglycemia
  - Polycythemia
  - Seizures
  - Cold stress

● **Pathophysiology**
- The cause isn't well understood
- Postmaturity is associated with primigravida mother, anencephalic fetus, history of postmaturity, and delayed ovulation and fertilization

● **Assessment findings**
- Alert, wide-eyed look
- Absence of vernix caseosa
- Long fingernails
- Profuse scalp hair
- Long, thin body
- Decreased or absent subcutaneous fat
- Loose, dry skin
- Meconium

Key findings associated with LGA neonates

- Generally weigh more than 4,000 g
- Plump and full faced
- Fractures or intracranial hemorrhage
- Immature reflexes
- Possible asymmetry of chest

Potential complications for postmature neonates

- Meconium aspiration
- Placental insufficiency
- Hypoxia
- Hypoglycemia
- Polycythemia
- Seizures
- Cold stress

Key findings associated with postmaturity

- Alert, wide-eyed look
- Absence of vernix caseosa
- Long fingernails
- Profuse scalp hair
- Long, thin body
- Decreased or absent subcutaneous fat
- Loose, dry skin
- Meconium

● **Treatment**
  • Close observation
  • Supportive care (similar to that required for prematurity)
● **Nursing interventions** (see Nursing interventions for "Prematurity," page 302)

HUMAN IMMUNODEFICIENCY VIRUS INFECTION

● **Description**
  • An infectious disease caused by human immunodeficiency virus (HIV) that compromises the immune system
  • Acquired by the fetus transplacentally through contact with maternal blood and secretions; also transmitted in breast milk
  • Risk factors for perinatal transmission of HIV include the following neonatal factors:
    – First-born twin
    – Prematurity
    – Bacterial infection
    – Breast-feeding
  • Diagnosis is aided by laboratory test results and evidence of immunosuppression, wasting syndrome, encephalopathy, or opportunistic disease
  • A false-positive test result for HIV antibodies may result from transplacental transfer of maternal HIV antibodies to the fetus; final diagnosis may take up to 6 months
  • A neonate is considered uninfected with HIV under these conditions
    – No physical findings consistent with HIV are present
    – Immunologic test results are negative
    – Virologic tests are negative
    – After age 12 months, the infant tests negative for two or more HIV antibody tests
● **Assessment findings**
  • Recurrent infections
  • SGA
  • Oral candidiasis (thrush) or dermatitis
  • Lymphoid interstitial pneumonia
  • Lymphadenopathy
  • Hepatosplenomegaly
  • Failure to thrive
  • Positive enzyme-linked immunosorbent assay and Western blot test at age 18 months indicative of infection in the child
  • Positive HIV DNA polymerase chain reaction test by age 14 days

---

Risk factors for perinatal transmission of HIV

• First-born twin
• Prematurity
• Bacterial infection
• Breast-feeding

Assessment findings for HIV infection

• Recurrent infections
• Small for gestational age
• Oral candidiasis or dermatitis
• Lymphoid interstitial pneumonia
• Lymphadenopathy
• Hepatosplenomegaly
• Failure to thrive
• Positive enzyme-linked immunosorbent assay and Western blot test at age 18 months
• Positive HIV DNA polymerase chain reaction test by age 14 days

Treatment

- Postnatal administration of zidovudine dramatically reduces the risk of perinatal transmission
- PCP prophylaxis for all neonates born to HIV-infected women regardless of the neonate's initial test results; PCP infection usually occurs between ages 3 and 6 months, when many HIV exposed infants haven't yet been identified as being infected

● Nursing interventions

- Institute standard precautions when caring for the neonate
- Keep in mind that diagnosis of HIV infection in neonates is complicated by the presence of maternal anti-HIV immunoglobulin G antibody; cord blood, therefore, should never be used for HIV testing
- Administer drugs as ordered
    - Know that zidovudine may cause transient anemia
    - Obtain a complete blood count and differential leukocyte count at birth as a baseline and again at 4 and 6 weeks of age
    - Provide supportive care as indicated
    - Educate the parents about the infection, treatment including drug therapy, possible modifications in immunization administration, and need for follow-up
- Teach parents how to identify complications, such as recurrent or unusual infections, failure to thrive, hematologic problems, renal disease, and neurologic disturbances
- Provide emotional support and guidance
- Assist with referrals to appropriate community resources for support

Treatment for HIV infection

- Postnatal administration of zidovudine reduces the risk of perinatal transmission
- PCP prophylaxis for all neonates born to HIV-infected women regardless of the neonate's initial test results

HIV complications that parents should identify

- Recurrent or unusual infections
- Failure to thrive
- Hematologic problems
- Renal disease
- Neurologic disturbances

NCLEX CHECKS

It's never too soon to begin your NCLEX preparation. Now that you've reviewed this chapter, carefully read each of the following questions and choose the best answer. Then compare your responses to the correct answers.

1. The chest X-ray of a neonate with respiratory distress syndrome (RDS) would typically demonstrate which sign?

- ☐ **A.** Alveolar hyperinflation
- ☒ **B.** Ground-glass appearance
- ☐ **C.** Constricted bronchioles
- ☐ **D.** Clear lung fields

TOP 33

Items to study for your next test on the high-risk neonate

1. Assessment findings in respiratory distress syndrome (RDS)
2. Treatment for RDS
3. Nursing interventions for RDS
4. Assessment findings for transient tachypnea of the neonate (TTN)
5. Treatment options for TTN
6. Nursing interventions for TTN
7. Assessment findings in meconium aspiration syndrome (MAS)
8. Treatment for MAS
9. Assessment findings for sepsis in the neonate
10. Assessment findings for hyperbilirubinemia
11. Nursing interventions for hyperbilirubinemia
12. Steps in phototherapy
13. Assessment findings for hemolytic anemia
14. Nursing interventions for hemolytic anemia
15. Assessment findings for fetal alcohol syndrome (FAS)
16. Nursing interventions for FAS
17. Neonatal assessment findings in maternal drug addiction
18. Treatment for ophthalmia neonatorum
19. Assessment findings for hydrocephalus
20. Treatment for hydrocephalus

(continued)

2. The nurse would anticipate transient tachypnea of the neonate (TTN) to occur in which of the following cases? Select all that apply.

- ☐ **A.** Neonate delivered by cesarean birth
- ☐ **B.** Large for gestational age neonate
- ☐ **C.** Postmature neonate
- ☒ **D.** Neonate born rapidly
- ☒ **E.** Neonate with diabetic mother
- ☒ **F.** Premature neonate

3. Which of the following levels of bilirubin would suggest hyperbilirubinemia in a term neonate?

- ☐ **A.** 5.2 mg/100 ml
- ☐ **B.** 7.3 mg/100 ml
- ☐ **C.** 10.4 mg/100 ml
- ☒ **D.** 12.8 mg/100 ml

4. When performing phototherapy, which of the following interventions would the nurse do?

- ☐ **A.** Wrap the neonate snugly in a blanket
- ☒ **B.** Protect the eyes with a mask
- ☐ **C.** Turn the neonate every 4 to 6 hours
- ☐ **D.** Monitor the neonate's temperature rectally

5. Which finding would the nurse expect to assess in a neonate experiencing opiate withdrawal?

- ☐ **A.** Difficulty in arousing
- ☐ **B.** Depressed deep tendon reflexes
- ☒ **C.** Poor feeding
- ☐ **D.** Bradycardia

6. Which of the following test results, if positive, would confirm the diagnosis of phenylketonuria (PKU)?

- ☒ **A.** Guthrie test
- ☐ **B.** Ortolani's sign Hip
- ☐ **C.** Barlow's sign Hip Dysplasia
- ☐ **D.** VDRL

7. Which of the following interventions should the nurse do first for a neonate who becomes apneic?

- ☒ **A.** Flick the sole
- ☐ **B.** Begin cardiopulmonary resuscitation
- ☐ **C.** Administer oxygen
- ☐ **D.** Document the length of the apneic period

ANSWERS AND RATIONALES

1. CORRECT ANSWER: B

With RDS, chest X-ray reveals a diffuse granular pattern resembling ground glass over all the lung fields. Lung fields wouldn't be clear. X-rays would show alveolar atelectasis, not alveolar hyperinflation, and dilated, not constricted, bronchioles by dark streaks within the granular pattern.

2. CORRECT ANSWERS: A, D, E, AND F

TTN is common in neonates born by cesarean birth because these neonates don't receive the thoracic compression that helps to expel fluid during vaginal delivery. It also occurs in neonates who are premature (not postmature), small for gestational age (not large for gestational age), and were born rapidly by vaginal delivery.

3. CORRECT ANSWER: D

Hyperbilirubinemia is suggested with the following elevated serum bilirubin levels: greater than 12 mg/100 ml in a term neonate, 15 mg/100 ml in a preterm neonate, or increasing more than 5 mg/100 ml in 24 hours.

4. CORRECT ANSWER: B

When performing phototherapy, the neonate's eyes should be protected with a mask. The neonate should be completely undressed except for a diaper placed under him or her to absorb any urine voided. The neonate should be turned at least every 2 hours to expose all body surfaces to the light and to prevent head molding and skin breakdown from pressure. Axillary temperatures are monitored.

5. CORRECT ANSWER: C

The neonate experiencing opiate withdrawal typically exhibits poor feeding with uncoordinated sucking and swallowing, irritability and increased sensitivity to noise and surroundings, increased deep tendon reflexes, and tachycardia.

6. CORRECT ANSWER: A

A positive Guthrie test, a heelstick blood test that's required by most states, indicates PKU. Positive Ortolani's sign and Barlow's sign are indicative of developmental hip dysplasia. VDRL is used to diagnose congenital syphilis.

7. CORRECT ANSWER: A

When a neonate has an apneic episode, the nurse should first gently flick the neonate's sole or shake the neonate to stimulate respiratory effort. Usually this is enough to stimulate breathing. If not, then resuscitative measures are initiated, including administration of oxygen, and cardiopulmonary resuscitation. Documentation of the length of the apneic period and measures used is completed once the neonate is breathing again.

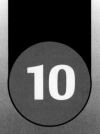

10

The normal postpartum period

LEARNING OBJECTIVES

After studying this chapter, you should be able to:

● Describe the physiologic changes that normally occur during the postpartum period.

● Trace the course of psychological adjustments made by the patient during the postpartum period.

● Name the steps to include in a postpartum teaching plan.

● Identify the needs of the patient and her family in adjusting to the neonate.

CHAPTER OVERVIEW

A new mother experiences many physiologic and psychological changes during the postpartum period. Knowledge of these changes is essential to guide appropriate nursing interventions. The nurse plays a key role in providing comprehensive postpartum teaching.

POSTPARTUM PHYSIOLOGIC CHANGES

● **Vascular system**
- Decreased blood volume (after vaginal delivery)
- Increased hematocrit (after vaginal delivery)

- Extensive activation of blood clotting factors
- Return of blood volume to prenatal levels within 3 weeks
- Receding of varicosities (although may never return to a completely prepregnant appearance)
- Return of vital signs to prepregnancy parameters

Reproductive system

- Rapid uterine involution and descent to its prepregnancy position in the pelvis
- Cervical and vaginal contraction
- Sloughing of the uterine lining and development of lochia
- Cessation of progesterone production until first ovulation
- Reduction in pregnancy hormones, such as human chorionic gonadotropin (HCG), human placental lactogen, progestin, estrone, and estradiol
- Permanent alteration of cervical external os shape from a circle to a jagged slit
- Endometrial regeneration within 6 weeks after delivery
- Recovery of vaginal and pelvic floor muscle tone
- Buildup of breast tissue for lactation

GI system

- Delayed bowel movement from decreased intestinal muscle tone and perineal discomfort
- Increased thirst from fluids lost during labor and delivery
- Increased hunger after labor and delivery
- Reactivation of digestion and absorption
- Gradual return of abdominal muscles, wall, and ligaments tone
- Weight loss due to rapid diuresis and lochial flow

Genitourinary system

- Increased urine output during the first 24 hours after delivery from puerperal diuresis
  - Rids the body of excess fluid accumulation
  - Reduces added blood volume of pregnancy
- Increased bladder capacity
- Proteinuria from the catalytic process of involution (in 50% of women)
- Decreased bladder-filling sensation from swelling and bruising of tissues
- Return of dilated ureters and renal pelvis to prepregnancy size by 6 weeks

Endocrine system

- Increased thyroid function
- Increased production of anterior pituitary gonadotropic hormones

Key postpartum physiologic changes

- Decreased blood volume (after vaginal delivery)
- Increased hematocrit (after vaginal delivery)
- Extensive activation of blood clotting factors
- Rapid uterine involution and descent to its prepregnancy position in the pelvis
- Cessation of progesterone production until first ovulation
- Permanent alteration of cervical external os shape from a circle to a jagged slit
- Increased urine output during the first 24 hours after delivery from puerperal diuresis
- Proteinuria from the catalytic process of involution (in 50% of women)

- Decreased production of estrogen, aldosterone, progesterone, HCG, corticoids, and 17-ketosteroids
- Rise in follicle-stimulating hormone production, resulting in the return of ovulation and menstrual cycles.

● **Integumentary system**
- Changes include eventual fading of striae gravidarum (stretch marks), chloasma (pigmentation on face and neck), and linea nigra (pigmentation on the abdomen)

POSTPARTUM PSYCHOLOGICAL CHANGES

● **General information**
- Mothers typically undergo psychological adjustments during the postpartum period
- Reva Rubin, a researcher who examined maternal adaptation to childbirth in the 1960s, identified three phases that can help the nurse understand maternal behavior after delivery (see *Highlighting the phases of the postpartum period*)
  - Historically, each phase encompassed a specific time span and women progressed through phases sequentially
  - Because of today's shorter hospitalizations for childbirth, women appear to move through the phases more quickly, possibly experiencing more than one phase at one time

● **Phases**
- Taking-in phase (maternal behavior 1 to 2 days after delivery)
  - Is passive and dependent
  - Directs energy toward herself instead of toward her neonate
  - May relive her labor and delivery to integrate the process into her life
  - May find difficulty in making decisions
- Taking-hold phase (maternal behavior 2 to 7 days after delivery)
  - Has more energy
  - Demonstrates independence and initiates self-care activities
  - Accepts increasing responsibility for her neonate
  - May be receptive to infant care and self-care education
  - May express lack of confidence in caring for the neonate
- Letting-go phase (maternal behavior about 7 days after delivery)
  - Readjusts relationships with family members such as assuming the mother role
  - Assumes responsibility for her dependent neonate
  - Recognizes the neonate as separate from the self and relinquishes the fantasized neonate
  - May experience depression

Highlighting the phases of the postpartum period

The chart below summarizes the three phases of the postpartum period as identified by Reva Rubin.

PHASE	MATERNAL BEHAVIOR AND TASKS
Taking in (1 to 2 days after delivery)	• Reflective time • Assumption of passive role and dependence on others for care • Verbalization about labor and birth • Sense of wonderment when looking at the neonate
Taking hold (2 to 7 days after delivery)	• Action oriented time of increasing independence in care • Strong interest in caring for neonate; commonly accompanied by feelings of insecurity about ability to care for neonate
Letting go (7 days after delivery)	• Ability to redefine new role • Acceptance of neonate's real image rather than fantasized image • Recognition of neonate as separate from herself • Assumption of responsibility for dependent neonate

NEONATE'S IMPACT ON THE FAMILY

● **Sibling reaction**
  • Siblings typically dislike the idea of sharing parents with the neonate
  • Reactions of siblings will depend on their age, the total number of siblings in the household, and the amount of preparation invested by the parents
  • Regression is a normal reaction to the neonate

● **Paternal reaction**
  • Fathers as well as mothers need to discuss the labor and delivery experience to integrate it into life experiences
  • The father may feel left out when attention is given to the neonate and mother
  • Fathers usually have less experience in and knowledge about infant care; thus, they need to be involved in the teaching plan

● **Mother-father relationship**
  • The time and effort devoted to infant care can strain the mother-father relationship
  • The father may become jealous of the mother-neonate bond
  • The parents should consider baby-sitting arrangements to allow private time for themselves

Key facts about a neonate's impact on the family

• Reactions of siblings will depend on their age, the number of other siblings, and the amount of preparation.
• Fathers usually have less experience in infant care and need to be involved in the teaching plan.
• The time and effort devoted to infant care can strain the parents' relationship.

When to monitor vital signs

- Every 15 minutes during the first hour after delivery
- Every 30 minutes during the second hour
- Every 4 hours for the remainder of the first postpartum day
- Every 8 hours thereafter

When to check the tone and location of the fundus

- Every 15 minutes for the first hour after delivery
- Every 30 minutes for the next 2 to 3 hours
- Every hour for the next 4 hours
- Every 4 hours for the rest of the first postpartum day

Key facts about the postpartum position of the fundus

- It's usually midway between the umbilicus and symphysis 1 to 2 hours after delivery.
- It's 1 cm above or at the level of the umbilicus 12 hours after delivery.
- It's about 3 cm below the umbilicus by the third day after delivery.
- It continues to descend about 1 cm/day.

POSTPARTUM NURSING CARE

● **Vital signs**
- Monitor vital signs every 15 minutes during the first hour after delivery, every 30 minutes during the second hour, every 4 hours for the remainder of the first postpartum day, then every 8 hours thereafter
  – Always take oral or axillary temperature to reduce risk of perineal contamination with rectal temperatures
  – Be aware that the patient's temperature may be elevated to 100.4° F (38° C) from dehydration and exertion of labor
  – Suspect a postpartum infection with any elevation in temperature above 100.4° F after the first 24 hours
- Evaluate pulse rate based on the woman's usual prepartum pulse rate
  – Be aware that bradycardia (50 to 70 beats/minute) is common during the first 6 to 10 days after delivery because of reductions in cardiac strain, stroke volume, and the vascular bed
  – Report a rapid, thready pulse, which could indicate hemorrhage
- Expect the respiratory rate to return to normal after delivery
- Compare postpartum blood pressure with the patient's prepregnancy blood pressure
  – Keep in mind that the woman's blood pressure is usually normotensive within 24 hours of delivery
  – Be alert for an increase in systolic blood pressure greater than 140 mm Hg or diastolic blood pressure greater than 90 mm Hg; these could suggest development of postpartum pregnancy-induced hypertension
  – Check for evidence of orthostatic hypotension, which may develop secondary to blood loss

● **Fundus**
- Check the tone and location of the fundus (the uppermost portion of the uterus) every 15 minutes for the first hour after delivery, every 30 minutes for the next 2 to 3 hours, every hour for the next 4 hours, every 4 hours for the rest of the first postpartum day, and then every 8 hours until the patient is discharged (see *Palpating the fundus*)
  – The involuting uterus should be at the midline
  – The fundus is usually midway between the umbilicus and symphysis 1 to 2 hours after delivery, 1 cm above or at the level of the umbilicus 12 hours after delivery, and about 3 cm below the umbilicus by the third day after delivery
  – The fundus will continue to descend about 1 cm/day until it isn't palpable above the symphysis (about 9 days after delivery)

Palpating the fundus

Before palpating the uterus, explain the procedure to the patient and provide privacy. Next, wash your hands, and put on gloves. Have the patient urinate. If she's unable to urinate, anticipate the need to catheterize her. Then lower the head of the bed until the patient is in a supine position or her head is slightly elevated, and expose the abdomen for palpation and the perineum for inspection. Watch for bleeding, clots, and tissue expulsion while massaging the uterus.

Follow these steps to palpate the uterine fundus:

- Gently compress the uterus between both hands to evaluate uterine firmness. A full-term pregnancy stretches the ligaments supporting the uterus, placing the uterus at risk for inversion during palpation and massage. To guard against this, place one hand against the patient's abdomen at the symphysis pubis level. This steadies the fundus and prevents downward displacement. Then place the other hand at the top of the fundus, cupping it.

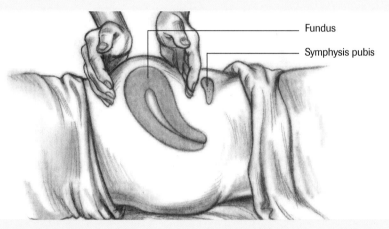

Fundus

Symphysis pubis

- Note the level of the fundus above or below the umbilicus in centimeters or fingerbreadths.
- If the uterus seems soft and boggy, gently massage the fundus with a circular motion until it becomes firm. Without digging into the abdomen, gently compress and release, always supporting the lower uterine segment with the other hand. Observe the vaginal drainage during massage.
- Massage long enough to produce firmness but not discomfort.

How to palpate the fundus

- Gently compress the uterus between both hands to evaluate firmness.
- To guard against inversion, place one hand against the patient's abdomen at the symphysis pubis. Place the other hand at the top of the fundus, cupping it.
- Note the level of the fundus above or below the umbilicus in centimeters or fingerbreadths.
- If the uterus seems soft, gently massage the fundus until it becomes firm.
- Observe for vaginal drainage during the massage.

- The uterus decreases to its prepregnancy size 5 to 6 weeks after delivery, not from a decrease in the number of cells but from a decrease in their size
- The fundus should feel firm to the touch
- Keep in mind that a firm uterus helps control postpartum hemorrhage by clamping down on uterine blood vessels
- If the fundus feels boggy (soft), massage it gently; if the fundus doesn't respond, a firmer touch should be used

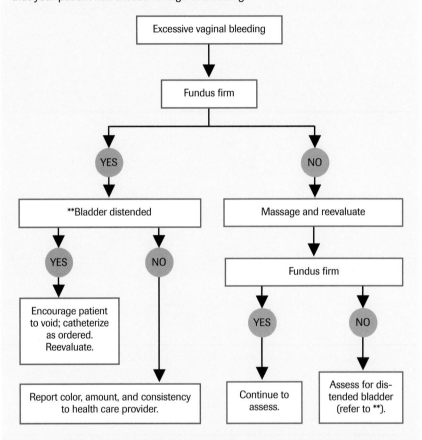

GO WITH THE FLOW

Assessing excessive vaginal bleeding

Use the flowchart below to help guide your interventions when you determine that your patient has excessive vaginal bleeding.

- Because the uterus and its supporting ligaments are tender after delivery, pain is the most common complication of fundal palpation and massage
- Excessive massage can stimulate premature uterine contractions causing undue muscle fatigue and leading to uterine atony or inversion
- Be prepared to administer oxytocin (Pitocin), ergonovine (Ergotrate), or methylergonovine (Methergine) to maintain uterine firmness as ordered
- Be alert for uterine relaxation, which may occur if the uterus relaxes from overstimulation because of massage or medication

- Suspect a distended bladder if the uterus isn't firm at the midline; a distended bladder can impede the downward descent of the uterus by pushing it upward and possibly to the side
- Evaluate any vaginal bleeding that's considered excessive (see *Assessing excessive vaginal bleeding*)
- Assess the patient for complaints of "afterpains"
    - A multipara is more prone to "afterpains" from uterine contractions
    - "Afterpains" generally last 2 to 3 days and may be intensified by breast-feeding

Lochia

- Assess lochia (discharge after delivery from sloughing of the uterine decidua) along with the fundus every 15 minutes during the first hour after delivery, every 30 minutes for the next 2 to 3 hours, every hour for the next 4 hours, every 4 hours for the rest of the first postpartum day, and then every 8 hours until the patient is discharged (see *Assessing lochia flow*)
    - Lochia rubra is the vaginal discharge for the first 3 days after delivery; it has a fleshy odor and is bloody with small clots
    - Lochia serosa is the vaginal discharge during days 4 to 9; it's pinkish or brown with a serosanguineous consistency and fleshy odor

When to assess lochia

- Every 15 minutes during the first hour after delivery
- Every 30 minutes for the next 2 to 3 hours
- Every hour for the next 4 hours
- Every 4 hours for the rest of the first postpartum day
- Every 8 hours thereafter until the patient is discharged

Assessing lochia flow

Use these guidelines when assessing a patient's lochia:

- Character: Lochia typically is described as lochia rubra, serosa, or alba, depending on the color of the discharge. Lochia should always be present during the first 3 weeks postpartum. The woman who has had a cesarean birth may have a scant amount of lochia; however, lochia is never absent.
- Amount: Although this varies, the amount can be compared to that of a menstrual flow. Saturating a perineal pad in less than 1 hour is considered excessive; the physician should be notified. Expect women who are breast-feeding to have less lochia. Lochia flow also increases with activity, for example when the patient gets out of bed the first several times (due to pooled lochia being released) or when the patient engages in strenuous exercise, such as lifting a heavy object or walking up stairs (due to an actual increase in amount).
- Color: Depending on the postpartum day, lochia typically ranges from red to pinkish brown, to creamy white or colorless. A sudden change in the color of lochia — for example, to bright red after having been pink — suggests new bleeding or retained placental fragments.
- Odor: Lochia has a similar odor to that of menstrual flow. Any foul or offensive odor suggests infection.
- Consistency: Lochia should be clot-free. Evidence of large clots indicates poor uterine contraction, which requires intervention.

Three types of lochia

- Lochia rubra — bloody with small clots and fleshy odor
- Lochia serosa — pinkish brown with serosanguineous consistency and fleshy odor
- Lochia alba — yellow to white discharge

Key steps in postpartum care

- Monitor vital signs.
- Be aware that bradycardia of 50 to 70 beats/minute is common during the first 6 to 10 days after delivery.
- Check the tone and location of the fundus.
- Assess lochia.
- Assess the breasts.

Postpartum changes in breasts

- On the first to second postpartum day, the breasts should be soft.
- By the third postpartum day, the breasts may feel warm and firm, indicating that they are filling.
- By the fourth or fifth postpartum day, the breasts may feel hard, tense, and tender and appear reddened and large, indicating engorgement.

Ensuring that the patient voids

- The patient should void within the first 6 to 8 hours after delivery.
- Check for a distended bladder.
- Use prescribed pain medication.
- Anticipate the need for urinary catheterization.

– Lochia alba is a yellow to white discharge that usually begins about 10 days after delivery; it may last from 2 to 6 weeks
- Note any foul odor; foul-smelling lochia may indicate an infection
- Watch for continuous seepage of bright red blood, which may indicate a cervical or vaginal laceration; additional evaluation is necessary
  – Lochia that saturates a sanitary pad within 45 minutes usually indicates an abnormally heavy flow
    · Weigh perineal pads to estimate the amount of blood loss
    · Be sure to look under the patient's buttocks where blood may pool
  – Lochial discharge may diminish after a cesarean delivery
- Be alert for an increase in lochia flow on arising; a heavier flow of lochia may occur when the patient first rises from bed because of pooling of the lochia in the vagina
- Evaluate amount of clots; numerous large clots require further evaluation because they may interfere with involution
- Remember that breast-feeding and exertion may increase lochia flow
- Know that lochia may be scant but should never be absent; this may indicate a postpartum infection

Breasts
- Assess the size and shape of the patient's breasts every shift, noting reddened areas, tenderness, or engorgement
  – On the first to second postpartum day, the breasts should be soft
  – By the third postpartum day, the breast may feel warm and firm, indicating that the breasts are filling
  – By the fourth or fifth postpartum day, the breasts may feel hard, tense, and tender and appear reddened and large; typically this indicates engorgement
- Check the nipples for cracking, fissures, or soreness
- Advise the patient to wear a support bra to maintain shape and enhance comfort; urge the woman to avoid bras with underwire

Elimination
- Assess the patient's elimination patterns
- Check to ensure that the patient voids within the first 6 to 8 hours after delivery
  – Check for a distended bladder within the first few hours after delivery; a distended bladder can interfere with uterine involution
  – Use prescribed pain medication before urination or pour warm water over the perineum to eliminate the fear of pain
  – Anticipate the need for urinary catheterization if the patient can't void

- · Check with the physician about the amount of urine to be removed from the bladder
  - · If catheterization yields greater than 1,000 ml of urine, expect to leave the catheter in place
  - · Too great a fluid loss at one time may lead to shock
  - · If catheter is left in place, check with the health care provider about clamping catheter and releasing every 2 hours to help improve bladder tone
- Encourage the patient to have a bowel movement within 2 days after delivery to avoid constipation
  - – Urge increased fluid and roughage intake
  - – Assist with alleviating maternal anxieties regarding pain from or damage to the episiotomy site
  - – If necessary, administer a laxative, a stool softener, a suppository, or an enema as ordered
  - – Be aware that nothing should ever be inserted into the rectum of a patient with a fourth-degree laceration

Episiotomy

- Assess the episiotomy site every shift to evaluate healing
  - – Be aware that the edges of an episiotomy are usually sealed 24 hours after delivery
  - – Note ecchymosis, hematoma, erythema, edema, drainage or bleeding from sutures, foul odor, or infection
- Position the patient comfortably when inspecting the episiotomy
  - – Position the patient with a mediolateral episiotomy on that side to provide better visibility and less discomfort
  - – Position the patient with a midline episiotomy on the side or the back during assessment

Rectal area

- Assess the rectal area
- Note the number and appearance of hemorrhoids

Medications

- Administer medications to relieve discomfort from the episiotomy, uterine contractions, incision pain, or engorged breasts, as prescribed
  - – Analgesics include propoxyphene (Darvocet-N), acetaminophen, aspirin, oxycodone with acetaminophen (Percocet), butalbital with aspirin (Fiorinal), ibuprofen (Motrin), and codeine
  - – Stool softeners and laxatives include docusate calcium (Surfak), docusate sodium (Colace), and magnesium hydroxide (milk of magnesia)

Encouraging a bowel movement

- Urge increased fluid and roughage intake.
- Assist with alleviating maternal anxieties regarding pain.
- Administer a laxative, a stool softener, a suppository, or an enema as ordered.
- Don't insert anything into the rectum of a patient with a fourth-degree laceration.

Indications of improper healing of the episiotomy site

- Ecchymosis
- Hematoma
- Erythema
- Edema
- Drainage
- Bleeding from sutures
- Foul odor
- Infection

Medications for postpartum nursing care

- Analgesics
- Stool softeners and laxatives
- Oxytocic agents

Topics for postpartum patient teaching

- Personal hygiene
- Sexual activity and contraception
- Weight loss
- Activity and exercise
- Nutrition
- Elimination
- Psychosocial adjustments

What the patient should know about lochia flow

- Look for flow to gradually reduce in amount and change color.
- Immediately report lochia with a foul smell, heavy flow, or clots. Also report lochia that changes to a bright red color.

What the patient should know about sexual activity and contraception

- Most couples can resume sexual activity 2 to 4 weeks after delivery.
- Sexual activity can resume after vaginal bleeding stops and the episiotomy heals.
- Sexual arousal can result in milk leakage from the breasts.
- Breast-feeding isn't a reliable form of contraception.
- Decreased intensity and rapidity of sexual response and vaginal dryness may occur; a water-based lubricant may be needed.
- Kegel exercises strengthen the pubococcygeal muscles.

– Oxytocic agents, such as methylergonovine (Methergine), oxytocin (Pitocin), and ergonovine (Ergotrate), help prevent or treat postpartum hemorrhage
  - Blood pressure is monitored closely for changes
  - Adjunctive therapy may be necessary because of the action of these drugs
- Monitor patient for therapeutic response and adverse reactions

POSTPARTUM PATIENT TEACHING

● Self-care instructions to the mother

- Personal hygiene
  – Change perineal pads frequently, removing from front to back
  – Monitor lochia flow
    - Look for flow to gradually reduce in amount and change color
    - Immediately report lochia with a foul smell, heavy flow, or clots; also report lochia that changes to a bright red color
  – Perform perineal care with each voiding, bowel movement, and pad change
  – Take a sitz bath three to four times daily as directed by the health care provider (see *Using a sitz bath*)
  – Take a daily shower to relieve discomfort of normal postpartum diaphoresis
  – Dispose of perineal pads in plastic bag
- Sexual activity and contraception
  – Follow the health care provider's instructions on sexual activity and contraception
    - Most couples can resume sexual activity 2 to 4 weeks after delivery
    - Cessation of vaginal bleeding and healing of the episiotomy are necessary before sexual activity can resume
    - Sexual arousal can result in milk leakage from the breasts
    - Breast-feeding isn't a reliable form of contraception
    - About 50% of bottle-feeding mothers ovulate during the first cycle after delivery; about 80% of breast-feeding mothers have several anovulatory cycles before ovulating
  – Use a water-based lubricant, if needed (steroid depletion may diminish vaginal lubrication for up to 6 months)
  – Expect decreased intensity and rapidity of sexual response (a normal response for about 3 months after delivery)
  – Perform Kegel exercises to help strengthen the pubococcygeal muscles

TIME-OUT FOR TEACHING

Using a sitz bath

Sitz bath therapy involves immersion of the perineal area in warm or hot water to relieve discomfort and promote wound healing by cleaning the perineum and anus, which helps increase circulation and reduce inflammation. It also helps relax local muscles.

In most cases, a commercial disposable sitz bath kit that includes a plastic basin that fits over a commode and an irrigation bag with tubing and clamp is used.

To ensure that your patient uses a sitz bath correctly, have her follow these steps:

- Assemble the equipment.
- Empty her bladder, and wash her hands.
- Fill the basin to the specified line with water at the prescribed temperature (usually 100° to 105° F [37.8° to 40.6° C]). Check water temperature frequently to ensure its therapeutic effects.
- Place the basin under the commode seat, clamp the irrigation tubing to block water flow, and fill the irrigation bag with water of the same temperature as that in the basin.
- To create flow pressure, hang the bag above her head on a hook, towel rack or edge of a door.
- Remove and dispose of her perineal pad, and then sit on the basin.
- If her feet don't reach the floor and the weight of her legs presses against the edge of the equipment, she should place a small stool under her feet. Also have her place a folded towel or small pillow against her lower back.
- Cover her shoulders and knees with blankets or robe to prevent chilling.
- Open the clamp on the irrigation tubing to allow a stream of water to flow continuously. Refill the bag with water of the correct temperature, as needed, and continue to regulate the flow.
- After 15 to 20 minutes, clamp the tubing and rest for a few minutes

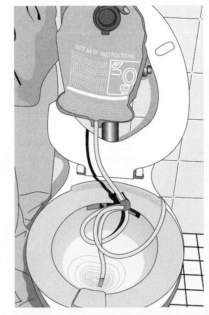

before arising to prevent dizziness and light-headedness.
- Pat the area dry from front to back, and apply a new perineal pad (by holding the bottom sides or ends).
- Properly dispose of soiled materials. Empty and clean the sitz bath according to manufacturer's directions.
- Report any changes in drainage amount or characteristics, complaints of light-headedness, diaphoresis, weakness, nausea, or irregular heart rate.
- Promptly dress afterward to prevent vasoconstriction.

Steps for using a sitz bath

- Fill the basin with water at the prescribed temperature (usually 100° to 105° F [37.8° to 40.6° C]).
- Place the basin under the commode seat.
- Clamp the irrigation tubing.
- Fill the irrigation bag with water of the same temperature as that in the basin.
- Hang the bag on a hook above your head.
- Remove the perineal pad and sit on the basin.
- Open the clamp on the irrigation tubing to allow a stream of water to flow continuously.
- After 15 to 20 minutes, clamp the tubing
- Rest for a few minutes before rising (prevents dizziness and light-headedness).
- Pat the area dry from front to back.
- Apply a new perineal pad.

What the patient should know about weight loss

- The patient should expect to lose about 5 lb (2.3 kg) from diuresis during the early puerperium.
- The patient should expect to lose 10 to 12 lb (4.5 to 5.5 kg) after delivery.
- The patient should expect to return to prepregnancy weight within 6 to 8 weeks.

What the patient should know about activity and exercise

- The patient should nap during the day and rest when the neonate rests.
- The patient should begin slowly; abdominal breathing exercises can be started on the first postpartum day.
- Chin-to-chest exercises may be allowed on the second postpartum day, and arm-raising exercises on the fourth postpartum days.
- Abdominal crunches are usually postponed for at least 1½ to 2 weeks.
- Lochia increase (or lochia rubra return) may indicate excessive activity.

What the patient should know about nutrition

- The patient should increase protein and caloric intake, especially if breast-feeding.
- The patient can expect to be thirsty and should drink plenty of fluids.
- The patient should eat foods high in fiber.

- Weight loss
  - Expect to lose about 5 lb (2.3 kg) from diuresis during the early puerperium (in addition to the 10 to 12 lb [4.5 to 5.5 kg] typically lost after delivery)
  - Expect to return to prepregnancy weight within 6 to 8 weeks after delivery (if weight gain during pregnancy was 25 to 30 lb [11.3 to 13.6 kg])
- Activity and exercise
  - Request assistance in getting out of bed the first several times after delivery to minimize dizziness and fainting from medications, blood loss, and decreased food intake
  - Be sure to get adequate amounts of rest
    - Take naps during the day
    - Rest when the neonate is resting
  - Begin exercising when allowed by the health care provider; start slowly and gradually increase the amount done
    - Abdominal breathing exercises can be started on the first postpartum day
    - Chin-to-chest exercises are typically allowed on the second postpartum day; arm-raising exercises can be included on the fourth postpartum day
    - Abdominal crunches are usually postponed for at least 1½ to 2 weeks after delivery
  - Sit with the legs elevated for about 30 minutes if lochia increases or lochia rubra returns, either of which may indicate excessive activity; if excessive vaginal discharge persists, notify the health care provider
  - Expect abdominal muscle tone to increase 2 to 3 months after delivery
- Nutrition
  - Increase protein and caloric intake to restore body tissues
  - If breast-feeding, increase daily caloric intake by 200 kcal over the pregnancy requirement of 2,400 kcal
  - Expect increased thirst because of postpartum diuresis
  - If breast-feeding, drink at least ten 8-oz (237-ml) glasses of water per day
  - Drink plenty of fluids, especially water, and eat foods that are high in fiber to prevent constipation
- Elimination
  - Don't ignore the urge to defecate or urinate
  - Notify the health care provider of complaints of burning or pain on urination
  - Use stool softeners as prescribed

– Use witch hazel compresses, sitz baths, or anesthetic sprays to help relieve discomfort of hemorrhoids

– Lie on the left side with the upper leg flexed to help reduce the discomfort of hemorrhoids

- Comfort measures
  – To relieve perineal discomfort, use ice packs for the first 8 to 12 hours to minimize edema
  – Perform perineal care using peri bottles, sitz baths as ordered
  – Use anesthetic sprays, creams, and pads and prescribed pain medications to help relieve pain and discomfort
  – To relieve discomfort from engorged breasts, wear a supportive bra, apply ice packs, and take prescribed medications
  – If breast-feeding, eat frequent meals, apply warm compresses, and express milk manually from the breasts
- Psychosocial adjustments
  – Don't be alarmed by mood swings and bouts of depression; these are normal postpartum responses
    - More than half of postpartum women experience transient mood alterations called "baby blues"
    - Common signs and symptoms include sadness, crying, fatigue, and low self-esteem
    - Possible causes include hormonal changes, genetic predisposition, and altered role and self-concept
  – Know that mood swings typically occur within the first 3 weeks after delivery and usually subside within 1 to 10 days
- Make a follow-up appointment for 4 to 6 weeks after delivery

● Neonatal care instructions for the parents
- Cord care
  – Wipe the umbilical cord with alcohol, especially around the base, at every diaper change
  – Report promptly any odor, discharge, or signs of skin irritation around the cord
  – Fold the diaper below the cord until the cord falls off (7 to 10 days)
- Circumcised penis care
  – Gently clean the penis with water, and apply fresh petroleum gauze with each diaper change
  – Loosen petroleum gauze stuck to the penis by pouring warm water over the area
  – Don't remove yellow discharge that covers the glans about 24 hours after circumcision; this is part of normal healing
  – Report promptly any foul-smelling, purulent discharge
  – Apply diapers loosely until the circumcision heals (about 5 days)

Ways the patient can relieve discomfort

- Use ice packs, peri bottles, or sitz baths to minimize perineal edema and discomfort.
- Use anesthetic sprays, creams, and pads and prescribed pain medications to help relieve pain and discomfort.
- Wear a supportive bra, apply ice packs, and take prescribed medications to relieve discomfort from engorged breasts.
- If breast-feeding, eat frequent meals, apply warm compresses, and express milk manually.

Topics for neonatal care

- Cord care
- Circumcised or uncircumcised penis care
- Elimination
- Thermometer use
- Diapering and clothing
- Bathing
- Breast-feeding and breast care
- Bottle-feeding and formula preparation
- Health promotion and illness prevention

What parents should know about cord care

- Wipe the umbilical cord with alcohol.
- Report odor, discharge, or signs of skin irritation.
- Fold the neonate's diaper below the cord until the cord falls off.

What parents should know about neonatal elimination

- The first stool is called *meconium;* it's a thick, odorless, dark green substance.
- Transitional stools occur 2 to 3 days after ingestion of milk; they're greenish brown and thinner than meconium.
- The stool changes to a pasty, pungent, yellow stool (bottle-fed neonate) or to a loose, sweet-smelling yellow stool (breast-fed neonate) by the fourth day.

What parents should know about thermometer use

- Don't use a glass mercury bulb thermometer in the rectum.
- Obtain the temperature under the arm or via the ear (tympanic membrane).
- Hold an axillary thermometer in place for 10 minutes.

What parents should know about diapering

- Change diapers before and after every feeding.
- Change diapers frequently and dry skin thoroughly to prevent diaper rash.
- Apply ointment sparingly to prevent contact of urine and feces with skin.
- Don't use powders.

- Uncircumcised penis care
  - Don't retract the foreskin when washing the neonate because the foreskin is adhered to the glans
  - Understand that although natural loosening of the foreskin begins at birth, it's retractable in only about 50% of males age 1
- Elimination
  - Become familiar with the neonate's voiding patterns (usually six to eight wet diapers daily)
  - Become familiar with the neonate's bowel patterns (usually two to three stools daily; more frequently if breast-fed)
    - The first stool is called *meconium;* it's an odorless, dark green, thick substance containing bile, fetal epithelial cells, and hair
    - Transitional stools occur 2 to 3 days after ingestion of milk; they are greenish brown and thinner than meconium
    - The stool changes to a pasty, yellow, pungent stool (bottle-fed neonate) or to a sweet-smelling loose yellow stool (breast-fed neonate) by the fourth day
- Thermometer use
  - Refrain from using a glass mercury bulb thermometer in the neonate's rectum
  - Obtain the neonate's temperature under the arm (axillary) or via the ear (tympanic membrane)
    - Carefully place an axillary thermometer under the arm and hold in place for 10 minutes
    - Be aware of alternate devices for obtaining temperature, including a plastic temperature strip and pacifiers with a built-in thermometer
  - Report any temperature greater than 99° F (37.2° C)
- Diapering
  - Change diapers before and after every feeding
  - Avoid diaper rash with frequent diaper changes and thorough cleaning and drying of the skin; be sure to clean thoroughly between the skin folds
  - Expose the neonate's buttocks to the air and light several times per day for about 20 minutes to treat diaper rash
  - Apply ointment sparingly to prevent contact of urine and feces with skin
  - Avoid the use of powders; they irritate the pores of the skin and may cause respiratory difficulties in the neonate
- Bathing
  - Give the neonate sponge baths until the cord falls off; then wash him in a tub containing 4″ (10 cm) of warm water
  - Never leave the neonate unattended in the tub

– Place a washcloth on the bottom of the tub or sink to prevent slipping
– Use tepid bath water temperature because neonatal thermoregulation is unstable
– Avoid using perfumed or deodorant soap
– Organize supplies before the bath to avoid interruptions
– Keep room temperature between 68° and 72° F (20° to 22.2° C) and avoid drafts
– Avoid using soap on the face; clean the eye from the inner to outer canthus with plain water
– Vary the frequency of bathing with weather; a bath every other day during winter is sufficient

• Clothing
– Dress the infant appropriately according to indoor temperatures and outdoor weather conditions
– Layer clothing appropriately because infants don't shiver
– Provide the infant with a hat to avoid drafts and minimize heat loss through the scalp when outdoors

• Breast-feeding
– Initiate breast-feeding as soon as possible after delivery, and then feed the neonate on demand (see *Physiology of lactation,* page 326)
– Drink a beverage before and during or after breast-feeding to ensure adequate fluid intake and maintain milk production
– Be sure to attend to personal needs and change the neonate's diaper before breast-feeding begins so that feeding is uninterrupted
– Wash your hands before breast-feeding, and find a comfortable position (see *Breast-feeding positions,* page 327)
– Expose one breast, and rest the nape of the neonate's neck in the crook of the arm, supporting his back with the forearm
– Try to relax during breast-feeding because relaxation also promotes the letdown reflex
  • Be aware that you may feel a tingling sensation when it occurs and that milk may drip or spray from the breasts; it may also be initiated by hearing the neonate's cry
  • Remember that uterine cramping may occur during breast-feeding until the uterus returns to its original size
– Place thumb of free hand on top of the exposed breast's areola and first two fingers beneath it, forming a "C" with the hand
– Turn the neonate so that he faces the breast
– Stroke the neonate's cheek located nearest to the exposed breast or the neonate's mouth with the nipple, to stimulate the rooting reflex
– Avoid touching the neonate's other cheek because he may turn his head toward the touch and away from the breast

What parents should know about bathing

• Give the neonate a sponge bath until the cord falls off.
• Fill the tub or sink with 4" of water.
• Never leave the neonate unattended.
• Place a washcloth on the bottom of the tub or sink.
• Use tepid water.
• Avoid the use of perfumed or deodorant soaps.
• Don't use soap on the face; clean the eyes from the inner to the outer canthus with plain water.

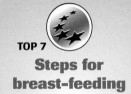

TOP 7

Steps for breast-feeding

1. Drink a beverage before and during or after breast-feeding.
2. Place thumb of free hand on top of the exposed breast's areola and first two fingers beneath it, forming a "C" with the hand.
3. Turn the neonate so that he faces the breast.
4. Stroke the cheek nearest to the breast or stroke the neonate's mouth with the nipple to stimulate the rooting reflex.
5. Position the neonate's mouth slightly differently at each feeding to reduce irritation.
6. Burp the neonate before switching to the other breast.
7. Follow a diet that ensures adequate nutrition.

Key facts about breast milk

- Produced in the acinar cells of the mammary glands
- Production stimulated by pro-lactin and neonate sucking
- Flows from acinar cells to lac-tiferous sinuses in nipple
- Movement of milk through the nipple is called the *let-down reflex*
- Two types of milk
- Foremilk: constantly forming
- Hind milk: forms after let-down reflex; has higher fat content than foremilk

Physiology of lactation

The acinar (also called alveolar) cells of the mammary gland are the site of milk production. After delivery of the placenta, the drop in progesterone and estrogen levels stimulates the production of prolactin. This hormone acts on the acinar cells stimulating milk production. Nerve impulses that result from the neonate sucking at the breast travel from the nipple to the hypothalamus resulting in the production of prolactin releasing factor. This leads to additional production of prolactin and subsequently, more milk production.

Milk flows from the acinar cells through small tubules to the lactiferous sinuses (small reservoirs), located behind the nipple. This milk, called *foremilk,* is constantly forming. When the infant sucks at the breast, oxytocin is released causing the sinuses to contract. Contraction pushes the milk forward, through the nipple to the neonate. In addition, release of oxytocin causes the smooth muscles of the uterus to contract.

Movement of the milk forward through the nipple is termed the *let-down reflex* and may be triggered by incidents other than the infant sucking at the breast. For example, women have reported that hearing a baby cry or thinking about a baby has led to this reflex. Once the let-down reflex occurs, new milk, called *hind milk* is formed. Hind milk has a higher fat content than foremilk. It's this milk that leads to rapid growth of the breast-fed neonate.

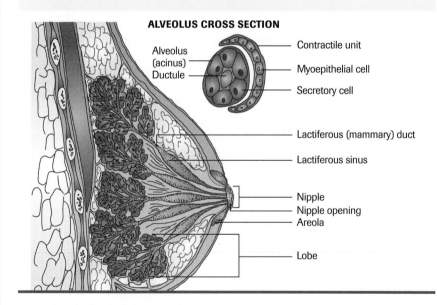

ALVEOLUS CROSS SECTION

Alveolus (acinus)
Ductule

Contractile unit
Myoepithelial cell
Secretory cell

Lactiferous (mammary) duct

Lactiferous sinus

Nipple
Nipple opening
Areola

Lobe

- When the neonate opens his mouth and roots for the nipple, in-sert the nipple and as much of the areola as possible into his mouth; this helps him to exert sufficient pressure with his lips, gums, and cheek muscles on the milk sinuses below the areola
- Check for blockage of the neonate's nostrils by the breast; if this happens, reposition the neonate to give him room to breathe
- Begin nursing the neonate for 15 minutes on each breast
- Switch to the other breast; slip a finger into the side of the neonate's mouth to break the seal and move him to the other breast; never just pull it because doing so can damage the areola

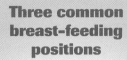

Breast-feeding positions

A breast-feeding position should be comfortable and efficient. By changing positions periodically, the woman can alter the neonate's grasp on the nipple, thereby avoiding contact friction on the same area. As appropriate, suggest these three common positions.

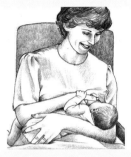 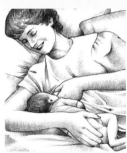 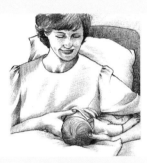

CRADLE POSITION
The mother cradles the neonate's head in the crook of her arm.

SIDE-LYING POSITION
The mother lies on her side with her stomach facing the neonate's. As the neonate's mouth opens, she pulls him or her toward the nipple.

FOOTBALL POSITION
Sitting with a pillow under her arm, the mother places her hand under the neonate's head. As the neonate's mouth opens, she pulls the neonate's head near her breast. This position may be helpful for the woman who has had a cesarean birth.

Three common breast-feeding positions

- Cradle — the neonate's head is placed in the crook of the mother's arm
- Side-lying — the mother is on her side with neonate next to her
- Football — the mother sits with a pillow and the neonate's body under her arm; the neonate's head is pulled to the breast

- Expect about 90% of breast milk to be emptied from the breasts within the first 7 minutes of feeding
- Position the neonate's mouth slightly differently at each feeding to reduce irritation at one site
- Burp the neonate before switching to the other breast by placing him over one shoulder and gently patting or rubbing the back to help expel any digested air; alternatively hold the neonate in a sitting position on the lap, leaning him forward against one hand and supporting his head and neck with the index finger and thumb of that same hand or placing the neonate in a prone position across the lap
- Experiment with various breast-feeding positions (cradle, football hold, side-lying, and Australian or back-lying) to find the most comfortable one
– Perform thorough breast care to promote cleanliness and comfort
- After each feeding, wash the nipples and areolae with plain warm water and air dry during the first 2 to 3 weeks to prevent

Breast care after breast-feeding

- After each feeding, wash the nipples and areolae with plain warm water and let them air dry during the first 2 to 3 weeks to prevent nipple soreness.
- Avoid using soap, which can dry and crack the nipples and also leaves an undesirable taste for the neonate.
- Apply nonalcoholic cream to the nipple and areola to prevent drying and cracking.

Dietary recommendations for a breast-feeding mother

- Drink at least four 8-oz glasses of fluid daily.
- Increase daily caloric intake by 500 kcal above the pregnancy requirement of 2,500 kcal.
- Limit intake of caffeine and alcohol.
- Avoid foods that cause irritability, gas, or diarrhea.
- Consult with the primary health care provider before taking any medications.

Tips for formula feeding

- Make sure the seal on the formula bottle wasn't previously broken.
- Screw on the nipple and cap, keeping the protective sterile cap over the nipple until the neonate is ready to feed.
- Place the nipple on the neonate's mouth while making sure the tongue is down.
- Administer the formula at room temperature or slightly warmer.
- Invert the bottle and shake some formula onto your wrist to test the patency of the nipple and the formula's temperature.
- Always hold the bottle for the neonate.
- As the neonate feeds, tilt the bottle upward.
- Burp the neonate after each ½ to 1 oz of formula.

nipple soreness; after that, daily washing is adequate for cleanliness
  - Avoid using soap, which can dry and crack the nipples and leave an undesirable taste for the neonate
  - Apply nonalcoholic cream to the nipple and areola to prevent drying and cracking
- Wear a well-fitted nursing bra that provides support and contains flaps that can be loosened easily before feeding
- Use breast pads to avoid staining clothes from leakage, and change wet pads promptly to avoid skin breakdown
- Begin the next feeding using the breast on which the neonate finished this feeding; place a safety pin on the strap of the bra on the side last used as a reminder to begin on this breast for the next feeding
- Use the neonate's behavior as cues to determine if he's getting enough breast milk; a neonate who's content between feedings, wetting 6 to 8 diapers per day, and gaining weight is getting adequate nutrition
- Empty engorged breasts manually or with a breast pump
  - Expressed breast milk can be placed in a sterile bottle and stored in the refrigerator for 24 hours
  - Expressed breast milk can be frozen for up to 3 months
- Follow a diet that ensures adequate nutrition for both mother and neonate
  - Drink at least four 8-oz (237-ml) glasses of fluid daily
  - Increase daily caloric intake by 500 kcal above the pregnancy requirement of 2,500 kcal
  - Be aware that ingested substances (caffeine, alcohol, and medications) can pass into breast milk
  - Avoid foods that cause irritability, gas, or diarrhea
- Consult the **health care provider before taking any medications**
- Consider joining a breast-feeding support group, if desired
- Bottle-feeding and formula preparation
  - Follow the health care provider's instructions
  - Investigate various forms of formula available (ready-to-feed, concentrated, and powder) and preparation methods
    - If using commercially prepared formula, uncap the formula bottle, making sure the seal wasn't previously broken to ensure sterility and freshness
    - Then screw on the nipple and cap, keeping the protective sterile cap over the nipple until the neonate is ready to feed
    - If preparing formula, follow the manufacturer's instructions or the health care provider's prescription

- Administer the formula at room temperature or slightly warmer
- After properly preparing the formula and washing hands, invert the bottle and shake some formula onto the wrist to test the patency of the nipple hole and the formula's temperature
- Watch so that the formula drips freely but doesn't stream out
  - This indicates that the nipple hole is an appropriate size
  - If the hole is too large, the neonate may aspirate formula
  - If the hole is too small, the extra sucking effort he expends may tire him before he can empty the bottle
- Sit comfortably in a semireclining position, and cradle the neonate in one arm to support his head and back
  - This position allows swallowed air to rise to the top of the stomach where it's more easily expelled
  - If he can't be held, sit by him and elevate his head and shoulders slightly
- Place the nipple in the neonate's mouth while making sure the tongue is down, but don't insert it so far that it stimulates the gag reflex
  - The neonate should begin to suck, pulling in as much nipple as is comfortable
  - If he doesn't start to suck, stroke him under the chin or on his cheek, or touch his lips with the nipple to stimulate his sucking reflex
- As the neonate feeds, tilt the bottle upward to keep the nipple filled with formula and to prevent him from swallowing air
  - Watch for a steady stream of bubbles in the bottle
  - This indicates proper venting and flow of formula
- If the neonate pushes out the nipple with his tongue, reinsert the nipple
  - Expelling the nipple is a normal reflex
  - It doesn't necessarily mean that the neonate is full
– Always hold the bottle for a neonate; never leave a bottle propped in the neonate's mouth
  - If left to feed himself, he may aspirate formula or swallow air if the bottle tilts or empties
  - Experts link bottle propping with an increased incidence of otitis media and dental caries in older infants
– Burp the neonate after each ½ to 1 oz (15- to 30-ml) of formula (more frequently if the neonate spits up); hold him upright against the shoulder for burping
  - Holding the neonate across the lap for burping may bring up milk along with the air
  - Holding the neonate in a sitting position may prove ineffective because the air can't easily exit the stomach

Using the right size nipple hole

- If the formula drips freely but doesn't stream out, the nipple hole is an appropriate size.
- If the hole is too large, the neonate may aspirate formula.
- If the hole is too small, the extra sucking effort the neonate expends may tire him before he can empty the bottle.

Why a bottle shouldn't be propped in the neonate's mouth

- If the neonate is left to feed himself, he may aspirate formula or swallow air if the bottle tilts or empties.
- Experts link bottle propping with an increased incidence of otitis media and dental caries in older infants.

- A neonate who hasn't burped after 3 minutes of gentle patting and rubbing may not need to burp
  - Handling
    - Be aware that neonates have an inborn fear of falling and become upset if left unsupported or if their position is abruptly changed
    - Don't startle the neonate; talk softly and touch gently before picking him up
    - Support the neonate's head; he can't control it
  - Health promotion and illness prevention
    - Don't expose the neonate to persons with communicable illnesses
    - Minimize the neonate's exposure to crowds
    - Provide adequate covering and clothing
    - Use a reliable car seat (legally required)
    - Immediately report signs and symptoms of illness to the health care provider
      - Temperature greater than 101° F (38.3° C) or below 97° F (36.1° C)
      - Projectile vomiting
      - Lethargy
      - Cyanosis
      - Change in normal feeding pattern
      - Change in normal elimination pattern

Tips for promoting neonatal health and preventing illness

- Don't expose the neonate to persons with communicable illnesses.
- Minimize the neonate's exposure to crowds.
- Provide adequate covering and clothing.
- Use a reliable car seat.
- Immediately report signs and symptoms of illness, including a temperature > 101° F (38.3° C) or < 97° F (36.1° C), projectile vomiting, lethargy, and cyanosis.

NCLEX CHECKS

It's never too soon to begin your NCLEX preparation. Now that you've reviewed this chapter, carefully read each of the following questions and choose the best answer. Then compare your responses to the correct answers.

1. Which changes occur in the woman during the postpartum period? Select all that apply.

☑ **A.** Increased hematocrit
☑ **B.** Increased hunger
☑ **C.** Increased urine output
☐ **D.** Increased progesterone production
☐ **E.** Increased blood volume

2. Which behavior would the postpartum woman demonstrate during the taking-in phase?

☑ **A.** Passive dependent role *taking in phase energy towards self*
☐ **B.** Increased energy *Talking hold*
☐ **C.** Receptiveness to self-care education *Talking hold*
☐ **D.** Increased responsibility for neonate *Letting go phase*

3. On the second postpartum day, where would the nurse expect to palpate the fundus?

- ☐ **A.** 1 cm above the umbilicus
- ☐ **B.** At the level of the umbilicus
- ☐ **C.** 1 cm below the umbilicus
- ☒ **D.** 2 cm below the umbilicus

4. When assessing a woman's lochia on the fifth postpartum day, what would the nurse expect to find?

- ☐ **A.** Lochia rubra *1st 1–3*
- ☒ **B.** Lochia serosa *3rd 4–9*
- ☐ **C.** Lochia alba *2nd 10 day*
- ☐ **D.** Absence of lochia

5. Which instruction about neonatal care would the nurse include in the discharge-teaching plan for a woman and her male neonate?

- ☐ **A.** Pull the foreskin back from the head of the penis when bathing him.
- ☐ **B.** Report any foul odor coming from the circumcision or umbilical cord site.
- ☐ **C.** Be sure to check the child's rectal temperature every morning.
- ☐ **D.** Use soap and water to wash the neonate's face.

6. Which action is appropriate for a woman who's breast-feeding?

- ☒ **A.** Having the neonate begin the next feeding on the breast last used for the previous feeding
- ☐ **B.** Wearing a loose-fitting bra that can be closed in the front instead of the back
- ☐ **C.** Washing the breasts after each feeding with warm soapy water and then patting them dry
- ☐ **D.** Establishing a feeding schedule of every 2 hours initially and then every 3 to 4 hours

ANSWERS AND RATIONALES

1. CORRECT ANSWERS: A, B, AND C

After delivery, the woman experiences an increased urine output secondary to diuresis, increased hematocrit, and increased hunger. Progesterone production decreases until the first ovulation. Blood volume decreases after a vaginal delivery.

2. CORRECT ANSWER: A

During the taking-in phase, the woman typically demonstrates a passive dependent role, directing her energy toward herself instead of the neonate. Increased energy and receptiveness to self-care education are typical behaviors

---

TOP 7

Items to study for your next test on the normal postpartum period

1. The key postpartum physiologic changes
2. The three psychological phases of the postpartum period
3. The frequency with which vital signs should be monitored after delivery
4. The method for checking tone and position of the fundus
5. The interventions to institute for excessive vaginal bleeding
6. The three types of lochia as well as the character, amount, color, odor, and consistency of lochia
7. Postpartum teaching topics: episiotomy care, nutrition, breast-feeding, neonatal care, and formula preparation

of the taking-hold phase. Taking increased responsibility for the neonate is typical in the letting-go phase.

3. CORRECT ANSWER: D

For each postpartum day, the uterus descends about 1 cm. Therefore on the second postpartum day, the uterus would be 2 cm below the umbilicus. The uterus would be 1 cm above or at the level of the umbilicus approximately 12 hours after delivery and 1 cm below the umbilicus by the first postpartum day.

4. CORRECT ANSWER: B

From postpartum days 4 through about 9, lochia serosa is found. Lochia rubra is found during the first three postpartum days. Lochia alba typically begins on the 10th postpartum day, possibly lasting 2 to 6 weeks. Lochia should never be absent in the early postpartum period. However, it may be absent by the time the woman goes for her 6-week follow-up appointment.

5. CORRECT ANSWER: B

Parents need to be instructed to report any foul odor coming from the circumcision or umbilical cord site. This could indicate an infection, which requires prompt treatment. The foreskin shouldn't be pulled back on the neonate because it is adhered to the glans. Temperature should be monitored, but not rectally. The neonate's temperature should be checked via the axillary or tympanic route. It also isn't necessary to check the neonate's temperature every day. When washing the neonate's face, only water should be used and the eyes should be wiped with a clean corner of a washcloth from the inner to the outer canthus.

6. CORRECT ANSWER: A

When breast-feeding, the woman should have the neonate begin the next feeding using the breast on which the neonate finished the previous feeding to help ensure complete emptying of the breast. The woman should wear a well-fitting bra that provides support and contains flaps that can be loosened easily before feeding. After each feeding, the woman should wash her breasts with water, and allow them to air dry. Breast-feeding should be initiated as soon as possible after delivery, and then the neonate is fed on demand.

11

Complications and high-risk conditions of the postpartum period

---

LEARNING OBJECTIVES

After studying this chapter, you should be able to:

● Describe management of the patient with mastitis.
● Identify predisposing factors to uterine subinvolution and late postpartum hemorrhage.
● Give examples of various puerperal psychiatric disorders.
● Describe management of the HIV-positive patient throughout pregnancy.

CHAPTER OVERVIEW

During the postpartum period, women remain at risk for complications due to many factors, including fatigue, blood loss, trauma, and infection. Prevention or early detection is vital to minimize difficulties during this period of great physiologic and psychological stress. The patient with human immunodeficiency virus (HIV) needs special attention throughout the pregnancy, but especially during the postpartum period.

MASTITIS

● **Description**
  • Refers to the parenchymatous inflammation of the mammary glands
    • Occurs postpartum in about 1% of women, mainly in primiparas who are breast-feeding

TIME-OUT FOR TEACHING

Preventing mastitis

To help prevent mastitis, be sure to include these instructions in your teaching plan for a patient who's breast-feeding:

- Always wash your hands before and after breast-feeding.
- If necessary, apply warm compresses or take a warm shower to help facilitate milk flow.
- Make sure the neonate is positioned properly at the breast and grasps the nipple and entire areola area when feeding.

- Empty the breasts as completely as possible with each feeding.
- Alternate feeding positions, and rotate pressure areas.
- Release the neonate's grasp on the nipple before removing him from the breast.
- Expose your nipples to the air for at least a portion of each day.
- Drink plenty of fluids, eat a balanced diet, and get sufficient rest to enhance the breast-feeding experience.

Predisposing factors for mastitis

- Fissure or abrasion on the nipple
- Blocked milk ducts — for example, from a constrictive bra or prolonged intervals between breast-feeding sessions
- Incomplete let-down reflex, usually due to emotional trauma

- Occurs occasionally in nonlactating females and rarely in males
- Predisposing factors
  - Fissure or abrasion on the nipple
  - Blocked milk ducts — for example, from a constrictive bra or prolonged intervals between breast-feeding sessions
  - Incomplete let-down reflex, usually due to emotional trauma
- Is generally preventable with good breast hygiene and hand washing

● **Pathophysiology**
- Causative organism is usually *Staphylococcus aureus* from the neonate's throat or nose, from the mother, or an organism carried by facility personnel such as methicillin-resistant *S. aureus*
- The pathologic organism usually enters through a crack or fissure in the nipples
- After it enters, the organism travels to the milk ducts where breast milk provides an excellent medium for growth

● **Assessment findings**
- Temperature is elevated, typically 101° F (38.3° C) or higher in those with acute mastitis
- The patient may complain of chills, general malaise, and headache
- Breast is red, warm, and tender — typically occurring 2 to 4 weeks after delivery
- Mastitis is usually unilateral and breast milk may become scant
- Cultures of expressed breast milk are used to confirm generalized mastitis and cultures of breast skin to confirm localized mastitis; such cultures are also used to determine antibiotic therapy

What to look for in mastitis

- Elevated temperature
- Chills
- Malaise
- Headache
- Red, warm, tender breast
- Scant breast milk

TIME-OUT FOR TEACHING

Patient with mastitis

Be sure to include these topics in your teaching plan for the patient who has mastitis:
- underlying cause of mastitis
- hand-washing procedure

- heat application, including technique, frequency, and duration
- breast-emptying techniques, if appropriate
- medication regimen
- follow-up appointment.

Treatment
- Administration of an antibiotic for 10 days
- Administration of an analgesic
- Application of local heat
- Possible cessation of breast-feeding (medical opinions vary concerning continuation or stoppage of breast-feeding during the acute phase)
- Incision and drainage, if mastitis progresses to breast abscess

Nursing interventions
- Institute measures to prevent mastitis (see *Preventing mastitis*)
- Institute infection-control measures for the patient and her infant to prevent the spread of infection to other nursing mothers; also, explain mastitis to the patient and why these measures are necessary
- Administer antibiotic therapy as ordered
- Assess and record the cause and amount of discomfort; give an analgesic as needed
- If breast-feeding is allowed to continue, tell the mother to offer the infant the affected breast first to promote complete emptying of the breast and prevent clogged ducts; however, if an open abscess develops, advise her to stop breast-feeding with this breast and continue to breast-feed on the unaffected side, using a breast pump until the abscess heals
- Suggest applying a warm, wet towel to the affected breast or taking a warm shower to relax and improve her ability to breast-feed
- Use meticulous hand-washing technique, and provide good skin care
- Tell the patient to take the antibiotic *exactly* as prescribed, even if her symptoms subside
- Show how to position the infant properly to prevent cracked nipples
- To relieve symptoms of mastitis, teach the patient good health care, breast care, and breast-feeding habits; advise her to always wash her hands before touching her breasts
- Instruct the patient to combat fever by getting plenty of rest, drinking sufficient fluids, and following prescribed antibiotic therapy (see *Patient with mastitis*)

Treatment for mastitis
- Administration of antibiotic
- Administration of analgesic
- Application of local heat
- Possible cessation of breast-feeding
- Incision and drainage (if mastitis progresses to abscess)

Nursing interventions for mastitis
- Institute prevention measures.
- Institute infection-control measures.
- Administer antibiotic therapy as ordered.
- Give an analgesic as needed.
- If breast-feeding is to continue, tell the mother to offer the affected breast first.
- Suggest applying a warm, wet towel to the affected breast or taking a warm shower.
- Use meticulous hand-washing technique.
- Show how to position the infant properly.
- Teach the patient good health care, breast care, and breast-feeding habits.
- Instruct the patient to get plenty of rest, drink fluids, and follow the prescribed antibiotic therapy.

LATE POSTPARTUM HEMORRHAGE

Description
- Defined as uterine blood loss in excess of 500 ml occurring after the first postpartum day, anytime during the remaining 6-week postpartum period
- Sometimes it may not occur until 5 to 15 days after delivery
- Predisposing factors
  - Delivery of a large infant
  - Hydramnios
  - Dystocia
  - Grand multiparity
  - Trauma during delivery

Pathophysiology
- May stem from various causes
  - Uterine atony
  - Incomplete placental separation
  - Retained placental fragments
- As a result, the uterus can't contract firmly, allowing the opened vessels at the site of placental attachment to continue to bleed
- Lacerations of the birth canal also may lead to late postpartum hemorrhage as the site of tearing fails to form a clot, thereby sealing the area
- Disseminated intravascular coagulation (DIC) may cause postpartum hemorrhage
- Any woman is at risk for DIC postpartally; however, it's more common in women with abruptio placenta, missed abortion, or intrauterine fetal death

Assessment findings
- Bleeding that can occur suddenly in large amounts or gradually as seeping or oozing of blood
- Frequent saturation of perineal pads
- Soft uterus on palpation if the cause is retained placental fragments
- If the bleeding continues or is large in amount, signs and symptoms of hypovolemic shock
  - Pallor
  - Decreased sensorium
  - Rapid, shallow respirations
  - Drop in urine output to below 25 ml/hour
  - Rapid, thready peripheral pulses
  - Cold, clammy skin
  - Mean arterial pressure below 60 mm Hg
  - Narrowing pulse pressure

Risk factors for late postpartum hemorrhage
- Delivery of a large infant
- Hydramnios
- Dystocia
- Grand multiparity
- Trauma during delivery

Causes of late postpartum hemorrhage
- Uterine atony
- Incomplete placental separation
- Retained placental fragments
- Lacerations of the birth canal
- Disseminated intravascular coagulation

What to look for in late postpartum hemorrhage
- Bleeding that can occur suddenly in large amounts or gradually as seeping or oozing of blood
- Frequent saturation of perineal pads
- Soft uterus on palpation
- Signs and symptoms of hypovolemic shock

● Treatment

- Treatment focuses on correcting the underlying cause of the hemorrhage and instituting measures to control blood loss and minimize the extent of hypovolemic shock
- Emergency treatment relies on prompt and adequate blood and fluid replacement to restore intravascular volume and to raise blood pressure and maintain it above 60 mm Hg; rapid infusion of normal saline or lactated Ringer's solution and, possibly, albumin or other plasma expanders to expand volume adequately until whole blood can be administered
- If uterine atony is the cause of bleeding, uterine massage is initiated
  - Oxytocin may be administered if massage is ineffective or the uterus can't be maintained in a contracted state
  - Bimanual massage may be performed if other measures prove ineffective
  - I.M. administration of prostaglandins may be ordered to promote strong, sustained uterine contractions
  - Hysterectomy may be indicated, but only as a last resort
- Lacerations, if present, are surgically repaired
- Retained placental fragments typically are removed by dilatation and curettage (D&C)
- Treatment of the underlying cause of DIC is indicated

● Nursing interventions

- Assess the patient's fundus and lochia frequently to detect changes; notify the physician if the fundus doesn't remain contracted or if lochia increases
- Perform fundal massage as indicated to assist with uterine involution (for more information, see chapter 7)
  - Remain with the patient, frequently reassessing the fundus to ensure that it remains firm and contracted
  - Keep in mind that the uterus may relax quickly after massage is completed, placing the patient at risk for continued hemorrhage
- Weigh perineal pads
- Turn the patient to the side and inspect under the buttocks for pooling of blood; if necessary, weigh disposable bed linen pads, adding this to the weight of the perineal pads to estimate blood loss
- Inspect perineal area closely for oozing from any lacerations
- Monitor vital signs frequently for changes, noting any trends such as a continuously rising pulse rate; report any changes immediately
- Assess intake and output; report urine output less than 30 ml/hour
  - Encourage the patient to void frequently to prevent bladder distention from interfering with uterine involution

Treatment for uterine atony

- Oxytocin may be administered if massage is ineffective.
- Bimanual massage may be performed.
- I.M. administration of prostaglandins may be ordered to promote strong, sustained contractions.
- Hysterectomy may be indicated.

Nursing interventions for late postpartum hemorrhage

- Perform fundal massage.
- Turn the patient to the side and inspect under the buttocks for pooling of blood.
- Inspect perineal area closely for oozing from any lacerations.
- Monitor vital signs frequently for changes.
- Assess intake and output.

What to do if the patient develops hypovolemic shock

- Begin an I.V. infusion.
- Record blood pressure and pulse, respiratory, and peripheral pulse rates.
- Monitor cardiac output and central venous, right atrial, pulmonary artery, and pulmonary artery wedge pressures.
- Administer oxygen.
- Obtain venous blood samples.

What to do if the patient's systolic blood pressure drops below 80 mm Hg

- Increase oxygen flow rate.
- Notify the health care provider.
- Increase the infusion rate if the patient's pulse is thready.

– If the patient can't void, anticipate the need for an indwelling urinary catheter
- Teach the patient the signs and symptoms of hemorrhage, and advise her to contact her physician if she develops any
- If the patient develops signs and symptoms of hypovolemic shock
  – Begin an I.V. infusion with normal saline solution or lactated Ringer's solution delivered through a large-bore (14G to 18G) catheter; assist with insertion of central venous line and pulmonary artery catheter for hemodynamic monitoring
  – Record blood pressure and pulse, respiratory, and peripheral pulse rates every 15 minutes until stable
  – Continuously monitor heart rhythm
  – Monitor cardiac output and central venous, right atrial, pulmonary artery, and pulmonary artery wedge pressures at least hourly or as ordered
  – During therapy, assess skin color and temperature, and note any changes — cold, clammy skin may signal continuing peripheral vascular constriction, indicating progressive shock
  – Watch for signs of impending coagulopathy (such as petechiae, bruising, bleeding, or oozing from gums or venipuncture sites)
  – Anticipate the need for fluid replacement and blood component therapy as ordered
  – Obtain arterial blood samples to measure arterial blood gas (ABG) levels
  – Administer oxygen by nasal cannula, face mask, or airway to ensure adequate tissue oxygenation, adjusting the oxygen flow rate as ABG results indicate
  – If the patient's systolic blood pressure drops below 80 mm Hg
    · Increase the oxygen flow rate, and notify the health care provider immediately because systolic blood pressure below 80 mm Hg usually results in inadequate coronary artery blood flow, cardiac ischemia, arrhythmias, and further complications of low cardiac output
    · Notify the health care provider, and increase the infusion rate if the patient experiences a progressive drop in blood pressure accompanied by a thready pulse; this usually signals inadequate cardiac output from reduced intravascular volume
  – Obtain venous blood samples as ordered for a complete blood count, electrolyte levels, typing and crossmatching, and coagulation studies
  – If the patient has received oxytocin I.V. for treatment of uterine atony, continue to assess the fundus closely, because although

oxytocin has an immediate onset of action, the duration of action is short, so the atony may reoccur
  – If the health care provider orders I.M. prostaglandin, be alert for possible adverse reactions (such as nausea, diarrhea, tachycardia, and hypertension), and alert the patient to them to help alleviate fear and anxiety
  – Prepare the patient for possible treatments such as bimanual massage, surgical repair of lacerations, or D&C as indicated

SUBINVOLUTION OF THE UTERUS

● **Description**
  • Refers to failure of the uterus to return to its normal size after childbirth
  • Diagnosis usually made at the postpartum checkup, 4 to 6 weeks after delivery
  • Predisposing factors include retained placental fragments and infection
  • *Chlamydia trachomatis* accounts for about one-third of the cases

● **Pathophysiology**
  • Retained placenta fragments or infection interferes with the ability of the uterus to contract effectively
  • As a result, the uterus remains enlarged and soft
  • Lochia also is present.

● **Assessment findings**
  • Displacement of the uterus in the abdominal cavity
  • Persistent lochia rubra, leukorrhea, and backache
  • Irregular or excessive uterine bleeding

● **Treatment**
  • Administration of an oxytocic such as methylergonovine (Methergine) and an antibiotic
  • Possibly a D&C

● **Nursing interventions**
  • Administer an oxytocic such as methylergonovine as ordered
    – Warn the patient that the drug may cause menstrual-like cramps
    – Use I.V. route only in emergency situations, and administer dose over at least 60 seconds; monitor blood pressure closely because severe hypotension can occur
    – Monitor the woman for possible adverse reactions, including nausea, vomiting, dizziness, headache, and ringing in the ears
  • Frequently assess uterine fundus for changes, including increasing firmness

What to look for in subinvolution of the uterus

- Displacement of the uterus in the abdominal cavity
- Persistent lochia rubra, leukorrhea, and backache
- Irregular or excessive uterine bleeding

Nursing interventions for subinvolution of the uterus

- Administer an oxytocic.
- Frequently assess uterine fundus for changes.
- Monitor vital signs closely.

- Monitor vital signs closely for changes suggesting excessive blood loss
- Provide emotional support and guidance to the patient and her family
- Instruct the woman to notify the health care provider if bleeding, including lochial discharge, continues
- Advise the woman to complete the full regimen of antibiotic therapy if ordered

PUERPERAL PSYCHIATRIC DISORDERS

Types of puerperal psychiatric disorders

- Depression
- Mania
- Schizophrenia
- Psychosis

Description

- Include depression, mania, schizophrenia, and psychosis
- Occur in 1% to 2% of all normal childbirths
- Between 15% and 20% of pregnant women have mental health issues
- *Postpartum depression* and *psychosis* are recognized by the *Diagnostic and Statistical Manual of Mental Disorders,* Fourth Edition, Text Revision (*DSM-IV-TR*) as psychiatric disorders occurring during the postpartum period
- Other psychiatric disorders may occur during the postpartum period (see *Highlighting psychiatric disorders in the postpartum period*)

Nursing interventions

- Be alert for signs and symptoms suggesting problems
- Provide emotional support and guidance for the woman and her family
- Assist with therapeutic interventions as appropriate; ensure adequate follow-up after discharge
- Administer drug therapy as ordered
- Teach the woman and her family about possible adverse effects and danger signs and symptoms to report to the health care provider

Nursing interventions for puerperal psychiatric disorders

- Watch for signs and symptoms that suggest problems.
- Provide emotional support and guidance.

PERINEAL HEMATOMA

Description

- Refers to a collection of blood in the soft subcutaneous tissue layer of the perineum
- The collection of blood can range from 25 to 500 ml
- Hematomas are usually seen in the vulva and vagina

Facts about perineal hematoma

- It's a collection of blood in the subcutaneous tissue layer of the perineum.
- It's usually seen in the vulva and vagina.
- The collection of blood can range from 25 to 500 ml.

Pathophysiology

- Hematomas are related to vascular injury during a spontaneous or assisted delivery
- They also may occur at the site of a laceration repair if a vessel was punctured during the repair
- Injury to the vessel leads to blood collecting in the subcutaneous tissue
- Hematomas are associated with minimal bleeding

Highlighting psychiatric disorders in the postpartum period

DISORDER	ASSESSMENT FINDINGS	TREATMENT
Depression (most common)	● Usually occurring within 4 to 6 weeks with symptoms possibly lasting several months ● Suicidal thinking ● Feelings of failure ● Exhaustion	● Psychotherapy ● Drug therapy such as antidepressants
Mania	● Occurring 1 to 2 weeks after delivery; possibly after a brief period of depression ● Agitation ● Excitement possibly lasting 1 to 3 weeks	● Psychotherapy ● Medication therapy with antimanic drugs
Schizophrenia	● Possibly occurring by the 10th postpartum day ● Delusional thinking ● Gross distortion of reality ● Flight of ideas ● Possible rejection of the father, infant, or both	● Antipsychotic drugs ● Psychotherapy ● Possible hospitalization
Psychosis	● Possibly appearing from 2 weeks to 12 months after delivery; more commonly seen within first month after delivery ● Sleep disturbances ● Restlessness ● Depression ● Indecisiveness progressing to bewilderment, perplexity, a dreamy state, impaired memory, confusion, and somatic delusion	● Antipsychotic drugs ● Psychotherapy ● Hospitalization

● **Assessment findings**
  • Severe vulvar pain (requires immediate investigation to rule out hematoma)
  • Unilateral purplish discoloration of the perineum and buttocks; discoloration firm and tender
  • Feeling of fullness in the vagina

● **Treatment**
  • Application of small ice packs
  • An analgesic
  • Surgical ligation and evacuation

● **Nursing interventions**
  • Inspect the perineal area closely for swelling or discoloration
  • If any is noted, measure the size of the area and report; monitor the size of the hematoma for changes
    – The hematoma should gradually decrease in size over several days
    – Any increase or failure to decrease in size may necessitate surgical ligation and evacuation

What to look for in perineal hematoma

● Severe vulvar pain
● Unilateral purplish discoloration of the perineum and buttocks
● Feeling of fullness in the vagina

Treatment for perineal hematoma

● Application of small ice packs
● Analgesic
● Surgical ligation and evacuation

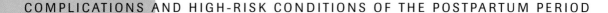

- Assess the patient's degree of discomfort, and administer an analgesic as ordered
- Help the patient apply ice to the area to minimize discomfort; make sure that the ice pack is covered to prevent thermal injury
- Instruct the woman in perineal hygiene measures, including measures to reduce the risk of infection

PUERPERAL INFECTION

● Description
- A postpartum infection of the uterus and higher structures, with a characteristic pattern of fever
- According to the Joint Committee on Maternal Welfare, puerperal morbidity may be defined in the following way:
  - Temperature of 100.4° F (38° C) or above
  - Such a rise in temperature may occur on any 2 of the first 10 postpartum days, exclusive of the first 24 hours
  - Temperature should be measured orally by a standard technique at least four times per day
- Puerperal infection can result in endometritis, parametritis, pelvic or femoral thrombophlebitis, or peritonitis
- It can remain localized (in the form of endometritis or salpingitis, for example) or extend to other parts of the body (in the form of peritonitis or pelvic cellulitis, for example)

● Pathophysiology
- Puerperal infection results from the introduction of vaginal microorganisms into the sterile uterine cavity via premature rupture of membranes, operative incisions, hematomas, damaged tissues, or lapses in sterile technique
- Microorganisms that commonly cause puerperal infection include group B hemolytic streptococci, coagulase-negative staphylococci, *Clostridium perfringens, Bacteroides fragilis, Klebsiella, Proteus mirabilis, Pseudomonas, Staphylococcus aureus,* and *Escherichia coli*
- Most of these organisms are considered normal vaginal flora but are known to cause puerperal infection in the presence of certain predisposing factors
  - Prolonged and premature rupture of the membranes (over 24 hours, allowing bacteria to enter while the fetus was still in utero)
  - Prolonged (more than 24 hours) or difficult labor
  - Frequent or unsterile vaginal examinations or unsterile delivery
  - Delivery requiring the use of instruments that may traumatize the tissue providing a portal of entry for microorganism invasion
  - Internal fetal monitoring use allowing introduction of organisms with placement of electrodes

Key facts about puerperal infection

- It's a postpartum infection of the uterus and higher structures.
- It can result in endometritis, parametritis, pelvic or femoral thrombophlebitis, or peritonitis.
- It can remain localized or extend to other body parts.

Predisposing factors for puerperal infection

- Premature rupture of membranes
- Prolonged or difficult labor
- Frequent or unsterile vaginal examinations or unsterile delivery
- Delivery requiring the use of instruments
- Internal fetal monitoring

Assessing puerperal infection

Accompanying signs and symptoms of a puerperal infection depend on the extent and site of infection and may include:

- localized perineal infection: pain, elevated temperature, edema, redness, firmness, and tenderness at the site of the wound; sensation of heat; burning on urination; and discharge from the wound
- endometritis: heavy, sometimes foul-smelling lochia; tender, enlarged uterus; backache; and severe uterine contractions persisting after childbirth
- parametritis (pelvic cellulitis): vaginal tenderness and abdominal pain and tenderness (pain may become more intense as infection spreads). The inflammation may remain localized, may lead to abscess forma-

tion, or may spread through the blood or lymphatic system. Widespread inflammation may cause:

- septic pelvic thrombophlebitis: severe, repeated chills and dramatic swings in body temperature; lower abdominal or flank pain; and, possibly, a palpable tender mass over the affected area, which usually develops during the second postpartum week
- peritonitis: body temperature usually elevated, accompanied by tachycardia (greater than 140 beats/minute), weak pulse, hiccups, nausea, vomiting, and diarrhea; constant and possibly excruciating abdominal pain; and a rigid, boardlike abdomen with guarding (commonly the first manifestation).

- Retained products of conception such as retained placental fragments, allowing tissue necrosis, which provides an excellent medium for bacterial growth
- Hemorrhage, which weakens the patient's overall defenses
- Maternal conditions, such as anemia or debilitation from malnutrition, which lower the woman's ability to defend against microorganism invasion
- Cesarean birth (20-fold increase in the risk of puerperal infection)
- Existence of localized vaginal infection at delivery allowing direct infection transmission

● Assessment findings

- Depend on the site and extent of infection (see *Assessing puerperal infection*)
- Fever, at least 100.4° F (38° C), that occurs after first 24 hours and lasts for 2 consecutive days during the first 10 days postpartum
  - Fever possibly as high as 105° F (40.6° C)
  - Commonly associated with chills, backache, malaise, restlessness, and anxiety
- Foul-smelling lochia
- Lethargy
- Abdominal pain
- Subinvolution of the uterus

Signs and symptoms of puerperal infection

- Fever, at least 100.4° F (38° C), that occurs after first 24 hours postpartum and lasts for 2 consecutive days during the first 10 days
- Foul-smelling lochia
- Lethargy
- Abdominal pain
- Subinvolution of the uterus

Treatment for puerperal infection

- Broad-spectrum antibiotic therapy
- Analgesics for pain
- Sitz baths
- Infection-control precautions
- Positioning to enhance drainage
- Maintenance of fluid and electrolyte balance
- Monitoring of vital signs and symptoms
- Surgery

Ways to prevent infection

- Use standard precautions.
- Maintain sterile technique during vaginal examination.
- Limit number of vaginal examinations during labor.
- Thoroughly wash your hands after each patient contact.
- Instruct the patient to immediately report rupture of her membranes.
- Keep the episiotomy site clean.
- Keep persons with active infections away from patient.

What to do if the patient develops an infection

- Monitor vital signs every 4 hours.
- Closely assess intake and output.
- Enforce strict bed rest.
- Frequently inspect the perineum.
- Administer an antibiotic or analgesic as ordered.
- Assess and document the type, degree, and location of pain.

● Treatment

- Broad-spectrum antibiotic therapy
- Analgesics for pain
- Sitz baths
- Infection-control precautions
- Positioning to enhance drainage
- Maintenance of fluid and electrolyte balance
- Monitoring of vital signs and symptoms
- Surgery to remove any remaining products of conception or retained placental fragments, or to drain local lesions such as an abscess in parametritis

● Nursing interventions

- Institute measures to prevent infection
  - Always adhere to standard precautions
  - Maintain sterile technique when assisting with or performing a vaginal examination
  - Limit the number of vaginal examinations performed during labor
  - Thoroughly wash your hands after each patient contact
  - Instruct the pregnant patient to call her health care provider immediately when her membranes rupture
  - Warn the patient to avoid intercourse after rupture or leak of the amniotic sac
  - Keep the episiotomy site clean, and teach the patient how to maintain good perineal hygiene
  - Screen personnel and visitors to keep persons with active infections away from maternity patients
- If the postpartum patient develops an infection
  - Monitor vital signs every 4 hours (or more frequently depending on the patient's condition)
  - Closely assess intake and output, and enforce strict bed rest
  - Frequently inspect the perineum
    - Assess the fundus, and palpate for tenderness (subinvolution may indicate endometritis)
    - Note the amount, color, and odor of vaginal drainage, and document your observations
  - Encourage the patient to change bed linen and perineal pads frequently, removing them from front to back; wear gloves when helping the patient change pads
  - Administer antibiotics and analgesics as ordered
  - Assess and document the type, degree, and location of pain as well as the patient's response to analgesic
  - Give the patient an antiemetic to relieve nausea and vomiting as needed

– Provide sitz baths or warm compresses for local lesions

– Keep the patient warm

– Offer reassurance and emotional support, and thoroughly explain all procedures to the patient and her family

– If the mother must be separated from her neonate, provide reassurance and frequently update her about his progress; encourage the father to reassure the mother about the neonate's condition as well

DEEP VEIN THROMBOSIS

● Description

* Also called *deep vein thrombophlebitis,* or *DVT*
* Refers to an inflammation of the lining of a blood vessel in conjunction with the formation of clots
* Typically occurs at the valve cusps because venous stasis encourages the accumulation and adherence of platelets and fibrin
* Thrombophlebitis usually begins with localized inflammation alone (phlebitis), but such inflammation rapidly provokes thrombus formation
* DVT can affect small veins, such as the lesser saphenous vein, or large veins, such as the iliac, femoral, pelvic, and popliteal veins and the venae cavae
* DVT is more serious than superficial vein thrombophlebitis because it affects the veins deep in the leg musculature that carry 90% of the venous outflow from the leg
* During the postpartum period, two major types of DVT may occur: femoral or pelvic; pelvic DVT runs a long course, usually 6 to 8 weeks (see *Comparing femoral and pelvic DVT,* page 346)

● Pathophysiology

* DVT may be idiopathic, but it's more likely to occur in the presence of certain diseases, treatments, injuries, or other factors
* In the postpartum woman, DVT most commonly results from an extension of endometritis
* Risk factors associated with the development of DVT in the postpartum period
  – History of varicose veins
  – Obesity
  – History of previous DVT
  – Increased parity and age (older than age 30)
  – Familial history of DVT
* Risk factors are further compounded by specific occurrences associated with labor and delivery

Comparing femoral and pelvic DVT

	FEMORAL DVT	PELVIC DVT
Vessels affected	• Femoral • Saphenous • Popliteal	• Ovarian • Uterine • Hypogastric
Onset	• Around 10th day postpartum	• Around the 14th to 15th day postpartum
Assessment findings	• Associated arterial spasm making leg appear milky white or drained • Edema • Fever • Chills • Pain • Redness of affected leg • Shiny white skin on extremity	• Extremely high fever • Chills • General malaise • Possible pelvic abscess
Treatment	• Bed rest • Elevation of affected extremity • Anticoagulants • Moist heat applications • Analgesics	• Complete bed rest • Anticoagulants • Antibiotics • Incision and drainage of abscess (if develops)

What to look for in superficial thrombophlebitis

- Pain in the midcalf area
- Tenderness
- Redness along the vein

What to look for in femoral DVT

- Pain
- Stiffness or swelling in a leg or the groin
- Increase in temperature around the 10th day postpartum
- Affected extremity appearing reddened or inflamed, edematous below the level of the obstruction, and possibly shiny and white
- Thigh and calf diameter typically greater than that of the unaffected extremity
- Malaise and chills
- Positive Homans' sign
- Palpable veins inside the thigh and calf
- Pain in the calf when pressure is applied on the inside of the foot

– Postpartally, blood clotting is increased because the elevated fibrinogen levels of pregnancy are still elevated

– Pressure from the fetal head during pregnancy and delivery causes the lower-extremity veins to dilate, leading to venous stasis

– The period of inactivity and time in the lithotomy position with the lower extremities in stirrups promotes venous pooling and stasis

Assessment findings

- Superficial thrombophlebitis
  – Pain in the midcalf area
  – Tenderness
  – Redness along the vein
- Femoral DVT
  – Pain
  – Stiffness or swelling in a leg or the groin
  – Increase in temperature around the 10th day postpartum
  – Affected extremity appearing reddened or inflamed, edematous below the level of the obstruction, and possibly shiny and white (possibly because of an accompanying arterial spasm, which results in a decrease in arterial circulation to the area)
  – Thigh and calf diameter typically greater than that of the unaffected extremity

– Malaise and chills

– Positive Homans' sign

– Palpable veins inside the thigh and calf

– Pain in the calf when pressure is applied on the inside of the foot

• Pelvic DVT

– Onset of a high fever with wide swings in body temperature

– Severe repeated chills

– General malaise

– Lower-abdominal or flank pain

– Possible palpable tender mass over the affected area.

– Palpable veins inside the thigh and calf

– Pain in the calf when pressure is applied on the inside of the foot

● **Treatment**

• Bed rest

• Elevation of the affected arm or leg

• Application of warm, moist compresses to the affected area

• Analgesic administration

• Anticoagulant therapy

• Ambulation with antiembolism stockings when acute episode subsides

• Antibiotic for pelvic thrombophlebitis

● **Nursing interventions**

• Institute measures to prevent DVT

– Assess the woman for risk factors that could predispose her to DVT

– Teach her about measures to reduce her risk (see *Preventing DVT,* page 348)

– Be alert to signs and symptoms of endometritis, notify the physician if any occur, and institute treatment promptly as ordered

– If the woman develops postpartum DVT, institute the following measures

  • Enforce bed rest as ordered, and elevate the patient's affected arm or leg (if you plan to use pillows for elevating the leg, place them so they support its entire length to avoid compressing the popliteal space)

  • Apply warm compresses or a covered aquathermia pad to increase circulation to the affected area and to relieve pain and inflammation

  • Give an analgesic to relieve pain as ordered

  • Assess uterine involution and note any changes in fundal consistency, such as inability to remain firm or contracted

TIME-OUT FOR TEACHING

Preventing DVT

Incorporate the instructions below in your teaching plan to reduce a woman's risk of developing deep vein thrombosis (DVT):

- Check with the health care provider about using a side-lying or back-lying (supine recumbent) position for birth instead of the lithotomy position (on back with legs in stirrups); these alternative positions reduce the risk of blood pooling in the lower extremities.
- If the lithotomy position must be used for birth, ask health care personnel to pad the stirrups well so that less pressure is put on the calves of legs.

- Avoid standing in one place for too long or sitting with knees bent or legs crossed. Elevate legs slightly to improve venous return.
- Avoid using garters or wearing constrictive clothing.
- Wiggle toes and perform leg lifts while in bed to minimize venous pooling and help increase venous return.
- Ambulate as soon as possible after delivery.
- Wear antiembolism or support stockings as ordered. Put them on before getting out of bed in the morning.

What to do if DVT develops

- Enforce bed rest.
- Apply warm compresses or a covered aquathermia pad.
- Give an analgesic to relieve pain.
- Assess uterine involution.
- Monitor vital signs closely.
- Administer an anticoagulant.
- Administer an antibiotic and antipyretic.
- Mark, measure, and record the circumference of the affected extremity at least daily.
- Obtain coagulation studies.
- Monitor the patient's lochia.
- Watch for signs and symptoms of bleeding.
- Assess the patient for signs and symptoms of pulmonary emboli.

- Monitor vital signs closely, at least every 4 hours or more frequently if indicated. Report any changes in pulse rate or blood pressure or temperature elevations
- Administer anticoagulant therapy, such as heparin, I.V. as ordered with an infusion monitor or pump to control the flow rate, if necessary; have anticoagulant antidote, such as protamine sulfate (for heparin therapy), readily available
- Administer antibiotic and antipyretic therapy for the patient with pelvic DVT
- Mark, measure, and record the circumference of the affected extremity at least daily
  - Compare this measurement with that of the other extremity
  - To ensure accuracy and consistency of serial measurements, mark the skin over the area and measure at the same spot daily
- Obtain coagulation studies, such as international normalized ratio, partial thromboplastin time, and prothrombin time, as ordered, and evaluate results based on established parameters for therapeutic anticoagulation
- Monitor the patient's lochia for increases in amount
  - Encourage patient to change perineal pads frequently
  - Weigh perineal pads to estimate the amount of blood lost.
- Watch for signs and symptoms of bleeding, and immediately report if the patient experiences any

- Look for tarry stools, coffee-ground vomitus, and ecchymoses
- Note any oozing of blood at I.V. sites
- Assess gums for excessive bleeding
- Assess the patient for signs and symptoms of pulmonary emboli such as crackles, dyspnea, hemoptysis, sudden changes in mental status, restlessness, and hypotension
- Provide emotional support to the patient and her family; explain all procedures and treatments; prepare her for surgery if indicated
- As appropriate, emphasize the importance of followup blood studies to monitor anticoagulant therapy
- If the patient will be discharged on heparin therapy, teach her or her family how to give subcutaneous injections; if additional assistance is required, arrange for a home health care referral and follow-up
- Teach the patient how to properly apply and use antiembolism stockings; tell her to report any complications, such as cold and blue toes
- To prevent bleeding, encourage the patient to avoid drugs that contain aspirin and to check with the physician before using any over-the-counter drugs; also, alert the patient to the signs and symptoms of bleeding

ACQUIRED IMMUNODEFICIENCY SYNDROME

● Description
- A life-threatening disease, caused by HIV, acquired immunodeficiency syndrome (AIDS) is a virus in which the body's immune system becomes susceptible to opportunistic infections
- Characterized by laboratory evidence of HIV infection coexisting with one or more indicator diseases, such as herpes simplex cytomegalovirus, *Pneumocystis carinii,* Kaposi's sarcoma, wasting syndrome
- Various women are at risk
  - I.V. drug users
  - Those with multiple sex partners
  - Partners of those considered high risk
  - Recipients of blood products (although this is relatively rare at present)

● Pathophysiology
- HIV, a retrovirus, selectively infects human cells containing a CD4+ antigen on their surface, most of which are T4 lymphocytes
- HIV infects the CD4+ T cells and when stimulated, HIV is rapidly produced, destroying and killing the CD4+ T cells

Signs and symptoms of pulmonary emboli

- Crackles
- Dyspnea
- Hemoptysis
- Sudden changes in mental status
- Restlessness
- Hypotension

Key facts about AIDS

- It's a life-threatening immune disease caused by HIV.
- It's characterized by laboratory evidence of HIV infection co-existing with one or more indicator diseases, such as herpes simplex cytomegalovirus, *Pneumocystis carinii,* or Kaposi's sarcoma.

Risk factors for AIDS

- Using I.V. drugs
- Having multiple sex partners
- Having a high-risk partner
- Being a recipient of blood products

Treatment for AIDS

- Continuation of antiretroviral therapy
- Antiretroviral therapy for the neonate
- Standard precautions
- Pharmacologic therapy for opportunistic infections
- Avoidance of breast-feeding

What to do if your patient has AIDS

- Know that circumcision should be avoided if the mother is HIV positive.
- Discuss birth control alternatives with the patient before discharge.
- Maintain standard precautions.

- HIV infection renders the patient immunodeficient and predisposes the patient to opportunistic infections, unusual cancers, and other characteristic abnormalities

● **Treatment**
- Continuation of antiretroviral therapy
- Antiretroviral therapy for the neonate
- Standard precautions
- Pharmacologic therapy for opportunistic infections
- Avoidance of breast-feeding

● **Nursing interventions**
- Keep in mind that circumcision should be avoided if mother is HIV positive
- Arrange follow-up care for neonate and mother before discharge
- Discuss birth-control alternatives before discharge
  - Advise patient to avoid intrauterine devices
  - Recommend a barrier method, such as a condom, as the best choice
  - Discourage pregnancy for a woman who's HIV positive
- Maintain standard precautions
- Provide psychosocial support and guidance
  - Allow direct mother-neonate contact unless open skin lesions are involved
  - Enforce strict category-specific infection-control precautions if the patient has tuberculosis, open lesions, or copious secretions or blood
  - Know that breast-feeding is contraindicated because HIV can be transmitted via breast milk

NCLEX CHECKS

It's never too soon to begin your NCLEX preparation. Now that you've reviewed this chapter, carefully read each of the following questions and choose the best answer. Then compare your responses to the correct answers.

1. Which of the following is the most common cause of mastitis?
- ☐ **A.** *Escherichia coli*
- ☐ **B.** *Neisseria gonorrhoeae*
- ☑ **C.** *Staphylococcus aureus*
- ☐ **D.** *Treponema pallidum*

2. Which of the following are risk factors for late postpartum hemorrhage? Select all that apply.

- ☒ **A.** Delivery of a large neonate
- ☒ **B.** Hydramnios
- ☐ **C.** Precipitate labor
- ☐ **D.** Primaparity
- ☒ **E.** Dystocia

3. Which drug would the nurse expect to administer to a woman experiencing subinvolution of the uterus?

- ☐ **A.** Heparin
- ☐ **B.** Methylergonovine
- ☐ **C.** Protamine
- ☐ **D.** Warfarin

4. Which assessment finding would lead the nurse to suspect that a woman with a puerperal infection has developed peritonitis?

- ☒ **A.** Rigid abdomen
- ☐ **B.** Edema of the area
- ☐ **C.** Burning on urination
- ☐ **D.** Site tenderness

5. Which finding is most characteristic of a perineal hematoma?

- ☐ **A.** Fever
- ☐ **B.** Lethargy
- ☐ **C.** Positive Homans' sign
- ☒ **D.** Severe vulvar pain

ANSWERS AND RATIONALES

1. CORRECT ANSWER: C

The most common cause of mastitis is *S. aureus. E. coli* is a common cause of urinary tract infection. *N. gonorrhoeae* causes gonorrhea. *T. pallidum* causes syphilis.

2. CORRECT ANSWERS: A, B, AND E

Risk factors for the development of late postpartum hemorrhage include the delivery of a large neonate, hydramnios, dystocia, and grand multiparity.

3. CORRECT ANSWER: B

To treat subinvolution, the physician may order methylergonovine to aid in uterine contraction. Neither heparin nor warfarin, which are anticoagulants, would be used because they would increase the risk of bleeding and do nothing to aid in uterine involution. They're more commonly used to treat deep vein thrombosis. Protamine is the antidote for heparin toxicity.

4. CORRECT ANSWER: A

Peritonitis is indicated by a rigid, boardlike abdomen with guarding (commonly the first manifestation) along with elevated body temperature, tachycardia (greater than 140 beats/minute), weak pulse, hiccups, nausea, vomiting, and diarrhea, and constant and possibly excruciating abdominal pain. Edema of the area, burning on urination, and site tenderness are associated with a localized perineal infection.

5. CORRECT ANSWER: D

With a perineal hematoma, the most characteristic finding is severe vulvar pain. Fever and lethargy are seen with any infection. A positive Homans' sign may suggest thrombophlebitis.

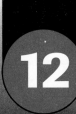

12

Infertility and genetics

CHAPTER OVERVIEW

A woman's ability to reproduce carries with it many uncertainties. The actual ability to reproduce as well as the possibility of transmitting genetic abnormalities are key concerns. Many of these concerns involve issues with ethical and legal implications. The nurse plays a key role in providing accurate information to allow patients to make an informed decision.

Key facts about infertility

- Inability to conceive after 1 year of trying
- Affects 15% to 20% of couples in the U.S.
- In primary infertility, no previous conceptions have occurred
- In secondary infertility, previous conceptions have occurred

Female factors that can cause infertility

- Endocrine disorders
- Genital tract obstruction
- Tubal transport problems
- Tubal and uterine problems
- Cervical problems
- Vaginal problems
- Absence of ovulation
- Emotional disorders
- Preexisting medical conditions
- Severe nutritional deficit

Male factors that can cause infertility

- Genital tract obstruction
- Spermatozoal problems
- Abnormal genital tract secretions
- Coital difficulties
- Testicular abnormalities from illness
- Sexual dysfunction
- Endocrine disorders

INFERTILITY

Description
- Refers to the inability to conceive after 1 year of consistent attempts without using contraceptives
- Affects 15% to 20% of the couples in the United States
- May be classified as primary or secondary
  - Primary infertility refers to the inability to impregnate or conceive; no previous conceptions have occurred
    - The man has never impregnated a woman
    - The woman has never been pregnant, despite consistent attempts
  - Secondary infertility refers to the woman's inability to conceive or sustain a pregnancy after an initial pregnancy

Causes
- Female factors
  - Endocrine disorders such as hypothyroidism
  - Genital tract obstruction
  - Anatomic abnormalities
    - Tubal transport problems, such as scarring from pelvic inflammatory disease (PID)
    - Tubal and uterine problems such as from endometriosis or inadequate endometrial development
    - Cervical problems such as too-thick cervical mucus
    - Vaginal problems, such as increased acidity of vaginal pH or sperm antibodies
    - Absence of ovulation
  - Emotional disorders
  - Preexisting medical conditions
  - Severe nutritional deficit
- Male factors
  - Genital tract obstruction
  - Spermatozoal problems
    - Reduced spermatozoa count
    - Decreased motility
    - Malformed spermatozoa
  - Abnormal genital tract secretions
  - Coital difficulties (for instance, failure to deposit sperm at the cervix, which may be linked to obesity)
  - Testicular abnormalities from illness, cryptorchidism, trauma, or irradiation
  - Sexual dysfunction
  - Endocrine disorders

● **Diagnostic evaluation**
  • In the female
    – Menstrual, medical, fertility, sexual, surgical, occupational, and family history
    – Physical examination
    – Review of personal habits
      · Medications
      · Use of tobacco and alcohol
      · Exercise
      · Weight history
      · Use of douches or vaginal deodorants
    – Laboratory examinations
      · Complete blood count (CBC)
      · Sedimentation rate
      · Serology
      · Urinalysis
      · Thyroid function tests
      · Glucose tolerance tests
      · Hormonal testing, such as prolactin, adrenal hormone, luteinizing hormone (LH), and follicle-stimulating hormone (FSH), insulin
      · C-peptide in polycystic ovarian syndrome
      · Blood type
      · Rubella status
      · Human immunodeficiency virus status
    – Basal body temperature monitoring or ovulation monitoring kit
    – Menstrual cycle mapping to track ovulatory and anovulatory cycles for 6 months
    – Cervical mucosal tests to assess elasticity and content
      · Fern test: done midcycle, just before ovulation when estrogen stimulation is greatest; cervical mucus thin, with low viscosity and cellularity appearing in a fernlike pattern when collected and allowed to dry on a slide
      · Spinnbarkeit test: done when estrogen stimulation high; mucus specimen appearing highly thin and stretchable indicating that ovulation is imminent
    – Postcoital sperm analysis to assess sperm mobility and morphology
    – Hysterosalpingography to assess tubular patency
    – Culdoscopy to assess tubular function
    – Laparoscopy to view pelvic organs directly
    – Endometrial biopsy to assess cyclic development of endometrium
  • In the male
    – Urologic, medical, sexual, surgical, and occupational history

---

Key diagnostic evaluations: Female

● Menstrual, medical, fertility, sexual, surgical, occupational, and family history
● Physical examination
● Review of personal habits, such as medications, use of tobacco and alcohol, use of douches or vaginal deodorants
● Laboratory examinations, such as sedimentation rate, serology, urinalysis, GTT, hormonal testing, C-peptide, HIV status
● Menstrual cycle mapping
● Cervical mucosal tests
● Postcoital sperm analysis
● Hysterosalpingography
● Culdoscopy
● Laparoscopy
● Endometral biopsy

Key diagnostic evaluations: Male

● Urologic, medical, sexual, surgical, and occupational histories
● Physical examination
● Review of personal habits (medications, tobacco and alcohol use, clothing preferences)
● Laboratory examinations (spermatozoa analysis, CBC, urinalysis, sedimentation rate, hormonal testing)

Key strategies for managing infertility

- Surgery
- Drug therapy

Treatments for female infertility

- Clomiphene (Clomid)
- Bromocriptine (Parlodel)
- Cabergoline (Dostinex)
- Levothyroxine (Synthroid)
- Menotropins (Pergonal)
- Estrogen and progesterone combinations
- Hydroxyprogesterone
- Insulin sensitizers
- Thyroid replacement

Treatments for male infertility

- Testosterone enanthate (Delatestryl)
- Testosterone cypionate (Depo-Testosterone)
- Chorionic gonadotropin (Pregnyl)
- Menotropins (Pergonal)

- – Physical examination
- – Review of personal habits
  - Medications
  - Use of tobacco and alcohol
  - Clothing preferences
  - Bathing habits
- – Laboratory examinations
  - Spermatozoa analysis
  - CBC
  - Urinalysis
  - Sedimentation rate
  - Hormonal testing, such as LH, FSH, and testosterone

● **Emotional reactions**
- The couple may demonstrate behaviors associated with loss: surprise, denial, anger, bargaining, depression, and finally acceptance
- Infertility can lower self-esteem and elicit feelings of inadequacy, loss of control over life, and rejection by society
- Medical investigations into infertility lead to embarrassment, decreased privacy, and disruption of normal, spontaneous sexual relations
- The infertile couple who ultimately conceives may exhibit the normal ambivalence associated with pregnancy

● **Management**
- Surgical management includes correction of anatomic defects and removal of obstructions in the reproductive tract
- Medications used when infertility is caused by anovulation
  - – Clomiphene (Clomid) for hypothalamic suppression
  - – Bromocriptine (Parlodel) or cabergoline (Dostinex) for increased prolactin levels
  - – Levothyroxine (Synthroid) for hypothyroidism
  - – Menotropins (Pergonal) for hypogonadotropic amenorrhea
- Medications used when infertility is caused by an endocrine disorder
  - – Estrogen and progesterone combinations for hypoestrogenic states
  - – Hydroxyprogesterone for luteal phase defects
  - – Insulin sensitizers for hyperinsulinemia
  - – Thyroid replacement for hypothyroidism
- Medications used with the male
  - – Testosterone enanthate (Delatestryl) and testosterone cypionate (Depo-Testosterone) to stimulate virilization
  - – Chorionic gonadotropin (Pregnyl) to virilize a hypogonadotropic male and to restore spermatogenesis
  - – Menotropins (Pergonal) to aid human chorionic gonadotropin in completing spermatogenesis

● Options for the infertile couple

- To fulfill their desire to become parents, an infertile couple may choose from various alternatives
    - Artificial insemination (AI)
        - Sperm from the partner or a donor instilled into the woman's cervix or uterus
        - Instillation on the day after ovulation
    - In vitro fertilization (IVF)
        - Removal of one or more eggs via laparoscopy
        - Fertilization of eggs in the laboratory
        - Reinsertion of fertilized eggs into woman's uterus about 40 hours after fertilization; called *embryo transfer* (ET)
    - Gamete intrafallopian tube transfer (GIFT)
        - Eggs obtained similar to that for IVF
        - Eggs and sperm transferred to woman's patent tube
        - Fertilization occurring in the tube, after implantation in the uterus
    - Zygote intrafallopian tube transfer (ZIFT)
        - Eggs retrieval via aspiration under ultrasonic guidance
        - Fertilization occurring in the laboratory
        - Fertilized eggs transferred to woman's patent tube via laparoscopy
    - Surrogate ET
        - Donor egg used
        - Menstrual cycles of donor and woman are synchronized using hormonal therapy
        - Donor egg obtained at ovulation and fertilized by sperm of woman's partner
        - Fertilized egg transferred to woman using ET or GIFT
    - Surrogate mothering
        - Another woman agreeing to carry pregnancy to term
        - Egg from the surrogate, woman, or another donor; sperm from woman's partner or a donor
    - Adoption (The decreased social stigma of out-of-wedlock and single-mother pregnancies has drastically reduced the number of infants available for adoption.)
- Many legal and ethical ramifications are associated with AI, IVF, GIFT, ZIFT, and surrogate mothering
- The advances in technology have improved success rates for IVF, GIFT, ZIFT, and surrogate embryo transfer
- However, the financial costs for many of these various alternatives is very high; reimbursement by third-party payers may be limited or absent
- The infertile couple also may choose a child-free life

Options for the infertile couple

- Artificial insemination
- In vitro fertilization
- Gamete intrafallopian tube transfer
- Zygote intrafallopian tube transfer
- Surrogate embryo transfer
- Surrogate mothering
- Adoption

What happens in IVF

- One or more eggs are removed via laparoscopy.
- Eggs are fertilized in the laboratory.
- The fertilized eggs are reinserted into the woman's uterus about 40 hours after fertilization.

What happens in surrogate embryo transfer

- Donor egg is used.
- Menstrual cycles of donor and woman are synchronized using hormonal therapy.
- Donor egg is obtained at ovulation and fertilized by sperm of the woman's partner.
- Fertilized egg is transferred to the woman using embryo transfer or gamete intrafallopian tube transfer.

Key facts about genes

- Genetic information is stored on chromosomes.
- Chromosomes contain thousands of genes, the smallest units of hereditary information.
- The normal number of chromosomes is 46 — 22 pairs of autosomes and 1 pair of sex chromosomes (XX for female and XY for male).
- A genetic disorder can be classified as congenital or hereditary.

Key facts about trait predominance

- Each parent contributes one set of chromosomes.
- Some traits are determined by one gene that may have many variants.
- Other traits, called *polygenic traits*, require the interaction of one or more genes.
- Environmental factors may affect how a gene or genes are expressed.

GENETIC DISORDERS

- **Description**
  - Genetic information is stored on chromosomes, tightly coiled strands of deoxyribonucleic acid (DNA)
  - Chromosomes are composed of DNA, histone proteins, and nonhistone proteins
  - Chromosomes contain thousands of genes; these are the smallest units of hereditary information, lined up in a specific pattern
  - The normal number of chromosomes is 46 — 22 pairs of autosomes and 1 pair of sex chromosomes (XX for female and XY for male)
  - A pictorial analysis of chromosomes (karyotype) can be performed most easily on the lymphocytes, but also on skin, bone marrow, or organ tissue
  - A genetic disorder can be classified as congenital or hereditary
- **Mendel's laws**
  - Principle of dominance
    - Genes aren't equal in strength
    - The stronger gene, producing an observable trait, is called *dominant*
    - The weaker gene, whose trait isn't seen, is called *recessive*
  - Principle of segregation
    - Paired chromosomes that contain genes from both parents separate during meiosis
    - Chance determines whether the maternal or paternal gene travels to a specific gamete
  - Principle of independent assortment is defined as pairs of genes that are distributed in the gametes in random fashion, unrelated to any other pairs
- **Trait predominance**
  - Each parent contributes one set of chromosomes, so every offspring has two genes for every location (locus) on the autosomal chromosome
  - Some traits are determined by one gene that may have many variants (alleles)
  - Other traits, called *polygenic traits,* require the interaction of one or more genes
  - Additionally, environmental factors may affect how a gene or genes are expressed (however, environmental factors don't affect the genetic structure)
  - Variations in a particular gene are called *alleles*

– A person with identical genes on each chromosome is homozygous for that gene

– If the alleles are different, they're said to be heterozygous

Inheritance patterns

- With autosomal inheritance, one allele on an autosomal chromosome may be more influential than the other in determining a specific trait
- The more powerful, or dominant, gene is more likely to be expressed in the offspring than the less influential, or recessive, gene
  - Offspring will express a dominant allele when one or both chromosomes in a pair carry it
  - A recessive allele won't be expressed unless both chromosomes carry alleles
- Sex-linked inheritance involves the X and Y chromosomes
  - Genes for disorders are located in and transmitted only by the female sex chromosome X
  - When the gene is dominant, it only needs to be present on one of the X chromosomes for the person to have symptoms
  - This type of inheritance is called *X-linked*
  - Majority of X-linked inheritance disorders are recessive
  - If a normal gene is present, it will block an abnormal gene
  - Some recessive genes on the X chromosomes act like dominants in females; one recessive allele will be expressed in some somatic cells and another in other somatic cells
- Environmental factors can affect the expression of some genes; this is called *multifactorial inheritance;* the gene for the problem is only expressed under certain environmental conditions

Categories of genetic disorders

- Single-gene disorders
  - An error occurs at a single gene site on the DNA strand
  - Such an error may occur in the copying and transcribing of a single codon (nucleotide triplet) through additions, deletions, or excessive repetitions
  - Single-gene disorders are inherited in clearly identifiable patterns that are the same as those seen in the inheritance of normal traits
  - Most hereditary disorders are caused by autosomal defects because every person has 22 pairs of autosomes and only 1 pair of sex chromosomes
- Autosomal dominant disorders
  - Usually affect males and females equally
  - If one parent is affected, each child has one chance in two of being affected
  - If both parents are affected, all children will be affected

---

Inheritance patterns

- With autosomal inheritance, one allele on an autosomal chromosome may be more influential than the other in determining a specific trait.
- The more powerful, or dominant, gene is more likely to be expressed in the offspring than the less influential, or recessive, gene.
- Sex-linked inheritance involves the X and Y chromosomes.
- Environmental factors can affect the expression of some genes; this is called *multifactorial inheritance.*

Key facts about single-gene disorders

- An error occurs at a single gene site on the DNA strand.
- Such an error may occur in the copying and transcribing of a single codon through additions, deletions, or excessive repetitions.

Key facts about autosomal dominant disorders

- They usually affect males and females equally.
- If one parent is affected, each child has one chance in two of being affected.
- If both parents are affected, all children will be affected.

- The disease trait in autosomal-dominant inheritance disorders is heterozygous
  - These disorders are caused by an abnormal dominant gene on an autosome
  - These include Marfan syndrome, osteogenesis imperfecta, and Huntington's disease
- Autosomal recessive disorders
  - Usually affect male and female offspring equally
  - If both parents are affected, all offspring will be affected
  - If both parents are unaffected but are heterozygous for the trait (carriers of the defective gene), each child has a one in four chance of being affected, but all will carry the defective gene
  - If one parent is affected and the other parent is a carrier, one-half of the children will be affected
  - The disease trait in autosomal-recessive inheritance disorders is homozygous
    - The normal gene is dominant, so the individual must have two abnormal genes to be affected
    - Examples include sickle cell anemia, Tay-Sachs disease, cystic fibrosis, and most metabolic diseases (see *Understanding autosomal inheritance*)
- Sex-linked disorders
  - Most are carried on the X chromosome
  - Because males have only one X chromosome, a single X-linked recessive gene can cause disease in a male
  - Females receive two X chromosomes, so they can be homozygous for a disease allele, homozygous for a normal allele, or heterozygous
- X-linked recessive disorders
  - Most commonly expressed in males who have parents who are unaffected
  - In rare cases, the father is affected and the mother is a carrier
  - All daughters of an affected male will be carriers
  - Sons of an affected male will be unaffected, and the unaffected sons aren't carriers
  - Unaffected male children of a female carrier don't transmit the disorder
  - The abnormal gene in X-linked recessive inheritance disorders is carried on the X chromosome
  - Examples include hemophilia, Duchenne's disease (pseudohypertrophic muscular dystrophy), and color blindness
- X-linked dominant disorders
  - X-linked dominant inheritance includes evidence of the inherited trait in the family history

Understanding autosomal inheritance

AUTOSOMAL DOMINANT INHERITANCE
The diagram shows the inheritance pattern of an abnormal trait when one parent has recessive normal genes (aa) and the other has a dominant abnormal gene (Aa). Each child has a 50% chance of inheriting A.

		Affected parent	
		A	a
Normal parent	a	Aa Affected	aa Normal
	a	Aa Affected	aa Normal

AUTOSOMAL RECESSIVE INHERITANCE
The diagram shows the inheritance pattern of an abnormal trait when both unaffected parents are heterozygous (Aa) for a recessive abnormal gene (a) on an autosome. As shown, each child has a one-in-four chance of having two normal genes (AA) and no chance of transmittal, and a 50% chance of being a carrier (Aa) who can transmit the gene.

		Heterozygous parent Aa	
		A	a
Heterozygous parent Aa	A	AA Normal	Aa Carrier
	a	Aa Carrier	aa Affected

- A person with the abnormal trait must have one affected parent
- If the father has an X-linked dominant disorder, all his daughters and none of his sons will be affected
- If a mother has an X-linked dominant disorder, each of her children has a 50% chance of being affected
- X-linked dominant inheritance disorders are similar to X-linked recessive disorders, except that heterozygous females are affected (see *A look at X-linked inheritance,* page 362)
  - Occurrence is rare
  - An example is vitamin D–resistant rickets
- Chromosomal aberrations (deviations in either the number or structure of chromosomes)
  - A structural defect can be caused by a loss, addition, or rearrangement of the genes on a chromosome or by the exchange of genes between chromosomes
  - Deviations in the number of chromosomes involve either the gain or loss of an entire chromosome during cell division; the suffix -*somy* is used in disorders with abnormal numbers
  - Nondisjunction is the failure of chromosomes to separate during cell division

Key facts about X-linked recessive disorders

- They're most commonly expressed in males who have parents who are unaffected.
- All daughters of an affected male will be carriers.
- Examples include hemophilia, Duchenne's disease (pseudohypertrophic muscular dystrophy), and color blindness.

Key facts about X-linked dominant disorders

- A person with the abnormal trait must have one affected parent.
- If the father has an X-linked dominant disorder, all his daughters and none of his sons will be affected.
- If a mother has an X-linked dominant disorder, each of her children has a 50% chance of being affected.

A look at X-linked inheritance

X-LINKED RECESSIVE INHERITANCE

The diagram shows the children of a normal parent and a parent with a recessive gene on the X chromosome (shown by an open dot). All daughters of an affected male will be carriers. The son of a female carrier may inherit a recessive gene on the X chromosome and be affected by the disease. Unaffected sons can't transmit the disorder.

Affected father	Normal mother	
	X	X
X	XX Carrier daughter	XX Carrier daughter
Y	XY Normal son	XY Normal son

Normal father	Carrier mother	
	X	X
X	XX Carrier daughter	XX Normal daughter
Y	XY Affected son	XY Normal son

X-LINKED DOMINANT INHERITANCE

The diagram shows the children of a normal parent and a parent with an abnormal, X-linked dominant gene on the X chromosome (shown by the dot on the X). When the father is affected, only his daughters have the abnormal gene. When the mother is affected, sons and daughters may be affected.

Affected father	Normal mother	
	X	X
X	XX Affected daughter	XX Affected daughter
Y	XY Normal son	XY Normal son

Normal father	Affected mother	
	X	X
X	XX Affected daughter	XX Normal daughter
Y	XY Affected son	XY Normal son

Key facts about multifactorial inheritance disorders

- Two types exist: In the first, genes and the environment interact to produce an aberration. In the second, no inheritance pattern is identifiable, but risk of recurrence is higher in certain families.
- Examples include cleft lip and palate, congenital dislocated hip, congenital heart defects, neural tube defects, and pyloric stenosis.

Categories of genetic disorders

- Single-gene disorders
- Autosomal dominant disorders
- Autosomal recessive disorders
- Sex-linked disorders
- X-linked recessive disorders
- X-linked dominant disorders
- Multifactorial inheritance disorders

– Translocation is the joining of two chromosomes to make one larger double chromosome
– The most common chromosomal disorder is Down syndrome (trisomy 21)
- Multifactorial inheritance disorders
  – Two types of multifactorial inheritance disorders exist
    • In the first type, genes and the environment interact to produce an aberration

- In the second type, no inheritance pattern is identifiable, but risk of recurrence is higher in certain families
    - Examples include cleft lip and palate, congenital dislocated hip, congenital heart defects, neural tube defects, and pyloric stenosis

Detection of genetic disorders

- Indications for preconception genetic counseling
    - Members of a high-risk group (for example, Tay-Sachs disease among Ashkenazic Jews)
    - Members of families with a history of genetic disorders
- Indications for prenatal genetic testing
    - Pregnant patient age 35 or older
    - Couple who previously produced a child with a genetic disorder
    - Couple who's heterozygous for a recessive disorder
    - Couple in which one or both partners have a genetic disorder
    - Female who's a carrier of an X-linked disorder
- Prenatal testing methods
    - Amniocentesis
    - Ultrasonography detects anencephaly, microcephaly, and hydrocephaly
    - Roentgenography detects bone abnormalities
- Postdelivery detection
    - Biochemical tests for phenylketonuria, hypothyroidism, and galactosemia
    - Cytologic studies for an infant whose appearance suggests a chromosomal aberration
    - Dermatoglyphics to determine chromosomal aberrations by evaluating dermal ridges

Nursing implications

- Understand genetic theory well enough to reinforce information given by the genetic counselor
- Be aware of factors necessitating genetic counseling, such as increased age and family history, when obtaining medical and obstetric history
- Prepare the patient by explaining the purpose of and procedure for each diagnostic test
- Assist with diagnostic testing as necessary
- Provide emotional support to those receiving genetic counseling
- Act as an advocate, counselor, and teacher; with advanced preparation and certification, the nurse can function as a genetic counselor
- Anticipate common responses to diagnoses of genetic disorders, such as apathy, denial, anger, hostility, fear, embarrassment, grief, and lowered self-esteem
- Be aware of new and controversial issues concerning genetics

---

Prenatal testing methods

- Amniocentesis
- Ultrasonography
- Roentgenography

Ways to detect genetic disorders after delivery

- Biochemical tests
- Cytologic studies
- Dermatoglyphics

Your role in genetic counseling

- Understand genetic theory well enough to reinforce information given by the genetic counselor.
- Be aware of factors necessitating genetic counseling when obtaining medical and obstetric history.
- Prepare the patient by explaining the purpose of and procedure for each diagnostic test.
- Provide emotional support to those receiving genetic counseling.

TOP 7

Items to study for your next test on infertility and genetics

1. The female factors that contribute to infertility
2. The male factors that contribute to infertility
3. Diagnostic evaluations used to determine female and male infertility
4. Treatment options for female and male infertility
5. Seven options for an infertile couple
6. Inheritance patterns
7. The categories of genetic disorders

NCLEX CHECKS

It's never too soon to begin your NCLEX preparation. Now that you've reviewed this chapter, carefully read each of the following questions and choose the best answer. Then compare your responses to the correct answers.

1. Which condition would be <u>least likely</u> to contribute to infertility?
- ☐ **A.** Pelvic inflammatory disease (PID)
- ☒ **B.** Alkalinity of vaginal pH
- ☐ **C.** Excessively thick cervical mucus
- ☐ **D.** Endometriosis

2. Which cervical mucus assessment finding suggests that a woman is about to ovulate?
- ☐ **A.** Thick cervical mucus
- ☐ **B.** Absence of ferning
- ☒ **C.** Highly stretchable mucus
- ☐ **D.** Highly viscous mucus

3. Which drug would the nurse expect to administer to a woman with infertility secondary to anovulation to suppress the hypothalamus?
- ☒ **A.** Clomiphene (Clomid)
- ☐ **B.** Bromocriptine (Parlodel)
- ☐ **C.** Levothyroxine (Synthroid)
- ☐ **D.** Testosterone cypionate (Depo-testosterone)

4. Which of the following conditions is an example of an autosomal recessive disorder? Select all that apply.
- ☑ **A.** Sickle cell anemia
- ☐ **B.** Marfan syndrome
- ☐ **C.** Huntington's disease
- ☒ **D.** Cystic fibrosis
- ☒ **E.** Tay-Sachs disease

5. Which disorder is an example of a chromosomal aberration?
- ☒ **A.** Down syndrome
- ☐ **B.** Color blindness — X linke recessive
- ☐ **C.** Hemophilia — x
- ☐ **D.** Vitamin D–resistant rickets — X linke dominat

ANSWERS AND RATIONALES

1. CORRECT ANSWER: B
An alkaline vaginal pH isn't likely to contribute to infertility because sperm can survive well in an alkaline environment. Rather, a highly acidic vaginal pH decreases the ability of sperm to survive. PID, which can lead to scarring of the fallopian tubes; excessively thick cervical mucus, which interferes with sperm motility; and endometriosis, which can cause obstructions in the reproductive tract are considered contributory factors for infertility.

2. CORRECT ANSWER: C
When estrogen stimulation is high, just before ovulation, cervical mucus is highly stretchable and thin, demonstrates ferning, and has low viscosity.

3. CORRECT ANSWER: A
Clomiphene (Clomid), which suppresses the hypothalamus, is the drug used to treat infertility due to anovulation. Bromocriptine (Parlodel) is used to increase prolactin levels in women with infertility who are anovulatory. Levothyroxine (Synthroid) is used to treat infertility secondary to hypothyroidism. Testosterone cypionate (Depo-testosterone), which increases virilization, is used to treat males with infertility.

4. CORRECT ANSWERS: A, D, AND E
Sickle cell anemia, cystic fibrosis, and Tay-sachs disease are examples of autosomal recessive disorders. Marfan syndrome and Huntington's disease are examples of autosomal dominant disorders.

5. CORRECT ANSWER: A
Down (trisomy 21) syndrome is an example of chromosomal aberration which involves a deviation in the number of chromosomes. Color blindness and hemophilia are examples of X-linked recessive disorders. Vitamin D–resistant rickets is an example of an X-linked dominant disorder.

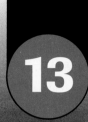

13

Family planning and contraception

LEARNING OBJECTIVES

After studying this chapter, you should be able to:

- Identify the goals of family planning.
- Describe how various methods of contraception prevent pregnancy.
- Discuss the nurse's role in family planning.
- Describe various emotional responses to an elective abortion.
- Discuss methods of pregnancy termination for each trimester.

CHAPTER OVERVIEW

A woman's ability to reproduce carries with it many options. Many of these choices may involve highly emotional issues. The nurse plays a key role, providing accurate information to allow patients to make an informed decision about reproductive choices along with nonjudgmental support to the patient and her partner.

FAMILY PLANNING

● **Description**
- Involves the decisions couples or individuals make about when (and if) they should have children, how many children to have, and how long to wait between pregnancies

- Also consists of choices to prevent or achieve pregnancy and to control the timing and number of pregnancies
- Has many ethical, physical, emotional, religious, and legal implications
- Can be achieved through various methods, such as the use of abstinence, natural methods for fertility awareness, mechanical barriers, pharmacologic agents, chemical barriers, and surgery
- Contraception is the deliberate prevention of conception, using a method or device to avert fertilization of an ovum
- With a 0% failure rate, abstinence, or refraining from sexual intercourse, is the most effective way to prevent conception
  - The most effective way to prevent the transmission of sexually transmitted diseases (STDs)
  - Not a popular option, especially among adolescents
  - Should always be presented as an option to the patient, along with information about other forms of contraception

Nursing implications

- Carefully evaluate own personal beliefs and attitudes about family planning
- Provide open, nonjudgmental counseling in a trusting setting
- If possible, include the woman's partner or significant other in teaching sessions
- Obtain a reproductive history, including the following information, to assess which method of family planning is most appropriate for the patient
  - Interval between menses
  - Duration and amount of flow
  - Problems that occur during menses
  - Number of previous pregnancies
  - Number of previous births (and date of each)
  - Duration of each pregnancy
  - Type of each delivery
  - Gender and weight of children when delivered
  - Problems that occurred during previous pregnancy
  - Problems that occurred after delivery
  - Potential risks of complications
- Include discussions about prevention and treatment of STDs when talking about family planning (see *Considerations for family planning,* page 368)
- Play different roles, including that of a teacher, counselor, advocate, and researcher
  - As a teacher, present information about various contraceptive methods as well as proper use

Family planning methods

- Abstinence
- Natural methods for fertility awareness
- Mechanical barriers
- Pharmacologic agents
- Chemical barriers
- Surgery

Information to obtain in a reproductive history

- Interval between menses
- Duration and amount of flow
- Problems that occur during menses
- Number of previous pregnancies
- Number of previous births (and date of each)
- Duration of each pregnancy
- Type of each delivery
- Gender and weight of children when delivered
- Problems that occurred during previous pregnancy
- Problems that occurred after delivery
- Potential risks of complications

TIME-OUT FOR TEACHING

Considerations for family planning

Be sure to include these topics in your teaching plan for the woman and her partner considering family planning:

- underlying reasons for family planning
- any physical, emotional, religious, or ethical concerns about family planning
- contraceptive methods available
- advantages and disadvantages of each
- information about sexually transmitted diseases and safer sex practices.

- As a counselor, help the woman select the method that best suits her lifestyle and needs
- As an advocate, support the woman's choice, regardless of personal beliefs
- As a researcher, participate in studies, and identify new avenues to be evaluated
- Evaluate the woman's (and partner's) understanding of the method chosen, including the following:
  - Correct use of the method
  - Possible adverse reactions and ability to report problems if any occur
  - The need to return for follow-up visit if indicated
  - Degree of acceptance of current method

NATURAL FAMILY PLANNING METHODS

Description
- Contraceptive methods that don't use chemicals or foreign material or devices to prevent pregnancy
- Religious beliefs may prevent some individuals from using hormonal or internal contraceptive devices
- Others just prefer a more natural method of planning or preventing pregnancy
- For most natural family planning methods, the woman's fertile days must be calculated so that she can abstain from intercourse on those days
  - Various methods are used to determine the woman's fertile period
  - The effectiveness of these methods depends on the patient's and partner's willingness to refrain from sex on the patient's fertile days
  - Failure rates vary from 10% to 20%

Quick guide to natural family planning methods

- **Rhythm method** – also known as *calendar method;* requires refraining from intercourse when the woman is likely to conceive
- **BBT** – requires the woman to take her temperature every morning; commonly combined with rhythm method
- **Cervical mucus** – also known as *Billings method;* relies on changes in the consistency of cervical mucus to predict when the woman is most likely to conceive
- **Symptothermal** – combines BBT method with cervical mucus method
- **Ovulation awareness** – use of over-the-counter ovulation detection kits to determine when the woman is most likely to conceive
- **Coitus interruptus** – withdrawal of the penis before ejaculation

– Natural family planning methods include the rhythm, or calendar, method; basal body temperature (BBT) method; cervical mucus, or Billings, method; symptothermal method; ovulation awareness; and coitus interruptus

Rhythm method

- Description
  - Also known as the *calendar method*
  - Requires that the couple refrain from intercourse on those days the woman is most likely to conceive based on her menstrual cycle
  - This fertile period usually lasts from 3 to 4 days before until 3 to 4 days after ovulation.
- Advantages
  - No drugs or devices are needed
  - It's free
  - It may be acceptable to members of religious groups that oppose birth control
  - It encourages couples to learn more about how the female body functions
  - It encourages communication between partners
  - It can also be used to plan a pregnancy
- Disadvantages
  - It requires meticulous record keeping as well as an ability and willingness for the woman to monitor her body changes
  - It restricts sexual spontaneity during the woman's fertile period
  - It requires extended periods of abstinence from intercourse
  - It's reliable only for women with regular menstrual cycles
  - It may be unreliable during periods of illness, infection, or stress
- Nursing implications
  - Teach the woman to keep a diary of her menstrual cycle (for six consecutive cycles) to determine when ovulation is most likely to occur
  - To calculate her safe periods, tell her to subtract 18 from the shortest cycle and 11 from the longest cycle that she has documented (see *Using the calendar method,* page 370)
    - For instance, if she had 6 menstrual cycles that lasted 26 to 30 days, her fertile period would be from the 8th day (26 minus 18) to the 19th day (30 minus 11)
    - To ensure that pregnancy doesn't occur, she and her partner should abstain from intercourse during days 8 to 19 of her menstrual cycle
    - During those fertile days, she and her partner may also choose to use contraceptive foam

The rhythm method: The pros

- No drugs or devices are needed.
- It's free.
- It can also be used to plan a pregnancy.

The rhythm method: The cons

- It requires meticulous record keeping.
- It restricts sexual spontaneity.
- It's reliable only for women with regular menstrual cycles.

Using the calendar method

This illustration demonstrates how the calendar method would be used to determine the woman's fertile period (ovulation) and when she should abstain from coitus.

			JULY			
S	M	T	W	T	F	S
			X̶1	X̶2	X̶3	X̶4
X̶5	X̶6	X̶7	⑧	⑨	⑩	⑪
⑫	⑬	⑭	⑮	16	⑰	⑱
⑲	20	21	22	23	24	25
26	27	28	X̶29	X̶30	X̶31	

X = Menstrual flow
O = Days of abstinence
▨ = Day of ovulation

Key facts about BBT

- It's lower during the first 2 weeks of the menstrual cycle, before ovulation.
- Immediately after ovulation, it rises until the next menses occur.
- The rise in BBT indicates that progesterone has been released and the woman has ovulated.
- To use the BBT method, a woman must take her temperature every morning before getting out of bed.
- The BBT method is typically combined with the calendar method.

● BBT

- Description
  - Lower during the first 2 weeks of the menstrual cycle, before ovulation
  - Immediately after ovulation, temperature begins to rise, continuing upward until it's time for the next menses
    - The rise in temperature indicates that progesterone has been released into the system
    - It also means that the woman has ovulated
  - Just before the day of ovulation, a woman's BBT falls about one-half degree
  - At the time of ovulation, her BBT rises a full degree because of progesterone influence
  - To use the BBT method of contraception, a woman must take her temperature every morning before getting out of bed and beginning her morning activity
  - By recording this daily temperature, she can see a slight dip and then an increase in body temperature; the increase in temperature indicates ovulation

- With the temperature increase, intercourse is avoided for the next 3 days, which is the life of a discharged ovum
- Because sperm can survive in the female reproductive tract for 4 days, the BBT method of contraception is typically combined with the calendar method so that the couple can abstain from intercourse a few days before ovulation as well
- BBT method can be affected by many variables, which may lead to mistaken interpretations of a fertile day as a safe day and vice versa
  - Forgetting to take the temperature or taking after arising may lead to a rise in temperature
  - Illness also may cause temperature to rise
  - Changes in daily routine or activities also could affect temperature
- Advantages
  - It's relatively inexpensive; only expense involved is the cost of a BBT thermometer, which is calibrated in tenths of a degree
  - No drugs are needed
  - It may be acceptable to members of religious groups that oppose birth control
  - It encourages couples to learn more about how the female body functions
  - It encourages communication between partners
  - It can also be used to plan a pregnancy
- Disadvantages
  - It requires meticulous record keeping and an ability and willingness to monitor the woman's body changes
  - It restricts sexual spontaneity during the woman's fertile period
  - It requires extended periods of abstinence from intercourse
  - It's reliable only for women with regular menstrual cycles
  - It may be unreliable during periods of illness, infection, or stress
  - It's contraindicated in women who have irregular menses
- Nursing implications
  - Advise the patient that charting BBT doesn't predict the exact day of ovulation; it just indicates that ovulation has occurred, allowing the patient to monitor her ovulatory pattern and giving her a time frame for planning
  - Advise the patient to chart the days of menstrual flow on a temperature graph; have her start with the first day of her menses (day 1) and then take her temperature each day after her menses ends
  - Tell the patient to use a thermometer that measures tenths of a degree

BBT: The pros

- It's relatively inexpensive.
- No drugs are needed.
- It can also be used to plan a pregnancy.

BBT: The cons

- It requires meticulous record keeping.
- It restricts sexual spontaneity.
- It requires extended periods of abstinence.
- It's reliable only for women with regular menstrual cycles.

Characteristics of cervical mucus at ovulation

- Thin
- Watery
- Transparent
- Copious
- Slippery
- Stretchable (up to 2.5 cm)

Cervical mucus method: The pros

- No drugs or devices are needed.
- It's free.
- It can also be used to plan a pregnancy.

Cervical mucus method: The cons

- It requires meticulous record keeping.
- It restricts sexual spontaneity.
- It may be unreliable during periods of illness, infection, or stress.

– Instruct the patient to take her temperature as soon as she wakes up—before she gets out of bed or does anything else; tell the patient to do this at the same time each morning
– Instruct the patient to place a dot on the graph's line that matches the temperature reading (Tell her not to be surprised if her waking temperature before ovulation is 96° to 97° F [35.6° to 36.1° C])
– If she forgets to take her temperature one day, instruct her to leave that day blank on the graph and not to connect the dots
– Instruct her to make notes on the graph if she misses taking her temperature, feels sick, can't sleep, or wakes up at a different time
– Advise her also that if she's taking any medicine—even aspirin— to note this on the graph, because it may affect her temperature
– Remind her also to mark the dates when she had sexual relations

● Cervical mucus method

- Description
  – Also known as the *Billings method*
  – Predicts changes in the cervical mucus during ovulation
  – Each month, before a woman's menses, the cervical mucus becomes thick and stretches when pulled between the thumb and forefinger
  – The normal stretchable amount of cervical mucus (also known as *spinnbarkeit*) is 8 to 10 cm
  – Just before ovulation, the cervical mucus becomes thin, watery, transparent, and copious
  – During the peak of ovulation, the cervical mucus becomes slippery and stretches at least 2.5 cm before the strand breaks
  – Breast tenderness and anterior tilt of the cervix also occur with ovulation
  – The fertile period consists of all the days that the cervical mucus is copious and the 3 days after the peak date.
  – During these days, the woman and her partner should abstain from intercourse to avoid conception
- Advantages
  – No drugs or devices are needed
  – It's free
  – It may be acceptable to members of religious groups that oppose birth control
  – It encourages couples to learn more about how the female body functions
  – It encourages communication between partners
  – It can also be used to plan a pregnancy
  – There are no contraindications

- Disadvantages
  - It requires meticulous record keeping and an ability and willingness to monitor the woman's body changes
  - It restricts sexual spontaneity during the woman's fertile period
  - It requires extended periods of abstinence from intercourse
  - It's reliable only for women with regular menstrual cycles
  - It may be unreliable during periods of illness, infection, or stress
- Nursing implications
  - Remind the woman to check her cervical mucus every day to note changes in the consistency and amounts so that she can recognize the changes that signify ovulation
  - Advise her to avoid checking cervical mucus after intercourse; doing so is unreliable because seminal fluid has a watery, postovulatory consistency, which can be confused with ovulatory mucus

Symptothermal method
- Description
  - Combines the BBT method with the cervical mucus method
  - The woman takes her daily temperature and watches for the rise in temperature that signals the onset of ovulation
  - She also assesses her cervical mucus daily
  - The couple abstains from intercourse until 3 days after the rise in basal temperature or the fourth day after the peak day (indicating ovulation) of cervical mucus because these symptoms indicate the woman's fertile period
  - Combining the two methods is more effective than if either is used alone
- Advantages
  - It's relatively inexpensive; the only expense involved is the cost of a BBT thermometer, which is calibrated in tenths of a degree
  - No drugs are needed
  - It may be acceptable to members of religious groups that oppose birth control
  - It encourages patients and their partners to learn more about how the female body functions
  - It encourages communication between partners
  - It can also be used to plan a pregnancy
- Disadvantages
  - It requires meticulous record keeping and ability and willingness of a woman to monitor body changes
  - It restricts sexual spontaneity during the woman's fertile period
  - It requires extended periods of abstinence from intercourse
  - It's reliable only for women with regular menstrual cycles
  - It may be unreliable during periods of illness, infection, or stress

Key facts about the symptothermal method
- It combines the BBT method with the cervical mucus method.
- The patient takes her daily temperature and watches for the rise in temperature that signals the onset of ovulation.
- The patient assesses her cervical mucus daily.

Symptothermal method: The pros
- It's relatively inexpensive.
- No drugs are needed.
- It can also be used to plan a pregnancy.

Symptothermal method: The cons
- It requires meticulous record keeping.
- It restricts sexual spontaneity.
- It's reliable only for women with regular menstrual cycles.

TIME-OUT FOR TEACHING

Performing a home ovulation test

A home ovulation test helps the patient determine the best time to try to become pregnant or to prevent pregnancy by monitoring the amount of leuteinizing hormone (LH) that's found in her urine. Normally, during each menstrual cycle, levels of LH rise suddenly, causing an egg to be released from the ovary 24 to 36 hours later. Ovulation test kits can be purchased over-the-counter.

Include the following topics in the teaching plan for the woman who will be using a home ovulation test.

Preparing for the test
- Read the kit's directions thoroughly before performing the test.
- Before testing, calculate the length of the menstrual cycle. Count from the beginning of one menses to the beginning of the next menses. (The patient should count her 1st day of bleeding as day 1. She can use the chart at right to determine when to begin testing.)
- Perform the test any time, day or night, but perform it at the same time every day.
- Avoid urinating for at least 4 hours before taking the test, and don't drink a lot of fluids for several hours before the test.

Taking the test
- After removing the test stick from the packet, sit on the toilet and direct the absorbent tip of the test stick downward and directly into the urine stream for at least 5 seconds or until it's thoroughly wet.
- Be careful not to urinate on the window of the stick.
- As an alternative method, urinate into a clean, dry cup or container and then dip the test stick (absorbent tip only) into the urine for at least 5 seconds.
- Make sure the stick is placed on a clean, flat, dry surface.

- Nursing implications
  - Make sure that the woman understands how to check cervical mucus and monitor temperature
  - Reinforce all instructions related to BBT monitoring and cervical mucus method

Ovulation awareness method
- Description
  - Over-the-counter ovulation detection kits determine ovulation by measuring luteinizing hormone (LH) in the urine
  - During each menstrual cycle, LH levels surge, causing an ovum to be released from the ovary 24 to 36 hours later (ovulation)
  - This method can be used to determine the midcycle surge of LH, which can be detected in the urine as early as 12 hours after ovulation
  - These kits are about 98% to 100% accurate, but they're fairly expensive to use as a primary means of birth control

Facts about ovulation

- During each menstrual cycle, LH levels surge, causing ovulation within 36 hours.
- The midcycle surge of LH can can be detected in the urine as early as 12 hours after ovulation.
- Over-the-counter ovulation detection kits can measure the amount of LH in urine.

Performing a home ovulation test (continued)

LENGTH OF CYCLE	START TEST THIS MANY DAYS AFTER YOUR LAST MENSES BEGINS	LENGTH OF CYCLE	START TEST THIS MANY DAYS AFTER YOUR LAST MENSES BEGINS
21	5	31	14
22	5	32	15
23	6	33	16
24	7	34	17
25	8	34	18
26	9	36	19
27	10	37	20
28	11	38	21
29	12	39	22
30	13	40	23

Reading the results
- Wait at least 5 minutes before reading the results. When the test is finished, a line appears in the small window (control window).
To determine ovulation:
- If there's no line in the large rectangular window (test window) or if the line is lighter than the line in the small rectangular window (control window), the patient hasn't begun an LH surge. She should continue testing daily.
- If she sees one line in the large rectangular window that's similar to or darker than the line in the small window, she's experiencing an LH surge. This means that ovulation should occur within the next 24 to 36 hours.
- After determining ovulation, use the knowledge that the patient is at the start of the most fertile time of her cycle to plan accordingly.

- Advantages
  - It's an easier way to determine ovulation than the BBT or cervical mucus methods
  - It may be less offensive to a woman than the cervical mucus method
  - It has a high rate of accuracy
  - There are no contraindications
- Disadvantages
  - It can be expensive
  - It requires extended periods of abstinence from intercourse
  - It's reliable only for women with regular menstrual cycles
- Nursing implications
  - Make sure that the woman understands how to use the ovulation test kit (see *Performing a home ovulation test*)
  - Instruct the patient in how to read the test correctly
  - Assist the patient with planning appropriately when ovulation is detected

Ovulation awareness method: The pros

- It's an easy way to determine ovulation.
- It has a high rate of accuracy.

Ovulation awareness method: The cons

- It can be expensive.
- It's reliable only for women with regular menstrual cycles.

Coitus interruptus: The pros and cons

- Pros
- It's free.
- It doesn't involve record keeping.
- It has no contraindications.
- Con
- It's unreliable.

Facts about oral contraceptives

- Also known as *birth control pills*, they consist of synthetic estrogen and progesterone.
- The estrogen suppresses ovulation.
- The progesterone decreases cervical mucus permeability, limiting sperm's access to the ova.

● **Coitus interruptus**

- Description
  - One of the oldest known methods of contraception
  - Involves withdrawal of the penis from the vagina during intercourse before ejaculation
  - However, because preejaculation fluid that's deposited outside the vagina may contain spermatozoa, fertilization can occur
- Advantages
  - It's free
  - It doesn't involve record keeping
  - There are no contraindications
- Disadvantage is that it's unreliable
- Nursing implications
  - Instruct the patient and her partner in the need to control ejaculation
  - Warn the couple that even with withdrawal, sperm may be deposited in the vagina, possibly leading to fertilization

PHARMACOLOGIC METHODS

● **Oral contraceptives**

- Description
  - Also known as *birth control pills* or *hormonal contraceptives*
  - Consist of synthetic estrogen and progesterone
  - The estrogen suppresses production of follicle-stimulating hormone (FSH) and LH, which, in turn, suppresses ovulation
  - The progesterone complements the estrogen's action by causing a decrease in cervical mucus permeability, which limits sperm's access to the ova
  - Progesterone also decreases the possibility of implantation by interfering with endometrial proliferation
  - Two types of oral contraceptives are available, dispensed in 21-day or 28-day packs
    - Monophasic oral contraceptives
      - Provide fixed doses of estrogen and progesterone throughout a 21-day cycle
      - Provide a steady dose of estrogen but an increased amount of progestin during the last 11 days of the menstrual cycle
    - Triphasic oral contraceptives
      - Maintain a cycle more like a woman's natural menstrual cycle because they vary the amount of estrogen and progestin throughout the cycle

- Have a lower incidence of breakthrough bleeding than monophasic oral contraceptives

- Advantages
  - Monophasic and triphasic oral contraceptives are 99.5% effective in providing contraception; failure rate, about 3%, usually occurs because the woman forgot to take the pill or because of other individual differences in the woman's physiology
  - They don't inhibit sexual spontaneity
  - They may reduce the risk of endometrial and ovarian cancer, ectopic pregnancy, ovarian cysts, and noncancerous breast tumors
  - They decrease the risk of pelvic inflammatory disease (PID) and dysmenorrhea.
  - They regulate the menstrual cycle and may diminish or eliminate premenstrual tension
- Disadvantages
  - They don't protect the woman or her partner from STDs
  - They must be taken daily
  - They can be expensive
  - Illnesses that cause vomiting may reduce their effectiveness
  - They're contraindicated in women who are breast-feeding or pregnant; those who have a family history of stroke, coronary artery disease, thrombohemolytic disease, or liver disease; and those who have undiagnosed vaginal bleeding, malignancy of the reproductive system, malignant cell growth, or hypertension
  - Women who are older than age 40 and those who have a history of or have been diagnosed with diabetes mellitus, elevated triglyceride or cholesterol level, breast or reproductive tract malignancy, high blood pressure, obesity, seizure disorder, sickle cell disease, mental depression, and migraines or other vascular-type headaches should be strongly cautioned about taking oral contraceptives for birth control
  - A patient older than age 35 is at increased risk for a fatal heart attack if she smokes more than 15 cigarettes per day and takes oral contraceptives
  - Adverse effects include nausea, headache, weight gain, depression, mild hypertension, breast tenderness, breakthrough bleeding, and candidal vaginal infections
  - When a woman wants to conceive, she may not be able to for up to 8 months after stopping oral contraceptives because the pituitary gland requires a recovery period to begin the stimulation of cyclic gonadotropins, such as FSH and LH, which help regulate ovulation

Types of oral contraceptives

- Monophasic oral contraceptives—fixed doses of estrogen and progesterone
- Triphasic oral contraceptives—varied doses of estrogen and progesterone

Oral contraceptives: The pros

- They're 99.5% effective in preventing pregnancy.
- They don't inhibit sexual spontaneity.
- They may reduce the risk of endometrial and ovarian cancer, ectopic pregnancy, ovarian cysts, and noncancerous breast tumors.
- They decrease the risk of PID and dysmenorrhea.

Oral contraceptives: The cons

- They don't protect the woman or her partner from STDs.
- They must be taken daily.
- They can be expensive.
- Illnesses that cause vomiting may reduce their effectiveness.

What to do for a patient taking an oral contraceptive

- Reinforce the need to take the medication every day.
- Explain how to take the medication.
- Reinforce the need to notify the health care provider of adverse reactions.
- Advise the woman to maintain yearly follow-up appointments for pelvic examinations, Pap smears, and breast examinations.
- Instruct the woman in breast self-examination techniques.

TIME-OUT FOR TEACHING

Oral contraceptives

Be sure to reinforce these points when teaching patients about oral contraceptives:

- possible adverse reactions, such as fluid retention, weight gain, breast tenderness, headache, breakthrough bleeding, chloasma, acne, yeast infection, nausea, and fatigue (it may be necessary to change the type or dosage of the contraceptive to relieve these adverse reactions)
- dietary needs, including increased intake of foods high in vitamin B_6 (wheat, corn, liver, meat) and folic acid (liver; green, leafy vegetables) because about 20% to 30% of oral contraceptive users have dietary deficiencies of vitamin B_6 and folic acid (some health care professionals contend that oral contraceptive users should increase their intake of

vitamins A, B_2, B_{12}, and C and niacin)
- use of an additional form of contraception for the first 7 days after starting the drug because it doesn't take effect for 7 days
- measures if patient misses one pill, including taking the pill as soon as remembered and continuing with the usual schedule the next day
- measures if patient misses two consecutive pills, including taking two pills as soon as remembered, two pills again on the following day, then continuing with the usual schedule
- measures if patient misses three or more consecutive pills, including discarding the remainder of the pack, then starting a new pack on the following Sunday.

  - Many health care providers recommend that women not become pregnant within 2 months of stopping the drug
- Nursing implications
  - Reinforce the need to take the medication every day
  - Instruct the patient how to take the medication, whether using a 21-day or 28-day pack
    - Advise the woman to take the first pill on the first Sunday after the start of her menses (or start oral contraceptives on any day)
    - If the woman has recently given birth, advise her to start oral contraceptives on the first Sunday 2 weeks after delivery
    - Instruct the woman to use an additional form of contraception for the first week after starting an oral contraceptive because the drug doesn't take effect for 7 days (see *Oral contraceptives*)
    - If the woman is using a 21-day pack, advise her to take a pill every day for 3 weeks, and then no pill for the next 7 days, with the expectation that her menstrual flow should start about 4 days after she takes a cycle of pills
    - If the woman is using a 28-day pill pack (which contains 3 weeks of hormonal agents and 1 week of placebos), instruct the woman to start a new pack of pills when she finishes the last

pack; using a 28 day pill pack helps to eliminate the risk of forgetting to start a new pack

- Reinforce the need to notify the health care provider of any adverse reactions
- Advise women using oral contraceptives to maintain yearly follow-up appointments for pelvic examination, Papanicolaou (Pap) test, and breast examination
- Instruct the woman in breast self-examination techniques, urging her to perform them every month

● **Transdermal patch**
  - Description
    - A highly effective, weekly hormonal birth control patch that's worn on the skin
    - Provides a combination of estrogen and progestin
    - The hormones are absorbed into the skin and then transferred into the bloodstream
    - The patch is very thin, beige, and smooth and measures 1¾" (4.4-cm) square
    - It can be worn on the upper outer arm, buttocks, abdomen, or upper torso
    - The patch is worn for 1 week and replaced on the same day of the week for 3 consecutive weeks. No patch is worn during the fourth week.
    - Studies have shown that the patch remains attached and effective when the patient bathes, swims, exercises, or wears it in humid weather
  - Advantages
    - It's 99% effective in preventing pregnancy if used exactly as directed
    - It's convenient
    - No preparation is needed before intercourse
    - It's a good alternative for patients who often forget to take oral contraceptives
  - Disadvantages
    - It doesn't protect the woman or her partner from STDs
    - It's contraindicated in women who are breast-feeding; those who have a family history of stroke, coronary artery disease, thrombohemolytic disease, or liver disease; those who have undiagnosed vaginal bleeding; and those who are sensitive to the adhesive used on the patch
    - It should be used cautiously by women who are older than 40; women who have a history of or have been diagnosed with diabetes mellitus, elevated triglyceride or cholesterol levels, breast or

reproductive tract malignancy, high blood pressure, obesity, seizure disorder, sickle cell disease, mental depression, and migraine or other vascular-type headaches; and women who smoke
- Nursing implications
  - Instruct the woman in how to apply the patch
  - Tell the woman to wear the patch for 1 week, replace it on the same day of the week for 3 consecutive weeks, and wear no patch during the fourth week.
  - Instruct the patient to report any danger signs, such as chest pain, shortness of breath, and pain or swelling in the lower extremities

Parenteral agents
- Description
  - Hormonal contraceptives may be given parenterally or as I.M. injections
  - I.M. injections of medroxyprogesterone (Depo-Provera) are administered every 12 weeks
    - Depo-Provera stops ovulation from occurring by suppressing the release of gonadotropic hormone
    - It also changes the cervical mucosa to prevent sperm from entering the uterus
- Advantages
  - Parenteral forms don't inhibit sexual response
  - Only abstinence is more effective than these methods
  - I.M. injection lasts for about 3 months; subdermal implants, for up to 5 years
  - Breast-feeding women may use the injection method
- Disadvantages
  - Insertion is invasive, either with I.M. injection or surgical insertion of rods
  - Either can be expensive
  - If the patient wants to become pregnant, it may take 9 to 10 months after the last I.M. injection to conceive
  - Neither method protects against STDs
  - Effects can't be reversed after injection or insertion
  - They may cause changes in the menstrual cycle, weight gain, headache, fatigue, and nervousness
  - Contraindications include pregnancy, liver disease, undiagnosed vaginal bleeding, breast cancer, blood clotting disorders, and cardiovascular disease
- Nursing implications
  - Instruct the patient in how these methods prevent pregnancy

Key facts about parenteral agents

- They're I.M. injections of medroxyprogesterone administered every 12 weeks.
- They stop ovulation from occurring by suppressing the release of gonadotropic hormone.
- They also change the cervical mucosa to prevent sperm from entering the uterus.

Parenteral agents: The pros

- They don't inhibit sexual response.
- They're fairly long-lasting.
- Breast-feeding women can use them.

Parenteral agents: The cons

- Insertion is invasive.
- They can be expensive.
- They don't protect against STDs.
- Their effects can't be reversed.

– Advise the patient with a subdermal implant to report any tenderness or bruising at the insertion site, or evidence of rods coming through the skin

– Remind the patient receiving I.M. injections to follow up every 3 months for repeat injections

– Advise the patient of danger signs and symptoms to report to the health care provider, such as chest pain, shortness of breath, pain or swelling in the extremities, or heavy vaginal bleeding

– Urge the woman with subdermal implants to notify the health care provider of any signs or symptoms of infection at the insertion site

BARRIER METHODS

● Description

- Involve insertion of a chemical or mechanical barrier between the cervix and the sperm to prevent the sperm from entering the uterus, traveling to the fallopian tubes, and fertilizing the ovum
- Because these methods don't use hormones, they're sometimes favored over hormonal contraceptives, which have many adverse effects
- However, failure rates for barrier methods are higher than those for hormonal contraceptives

● Male condom

- Description
  - A latex or synthetic sheath that's placed over the erect penis before intercourse
  - Prevents pregnancy by collecting spermatozoa in the tip of the condom, preventing them from entering the vagina
- Advantages
  - Many women favor the male condom because it puts the responsibility of birth control on the male
  - No health care visit is needed
  - Available over-the-counter in pharmacies and grocery stores
  - Easy to carry
  - Prevents the spread of STDs
- Disadvantages
  - A condom must be applied before any vulvar penile contact takes place because preejaculation fluid may contain sperm
  - It may cause an allergic reaction if the product contains latex and the patient or her partner is allergic
  - It may break during use if it's used incorrectly or is of poor quality
  - It can't be reused
  - Sexual pleasure may be affected

Quick guide to barrier methods

- **Male condom** – a latex or synthetic sheath that's placed over the erect penis before intercourse
- **Female condom** – a vaginal sheath made of polyurethane and lubricated with nonoxynol 9
- **Diaphragm** – a soft, latex dome that's supported by a round, metal spring
- **Cervical cap** – a thimble-shaped, soft rubber cup that fits over the cervix
- **Spermicides** – gels, creams, films, foams, and suppositories that act as chemical barriers

Male condom: The pros

- No health care visit is needed.
- It's readily available.
- It's easy to carry.
- It prevents the spread of STDs.

Male condom: The cons

- It can break during use.
- It may cause an allergic reaction.
- It can't be reused.
- Sexual pleasure may be affected.

Female condom: The pros

- It's 95% effective.
- It prevents the spread of STDs.
- It can be purchased over the counter.

Female condom: The cons

- It's more expensive than the male condom.
- It can be difficult to use.
- It can break or become dislodged.
- It may cause an allergic reaction.

- Nursing implications
  – Remind the patient and her partner that the condom must be positioned so that it's loose enough at the penis tip to collect ejaculate but not so loose that it comes off the penis
  – Reinforce that the penis must be withdrawn before it becomes flaccid after ejaculation, otherwise sperm may escape from the condom into the vagina

● **Female condom**
- Description
  – A vaginal sheath made of polyurethane and lubricated with nonoxynol 9
  – The inner ring (closed end) covers the cervix. The outer ring (open end) rests against the vaginal opening (see *Inserting a female condom*)
  – Intended for one-time use and shouldn't be used in combination with male condoms
- Advantages
  – It's 95% effective
  – It helps prevent the spread of STDs
  – It can be purchased over-the-counter
- Disadvantages
  – The female condom is more expensive than the male condom
  – It can be difficult to use and hasn't gained as much acceptance as a male condom
  – Pregnancy can occur as a result of failure to use or incorrect use
  – It may break or become dislodged
  – It's contraindicated in patients or partners with latex allergies
- Nursing implications
  – Instruct the patient in how to insert the female condom
  – Advise the patient that the condom may be inserted for up to 8 hours before intercourse
  – Reinforce that the condom is for one-time use only and must be discarded after use

● **Diaphragm**
- Description
  – A barrier-type contraceptive that mechanically blocks sperm from entering the cervix
  – Composed of a soft, latex dome that's supported by a round, metal spring on the outside
  – A diaphragm can be inserted up to 2 hours before intercourse
  – Optimum effectiveness is achieved by using it in combination with spermicidal jelly that's applied to the ring of the diaphragm before it's inserted
  – Diaphragms are available in various sizes and must be fitted to the individual

Inserting a female condom

A female condom is made of latex and lubricated with nonoxynol 9. It has an inner ring that covers the cervix and an outer ring that rests against the vaginal opening, as shown below.

To insert the condom, the inner ring should be folded in half with one hand pressing the opposite sides together, as shown below. When inserted, the inner ring covers the cervix.

After the condom is inserted, the outer ring (open end) should rest against the vaginal opening.

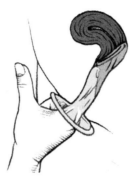

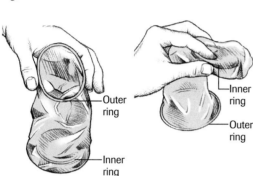

Outer ring

Inner ring

Inner ring

Outer ring

- Advantages
  - It's a good choice for women who choose not to use hormonal contraceptives or don't feel that they can be accurate in using natural family planning methods
  - When combined with spermicidal jelly, its effectiveness ranges from 80% to 93% for new users and increases to 97% for long-term users
  - It causes few adverse reactions
  - It helps protect against STDs when used with spermicide
  - It doesn't alter the body's metabolic or physiologic processes
  - It can be inserted up to 2 hours before intercourse
  - Providing it's correctly fitted and inserted, neither partner can feel it during intercourse
- Disadvantages
  - Some women dislike using a diaphragm because it must be inserted before intercourse
  - Although the diaphragm can be left in place for up to 24 hours, if intercourse is repeated before 6 hours (which is how long the diaphragm *must* be left in place after intercourse) more spermicidal gel must be inserted
  - The diaphragm can't be removed and replaced because this could cause sperm to bypass the spermicidal gel and fertilization could occur

The diaphragm: The pros

- When combined with spermicidal jelly, it's 80% to 93% effective.
- It helps protect against STDs when used with spermicide.
- It doesn't alter the body's metabolic or physiologic processes.
- It can be inserted up to 2 hours before intercourse.

The diaphragm: The cons

- It must be inserted before intercourse.
- It may cause more UTIs.
- It must be left in place for 6 hours after intercourse.

- It may cause more upper urinary tract infections (UTIs) due to the pressure of the diaphragm on the urethra
- The diaphragm must be refitted after birth, cervical surgery, miscarriage, dilatation and curettage (D&C), therapeutic abortion, or weight gain or loss of more than 15 lb (6.8 kg) because of cervical shape changes
- It's contraindicated in women who have a history of cystocele, rectocele, uterine retroversion, prolapse, retroflexion, or anteflexion because the cervix position may be displaced, making insertion and proper fit questionable
- It's contraindicated in patients with a history of toxic shock syndrome or repeated UTIs, vaginal stenosis, pelvic abnormalities, allergy to spermicidal jellies or rubber; it's also contraindicated in patients who show an unwillingness to learn proper techniques for diaphragm care and insertion
- It can't be used in the first 6 postpartum weeks

• Nursing implications
- Instruct the patient in proper insertion technique
- Urge the patient never to leave the diaphragm in place for longer than 24 hours
- Instruct the patient to leave the diaphragm in place for about 6 hours after intercourse
- Advise the patient to use additional spermicide for additional intercourse
- Urge the patient to adhere to medical follow-up and to have the diaphragm refitted after birth, cervical surgery, miscarriage, D&C, therapeutic abortion, or weight gain or loss of more than 15 lb because of cervical shape changes

● **Cervical cap**
• Description
- A barrier-type method of contraception, similar to the diaphragm but smaller
- A thimble-shaped, soft rubber cup that the patient places over the cervix
- Held in place by suction
- The addition of a spermicide creates an additional chemical barrier
- Women who aren't suited for diaphragms may use a cervical cap; failure of the cervical cap is commonly due to failure to use the device or inappropriate use of the device

• Advantages
- The cap requires less spermicide
- It has an efficacy rate of 85% for nulliparous women and 70% for parous women when used correctly and consistently

– It doesn't alter hormone levels

– It can be inserted up to 8 hours before intercourse

– It doesn't require reapplication of spermicide before repeated intercourse

– It can remain in place longer than diaphragms because it doesn't exert pressure on the vaginal walls or urethra

• Disadvantages

– It requires possible refitting after weight gain or loss of 15 lb (6.8 kg) or more, recent pregnancy, recent pelvic surgery, or cap slippage

– It is more likely to become dislodged during intercourse

– It may be difficult to insert or remove

– It may cause an allergic reaction or vaginal lacerations and thickening of the vaginal mucosa

– It may cause a foul odor if left in place for more than 36 hours

– It can't be used during menstruation or during the first 6 postpartum weeks

– It shouldn't be left in place longer than 24 hours

– It's contraindicated in patients with a history of toxic shock syndrome, a previously abnormal Pap test, allergy to latex or spermicide, an abnormally short or long cervix, history of PID, cervicitis, papillomavirus infection, cervical cancer, or undiagnosed vaginal bleeding

• Nursing implications

– Make sure the patient is properly fitted with the cap

· The gap or space between the base of the cervix and the inside of the cervical cap ring should be 1 to 2 mm (to reduce the possibility of dislodgment)

· The rim should fill the cervicovaginal fornix.

· If the cap is too small, the rim leaves a gap where the cervix remains exposed; if the cap is too large, it isn't snug against the cervix and is more easily dislodged

– Instruct the patient in how to insert the cap properly

– Remind the patient that the cap needs refitting after weight gain or loss of 15 lb or more, recent pregnancy, recent pelvic surgery, or cap slippage

● **Spermicides**

• Description

– Offer a chemical barrier method of contraception

– Available in gels, creams, films, foams, and suppositories

– Before intercourse, spermicidal products are inserted into the vagina with the goal of killing sperm before the sperm enter the cervix

---

Cervical cap: The pros

● It has an efficacy rate of 85% for nulliparous women and 70% for parous women.

● It doesn't alter hormone levels.

● It can be inserted up to 8 hours before intercourse.

Cervical cap: The cons

● It may be difficult to insert or remove.

● It can't be used during menstruation or during the first 6 postpartum weeks.

Cervical cap: A proper fit

● The gap or space between the base of the cervix and the inside of the cervical cap ring should be 1 to 2 mm.

● The rim should fill the cervicovaginal fornix.

● If the cap is too small, the rim leaves a gap where the cervix remains exposed.

● If the cap is too large, it isn't snug against the cervix and is more easily dislodged.

Spermicides: The pros

- They're inexpensive.
- They may be purchased over-the-counter.
- They don't require a visit to a health care provider.
- Spermicidal films wash away with natural body fluids.
- Nonoxynol 9, one of the most preferred spermicides, may also help prevent the spread of STDs.

Spermicides: The cons

- They need to be inserted 15 minutes to 1 hour before intercourse, so they may interfere with sexual spontaneity.
- Some spermicides may be irritating to the vagina and penile tissue.

– Spermicides also change the pH of the vaginal fluid to a strong acid, which isn't conducive to sperm survival

– The gels, foams, and creams are inserted using an applicator at least 1 hour before intercourse

– Spermicidal films, made of glycerin impregnated with nonoxynol 9, are folded and then inserted into the vagina; upon contact with vaginal secretions or precoital penile emissions, the film dissolves and carbon dioxide foam forms to protect the cervix against invading spermatozoa

– Spermicidal suppositories, consisting of cocoa butter and glycerin filled with nonoxynol 9, are inserted into the vagina where they dissolve to release the spermicide

- Advantages
  – They're inexpensive

  – They may be purchased over-the-counter, which makes them easily accessible

  – They don't require a visit to a health care provider

  – Spermicidal films wash away with natural body fluids

  – Nonoxynol 9, one of the most preferred spermicides, may also help prevent the spread of STDs

  – Vaginally inserted spermicides may be used in combination with other birth control methods to increase their effectiveness

  – They're useful in emergency situations such as when a condom breaks

  – They can be used as a backup contraceptive during the first several months of oral contraceptive or intrauterine device (IUD) use

- Disadvantages
  – They need to be inserted 15 minutes to 1 hour before intercourse, so they may interfere with sexual spontaneity

  – Some spermicides may be irritating to the vagina and penile tissue

  – Some women are bothered by the vaginal leakage that can occur, especially after using cocoa- and glycerin-based suppositories

  – The film form's effectiveness depends on vaginal secretions; therefore, it isn't recommended for women who are nearing menopause because decreased vaginal secretions make the film less effective

  – Spermicides may be contraindicated in women who have acute cervicitis because of the risk of further irritation

  – They're also contraindicated in individuals who must prevent contraception for medical reasons, such as those who are taking a medication that would be harmful to a fetus

- Nursing implications
  - Instruct the woman not to douche for 6 hours after intercourse to ensure that the agent has completed its spermicidal action in the vagina and cervix
  - Advise the woman using the suppository form to insert it 15 minutes before intercourse to ensure that the spermicide is dissolved; if using gel, cream, or foam form, advise woman to apply spermicide at least 1 hour before intercourse
  - Urge the woman to apply new spermicide before each act of intercourse

OTHER METHODS

● **IUD**
- Description: a plastic contraceptive device that's inserted into the uterus through the cervical canal
- Two types of IUDs are available in the United States
  - ParaGard T—a T-shaped, polyethylene device with copper wrapped around its vertical stem
    · Copper interferes with sperm mobility, decreasing the possibility of sperm crossing the uterine space
    · A knotted monofilament retrieval string is attached through a hole in the stem
  - Progestasert system—a T-shaped device made of an ethylene vinyl acetate copolymer with a knotted monofilament retrieval string attached through a hole in the vertical stem
    · Progesterone is stored in the hollow vertical stem, suspended in an oil base; drug gradually diffuses into the uterus and prevents endometrium proliferation
    · The IUD must be replaced annually to replenish the progesterone
    · The Progestasert system may relieve excessive menstrual blood loss and dysmenorrhea
- Advantages
  - They don't inhibit sexual spontaneity
  - Neither partner feels the device during intercourse
- Disadvantages
  - They're expensive
  - They may cause uterine cramping on insertion, especially in a nulliparous woman
  - They may cause infection, especially in the initial weeks after insertion
  - They're spontaneously expelled in the first year by 5% to 20% of women

– They don't protect against STDs
– The incidence of PID increases with IUD use
  · Most cases of PID occur during the first 3 months after insertion
  · After 3 months, the chance of PID is lower unless preinsertion screening failed to identify a person at risk for STDs
– They increase the risk of ectopic pregnancy
– IUDs are contraindicated in women who have Wilson's disease (because of inability to metabolize copper properly); and in women who have active, recent, or recurrent PID; infection or inflammation of the genital tract; an STD; a disease that suppresses immune function such as human immunodeficiency virus (HIV); unexplained cervical or vaginal bleeding; a history of problems with IUDs; cancer of the reproductive organs; or a history of ectopic pregnancy
– Insertion is also contraindicated in patients who have severe vasovagal reactivity, difficulty obtaining emergency care, valvular heart disease, anatomic uterine deformities, anemia, or nulliparity
• Nursing implications
– Know that IUD insertion is performed most easily during menses when the cervical canal is slightly dilated and the risk of pregnancy is reduced
– Assist with a bimanual examination as necessary for determining uterine position, shape, and size
– Before IUD insertion, make sure the procedure has been explained to the patient and that her questions have been addressed
– Ensure informed consent
– Keep in mind that if a woman becomes pregnant with an IUD in place, the device can be left; however, it's usually removed to prevent spontaneous abortion and infection
– Instruct the woman about signs and symptoms of PID including fever of 101° F (38.3° C); purulent vaginal discharge; dyspareunia (painful intercourse); abdominal or pelvic pain; suprapubic tenderness or guarding; pain with cervical motion; and adnexal tenderness

● **Hormonal ring**
• Description
– A combined hormonal (estrogen and progesterone) contraceptive that consists of a transparent plastic ring about 2″ (5.1 cm) in diameter
– Ring is inserted vaginally
– Ring is left in place for 3 weeks; after a 1-week ring-free period, a new ring is inserted
• Advantages
– More convenient than other methods
– As reliable as the contraceptive pill

– Exact position of the ring isn't important to effectiveness
– Easy to use
– Can be worn for 3 weeks
– Doesn't interrupt sexual play
– Affects fertility 1 month at a time
- Disadvantages
  – Adverse effects include vaginal discharge and irritation, headache, weight gain, nausea, irregular bleeding, breast changes, and mood changes
  – Doesn't protect against STDs, including HIV or acquired immunodeficiency syndrome
  – Requires a prescription
  – Increases the risk of heart attack and stroke
- Nursing implications
  – Instruct the woman how to insert the vaginal ring
  – Inform the patient that the effectiveness of the vaginal ring is lowered when used in combination with certain medications, such as St. John's wort, antiseizure drugs, antituberculotic medications, antibiotics, and antimigraine drugs

● **Emergency postcoital contraception**
- Description
  – Involves the use of hormonal agents to interfere with fertilization
  – Is used when a patient has had unprotected sexual intercourse within the last 72 hours
  – Various regimens may be used including two fixed-dose combination pills containing norgestrel and ethinyl estradiol (Ovral) followed by two additional doses 12 hours later , a commercial kit with a urine pregnancy test and four estrogen-progesterone pills, a two-pill progestin-only regimen, and mifepristone (an abortifacient)
- Advantages
  – It's 75% to 98% effective
  – It can prevent pregnancy in cases of sexual assault
- Disadvantages
  – It has numerous adverse effects, including nausea and vomiting
  – Because of hormonal components, it can be used only if the woman has no contraindications
  – The risk of congenital anomalies is increased if fertilization and, subsequently, pregnancy isn't prevented
- Nursing implications
  – Offer support and guidance to the patient
  – Instruct the patient in the prescribed regimen
  – Anticipate the need for administering an antiemetic to control nausea and vomiting

Hormonal ring: The cons

- It may cause vaginal discharge and irritation, irregular bleeding, and breast changes.
- It doesn't protect against STDs.
- It requires a prescription.
- It increases the risk of heart attack and stroke.

Emergency postcoital contraception: The pros

- It's 75% to 98% effective.
- It can prevent pregnancy in cases of sexual assault.

Emergency postcoital contraception: The cons

- It has numerous adverse effects, including nausea and vomiting.
- It can be used only if the woman has no contraindications to the hormonal components.
- The risk of congenital anomalies is increased if fertilization and pregnancy aren't prevented.

SURGICAL METHODS

● **Description**
- Include vasectomy (for men) and tubal ligation (for women)
- These procedures are the most commonly chosen contraceptive methods for couples older than age 30
- Although it's possible to reverse these procedures, doing so is expensive and in some cases ineffective
- Therefore, surgical sterilization should be chosen only when the patient and her partner, if applicable, have thoroughly discussed the options and know that these procedures are for permanent contraception

● **Vasectomy**
- Description
  - A procedure in which the pathway for spermatozoa is surgically severed
  - Incisions are made on each side of the scrotum, and the vas deferens is cut and tied and then plugged or cauterized, thus blocking the passage of sperm (see *Understanding a vasectomy*)
  - The testes continue to produce sperm as usual, but the sperm can't pass the severed vas deferens
- Advantages
  - It can be done as an outpatient procedure, with little anesthesia and minimal pain
  - It's 99.6% effective
  - It doesn't interfere with male erection and the male still produces seminal fluid—it just doesn't contain sperm
- Disadvantages
  - Misconceptions about the procedure may lead some men to resist it
  - Some reports indicate that vasectomy may be associated with the development of renal calculi
  - The procedure is contraindicated in individuals who aren't entirely certain of their decision to choose permanent sterilization and in those with specific surgical risks such as an anesthesia allergy
- Nursing implications
  - Ensure informed consent before the procedure
  - Perform all appropriate preoperative teaching
  - Caution the patient that sperm remaining in the vas deferens at the time of surgery may remain viable for as long as 6 months.
  - Advise the patient to use an additional form of contraception until two negative sperm reports have been obtained (These reports confirm that all of the remaining sperm in the vas deferens has been ejaculated.)

Understanding a vasectomy

In a vasectomy, the vas deferens is surgically altered to prohibit the passage of sperm. Here's how:

- The physician makes two small incisions on each side of the scrotum.

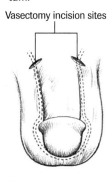

Vasectomy incision sites

- He then cuts the vas deferens with scissors.

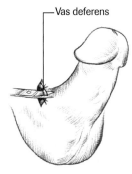

Vas deferens

- The vas deferens is then cauterized or plugged to block the passage of sperm.

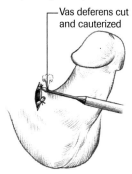

Vas deferens cut and cauterized

– To prevent your patients from making a rash decision regarding vasectomy, explain that this procedure should be viewed as irreversible, although reversal is possible in 95% of cases

- **Tubal ligation**
  - Description
    – A laparoscope is used to cauterize, crush, clamp, or block the fallopian tubes, thus preventing pregnancy by blocking the passage of ova and sperm
    – The procedure is performed after menses and before ovulation
    – It can also be performed 4 to 6 hours (although it's usually performed within 12 to 24 hours) after the birth of a baby or an abortion (see *Understanding tubal ligation,* page 392)
  - Advantages
    – It can be performed on an outpatient basis, and the patient is usually discharged within a few hours after the procedure
    – It's 99.6% effective
    – It has been associated with a decreased incidence of ovarian cancer
    – A woman can return to having intercourse 2 to 3 days after having the procedure
  - Disadvantages
    – Some woman may be reluctant to choose this type of procedure because it requires a small surgical incision and general anesthesia

Facts about tubal ligation

- In the procedure, the fallopian tubes are cauterized, crushed, clamped, or blocked to prevent the passage of ova and sperm.
- It's performed after menses and before ovulation.
- It can also be performed 4 to 24 hours after birth.

Tubal ligation: The pros

- It can be done as an outpatient procedure.
- The patient is usually discharged within a few hours.
- It has been associated with decreased incidence of ovarian cancer.

Understanding tubal ligation

In a laparoscopic tubal ligation, the surgeon inserts a laparoscope and occludes the fallopian tube by cauterizing, crushing, clamping, or blocking. This prevents the passage of ova and sperm.

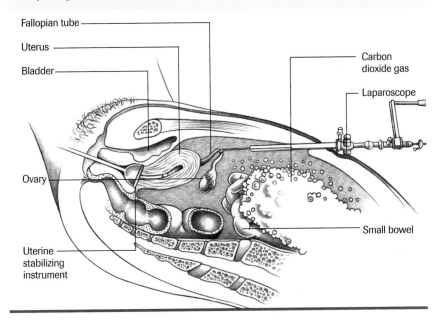

Fallopian tube
Uterus
Bladder
Carbon dioxide gas
Laparoscope
Ovary
Small bowel
Uterine stabilizing instrument

- Complications include a risk of bowel perforation and hemorrhage and the typical risks of general anesthesia (allergy, arrhythmia) during the procedure
- Contraindications include umbilical hernia and obesity
- Posttubal ligation syndrome may occur, which includes vaginal spotting and intermittent vaginal bleeding as well as severe lower abdominal cramping
- This form of contraception isn't recommended for individuals who aren't certain of their decision to choose permanent sterilization
- Nursing implications
  - Ensure informed consent before the procedure
  - Perform all appropriate preoperative teaching
  - Caution women not to have unprotected intercourse before the procedure because sperm that can become trapped in the tube could fertilize an ovum, resulting in an ectopic pregnancy
  - Help patients view this procedure as irreversible
  - Remember that although reversal is successful in 40% to 75% of patients, the process is difficult and could cause an ectopic pregnancy

---

Tubal ligation: The cons

- It requires general anesthesia and an incision.
- Complications include a risk of bowel perforation and hemorrhage.
- Vaginal spotting and severe lower abdominal cramping may occur.

ELECTIVE TERMINATION OF PREGNANCY

● Description
- Also called an *elective abortion*
- Refers to the willful termination of a pregnancy by mechanical or medical methods before the age of viability
- Although legally permitted, elected abortions remain a highly charged religious and social subject
- Different states have varying restrictions on timing, legality, counseling, and payment
- Women also experience varying emotional responses
  - Although some women may be relieved the pregnancy is terminated, many women feel guilt or remorse
  - Some women relive the experience each year on the anniversary of the abortion
  - Some women report imagining how their lost child would have looked or acted when they see other children

● Methods
- Dilatation and evacuation (D&E)
  - D&E is used in the first trimester
  - Cervix is dilated by mechanical means
  - Products of conception are removed by suction
- Prostaglandin suppositories
  - Prostaglandin suppositories are used in the second and third trimesters
  - Prostaglandin is inserted into the cervix, which causes dilation and initiation of contractions
- Menstrual extraction
  - Menstrual extraction is also called *suction evacuation*
  - It's typically done as an ambulatory surgery procedure usually 5 to 7 weeks after the patient's last menses
- Hysterotomy
  - Hysterotomy involves the removal of the fetus similar to the technique of cesarean birth
  - This procedure may be used when the fetus is more than 16 weeks' gestation
- Mifepristone
  - Mifepristone is an antiprogesterone agent taken as a single dose within the first 49 days of gestation
  - It interferes with implantation of the fertilized egg
  - If the drug is ineffective in expelling the pregnancy, misoprostol may be given to induce uterine contractions and aid in expulsion

TOP 6

Items to study for your next test on family planning and contraception

1. The six natural family planning methods
2. The three pharmacologic methods of contraception
3. The five barrier methods of contraception
4. The IUD, hormonal ring, and emergency postcoital methods of contraception
5. The two surgical methods of contraception
6. The methods of elective termination of pregnancy

- Nursing implications
  - Carefully explore own personal and religious beliefs about abortion
  - Know that any nurse can refuse to participate in an elective abortion because of moral or religious convictions
  - Present a nonjudgmental attitude when caring for the woman
  - Explain to the patient that she may experience grieving and a sense of loss
  - Instruct the patient in signs and symptoms to report to the physician, such as excessive vaginal bleeding, foul-smelling vaginal drainage, fever, and abdominal pain

NCLEX CHECKS

It's never too soon to begin your NCLEX preparation. Now that you've reviewed this chapter, carefully read each of the following questions and choose the best answer. Then compare your responses to the correct answers.

1. A woman chooses a family planning method that requires her to assess the quality of cervical mucus throughout the menstrual cycle. Which method is the woman using?

- ☐ **A.** Coitus interruptus
- ☐ **B.** Rhythm method
- ☐ **C.** Basal body temperature (BBT)
- ☒ **D.** Billings method

2. Which of the following would affect the accuracy of BBT readings?

- ☐ **A.** Taking the temperature immediately after awakening
- ☒ **B.** Measuring temperature after going to the bathroom to urinate
- ☐ **C.** Taking the temperature at the same time each morning
- ☐ **D.** Using a thermometer that registers temperature in tenths of degrees

3. Which method would be least effective in helping to prevent sexually transmitted diseases?

- ☒ **A.** Oral contraceptives
- ☐ **B.** Diaphragm
- ☐ **C.** Female condom
- ☐ **D.** Spermicidal cream

4. After intercourse, the patient is instructed to keep the diaphragm in place for at least what period of time?

- ☒ **A.** 6 hours
- ☐ **B.** 10 hours
- ☐ **C.** 18 hours
- ☐ **D.** 20 hours

5. Which of the following are contraindications for using an intrauterine device (IUD)? Select all that apply.

☐ **A.** Negative history of pelvic inflammatory disease (PID)
☒ **B.** Wilson's disease
☐ **C.** History of severe dysmenorrhea
☒ **D.** Unexplained cervical bleeding
☒ **E.** Human immunodeficiency virus (HIV)

ANSWERS AND RATIONALES

1. CORRECT ANSWER: D

The Billings method requires assessment of cervical mucus. At the time of ovulation, the cervical mucus is present in greater quantity, stretchy, and more favorable to penetration by sperm. Coitus interruptus involves withdrawing the penis before ejaculation. The rhythm method involves abstaining from sexual intercourse 3 to 4 days before and after ovulation. BBT involves monitoring the woman's body temperature for changes indicating ovulation (slight decrease in temperature followed by a rise) and abstaining from intercourse for the next 3 days.

2. CORRECT ANSWER: B

Various factors can affect the accuracy of BBT readings: changes in activities or daily routine, illness, forgetting to take the temperature, taking the temperature after arising. BBT is measured using a thermometer that registers temperatures in tenths of degrees.

3. CORRECT ANSWER: A

Oral contraceptives have no effect on the prevention of STDs. Barrier methods, such as the diaphragm, female condom, and spermicides, are associated with preventing STDs.

4. CORRECT ANSWER: A

After intercourse, a diaphragm should be left in place for 6 hours. Removing it before this time interferes with its effectiveness. A diaphragm can be left in place for up to 24 hours, but this is the maximum amount of time for placement.

5. CORRECT ANSWERS: B, D, AND E

IUDs are contraindicated in women with Wilson's disease, unexplained cervical bleeding, and any disease that suppresses the immune system, such as HIV. An IUD is an appropriate contraceptive choice for a woman who has no history of PID, dysmenorrhea, or previous IUD failures.

Glossary

aberration: deviation from what's typical or normal

acme: peak of a contraction

adnexal area: accessory parts of the uterus, ovaries, and fallopian tubes

agenesis: failure of an organ to develop

amnion: inner membrane of the two fetal membranes that form the amniotic sac and house the fetus and the fluid that surrounds it in utero

amniotic: relating to or pertaining to the amnion

amniotic fluid: fluid surrounding the fetus, derived primarily from maternal serum and fetal urine

amniotic sac: membrane ("bag of waters") that contains the fetus and fluid during gestation

analgesic: pharmacologic agent that relieves pain without causing unconsciousness

anesthesia: use of pharmacologic agents to produce partial or total loss of sensation, with or without loss of consciousness

anomaly: organ or structure that's malformed or in some way abnormal due to structure, form or position

artificial insemination: mechanical deposition of donor's or partner's spermatozoa at the cervical os

autosomes: any of the paired chromosomes other than the X and Y (sex) chromosomes

basal body temperature: temperature when body metabolism is at its lowest, usually below 98° F (36.7° C) before ovulation and above 98° F after ovulation

Bishop score: method of assessing cervical dilation, effacement, station, consistency, and position to determine readiness for induction of labor

c-peptide: an enzyme predictor of early hyperinsulinemia

cephalocaudal development: principle of maturation that development proceeds from the head to the tail (rump)

chorion: fetal membrane closest to the uterine wall; gives rise to the placenta and is the outer membrane surrounding the amnion

conduction: loss of body heat to a solid, cooler object through direct contact

congenital disorder: disorder present at birth that may be caused by genetic or environmental factors

convection: loss of body heat to cooler ambient air

corpus luteum: yellow structure, formed from a ruptured graafian follicle, that secretes progesterone during the second half of the menstrual cycle; if pregnancy occurs, the corpus luteum continues to produce progesterone until the placenta assumes that function

cotyledon: one of the rounded segments on the maternal side of the placenta, consisting of villi, fetal vessels, and an intervillous space

cryptorchidism: undescended testes

cul-de-sac: pouch formed by a fold of the peritoneum between the anterior wall of the rectum and the posterior wall of the uterus; also known as Douglas' cul de sac

decidua: mucous membrane lining of the uterus during pregnancy; shed after giving birth

dilation: widening of the external cervical os

dizygotic: proceeding from two fertilized ova, or zygotes (for example, dizygotic twins)

doll's eye phenomenon: movement of a neonate's eyes in a direction opposite to which the head is turned; this reflex typically disappears after 10 days of extrauterine life

Down syndrome: abnormality involving the occurrence of a third chromosome, instead of the normal pair (trisomy 21); characteristically results in mental retardation and altered physical appearance

dystocia: difficult labor

effleurage: gentle massage to the abdomen during labor for the purpose of relaxation and distraction

effacement: thinning and shortening of the cervix

embryo: conceptus from the time of implantation to 5 to 8 weeks

endometrium: inner mucosal lining of the uterus

engagement: descent of the fetal presenting part to at least the level of the ischial spines

Epstein's pearls: small white firm epithelial cysts on the neonate's hard palate

evaporation: loss of body heat when fluid on the body surface changes to a vapor

fetus: conceptus from 5 to 8 weeks until term

follicle-stimulating hormone: hormone produced by the anterior pituitary gland that stimulates the development of the graafian follicle

fontanel: space at the junction of the sutures connecting fetal skull bones

gamete intrafallopian tube transfer: placement of ovum and spermatozoa into the end of the fallopian tube via laparoscope; also called *in vivo fertilization*

gene: factor on a chromosome responsible for the hereditary characteristics of the offspring

general anesthesia: use of pharmacologic agents to produce loss of consciousness, progressive central nervous system depression, and complete loss of sensation

hematoma: collection of blood in the soft tissue

hereditary disorder: disorder passed from one generation to another

heterozygous: presence of two dissimilar genes at the same site on paired chromosomes

Homans' sign: calf pain on leg extension and foot dorsiflexion; an early sign of thrombophlebitis

homozygous: presence of two similar genes at the same site on paired chromosomes

human chorionic gonadotropin: hormone produced by the chorionic villi, serves as the biologic marker in pregnancy tests

hyperinsulinemia: a prediabetic state marked by insulin resistance and often seen in polycystic ovarian syndrome

hypoxia: reduced oxygen availability to tissues or fetus

increment: period of increasing strength of a uterine contraction

induction of labor: artificial initiation of labor

informed consent: written consent obtained by the doctor after the patient has been fully informed of the planned treatment, potential adverse effects, and alternative management choices

intensity: the strength of a uterine contraction, if measured externally a relative measurement may be used, if measured with an intrauterine pressure device measured and recorded in millimeters of mercury (mm Hg)

interval: period between the end of one uterine contraction and the beginning of the next uterine contraction

intervillous space: irregularly-shaped areas in the maternal portion of the placenta that are filled with blood and serve as the site for maternal-fetal gas, nutrient, and waste exchange

in vitro fertilization: fertilization of an ovum outside the woman's body, followed by reimplantation of the blastocyte into the woman

involution: reduction of uterine size after delivery; may take up to 6 weeks

karyotype: schematic display of the chromosomes within a cell arranged to demonstrate their numbers and morphology

lanugo: downy, fine hair that covers the fetus between 20 weeks of gestation and birth

lecithin and sphingomyelin: phospholipids (surfactants) that reduce surface tension and increase pulmonary tissue elasticity

leukorrhea: white or yellow vaginal discharge

lie: relationship of the long axis of the fetus to the long axis of the pregnant patient

linear terminalis: an imaginary line that separates the true pelvis from the false pelvis

local anesthesia: blockage of sensory nerve pathways at the organ level, producing loss of sensation only in that organ

lochia: discharge after delivery from sloughing of the uterine decidua

luteinizing hormone: hormone produced by the anterior pituitary gland that stimulates ovulation and the development of the corpus luteum

meiosis: process by which germ cells divide and decrease their chromosomal number by one half

mifepristone: progesterone antagonist that prevents implantation of fertilized egg; also called *RU486*

mitosis: process of somatic cell division in which a single cell divides but both of the new cells have the same number of chromosomes as the first

molding: shaping of the fetal head caused by shifting of sutures in response to pressure exerted by the maternal pelvis and birth canal during labor and delivery

myometrium: middle muscular layer of the uterus made up of three layers of smooth, involuntary muscles

neonate: an infant between birth and the 28th day

nevus pilosus: "hairy mole"; dermal sinus at the base of the spine, commonly associated with spina bifida

nidation: implantation of the fertilized ovum in the uterine endometrium

nitrazine paper: a treated paper used to detect pH when determining if amniotic fluid is present

Nuva Ring: a vaginal contraceptive ring that contains estrogen and progesterone

oligohydramnios: severely reduced and highly concentrated amniotic fluid

oocyte: incompletely developed ovum

oogenesis: formation and development of the ovum

Ortho Evra: a contraceptive topical patch that contains estrogen and progesterone

ovum: conceptus from time of conception until primary villi appear, approximately 4 weeks after the last menstrual period

perimetrium: outer serosal layer of the uterus

polyhydramnios: abnormally large amount (more than 2,000 ml) of amniotic fluid in the uterus

premonitory: forewarning, before the onset

primordial: existing in the most primitive form

puerperium: interval between delivery and 6 weeks after delivery

radiation: loss of body heat to a solid cold object without direct contact

regional anesthesia: blockage of large sensory nerve pathways in an organ and its surrounding tissue, producing loss of sensation in that organ and in the surrounding region

ripening: refers to the softening and thinning of the cervix in preparation for active labor

Ritgen maneuver: where manual pressure is applied through the perineum to the occiput of the head as the fetus is extending and emerging to extrauterine life

rugae: folds in the vaginal mucosa and scrotum

semen: white, viscous secretion of the male reproductive organs that consists of spermatozoa and nutrient fluids ejaculated through the penile urethra

smegma: whitish secretions around the labia minora and under the foreskin of the penis

sperm: male sex cell

spermatogenesis: formation and development of spermatozoa

station: relationship of the presenting part to the ischial spines

strabismus: condition characterized by imprecise muscular control of ocular movement

subinvolution: failure of uterus to return to normal size following delivery

surrogate mothering: conceiving and carrying a pregnancy to term with the expectation of turning the infant over to contracting, adoptive parents

sutures: narrow areas of flexible tissue on the fetal scalp that allow for slight adjustment during descent through the birth canal

teratogen: any drug, virus, irradiation, or other nongenetic factors that can cause fetal malformations

tocolytic agent: medication that stops premature contractions

tocotransducer: an external mechanical device that translates one physical quantity to another, most often seen in capturing fetal heart rates and transmitting and recording the value onto a fetal monitor

trisomy: condition where a chromosome exists in triplicate instead of in the normal duplicate pattern

vibroacoustic stimulation test: using shoulder stimulation to elicit acceleration of the fetal heart rate

Wharton's jelly: whitish, gelatinous material that surrounds the umbilical vessels within the cord

X chromosome: sex chromosome in humans that exist in duplicate in the normal female and singly in the normal male

Y chromosome: sex chromosome in the human male that's necessary for development of the male sex glands, or gonads

zygote intrafallopian tube transfer: fertilization of the ovum outside the mother's body, followed by reimplantation of the zygote into the fallopian tube via laparoscope

Selected references

Akert, J. "A New Generation of Contraceptives," *RN* 66(2):54-61, February 2003.

Association of Women's Health, Obstetric, & Neonatal Nurses. *Women's Health Nursing—Towards Evidence Based Practice.* Philadelphia: W.B. Saunders Co., 2003.

Becker R., et al. "Doppler Sonography of Uterine Arteries at 20-23 Weeks: Risk Assessment of Adverse Pregnancy Outcome by Quantification of Impedance and Notch," *Journal of Perinatal Medicine* 30(5):388-94, 2002.

Blackburn, S. *Maternal, Fetal and Neonatal Physiology—A Clinical Perspective,* 2nd ed. Philadelphia: W.B. Saunders Co., 2003.

Callister L.C., et al. "First Time Mothers' Views of Breastfeeding Support From Nurses," *American Journal of Maternal/Child Nursing.* 28(1):10-15, January-February 2003.

Hill, W.C. *Ambulatory Obstetrics.* Philadelphia: Lippincott Williams & Wilkins, 2002.

Mandeville, L.K., and Troiano, N.H. *AWHONN's High Risk and Critical Care Intrapartum Nursing,* 2nd ed. Philadelphia: Lippincott Williams & Wilkins, 1999.

Matteson, P.S. *Women's Health During the Childbearing Years—A Community-Based Approach.* Philadelphia: W.B. Saunders Co., 2001.

Mattson, S., and Smith, J.E. *Core Curriculum for Maternal-Newborn Nursing,* 2nd ed. Philadelphia: W.B. Saunders Co., 2000.

Moos, M.K. "Unintended Pregnancies: A Call for Nursing Action," *American Journal of Maternal/Child Nursing,* 28(1):24-30, January-February 2003.

Morgan, G., and Hamilton, C. *Practice Guidelines for Obstetrics & Gynecology,* 2nd ed. Philadelphia: Lippincott Williams & Wilkins, 2003.

Murphy, P.A. "New Methods of Hormonal Contraception," *Nurse Practitioner,* 28(2):11-21, February 2003.

Murray, S.S., et al. *Foundations of Maternal-Newborn Nursing,* 3rd ed. Philadelphia: W.B. Saunders Co., 2002.

Newman M.G., et al. "Perinatal Outcomes in Preeclampsia that is Complicated by Massive Proteinuria," *American Journal of Obstetrics & Gynecology* 188(1):264-68, January 2003.

Pillitteri, A. *Maternal & Child Health Nursing,* 4th ed. Philadelphia: Lippincott Williams & Wilkins, 2003.

Schiff M.A., and Holt V.L. "The Injury Severity Score in Pregnant Trauma Patients: Predicting Placental Abruption and Fetal Death," *Journal of Trauma* 53(5):946-49, November 2002.

Scott, J.R., et al. *Danforth's Obstetrics and Gynecology,* 9th ed. Philadelphia: Lippincott Williams & Wilkins, 2003.

Sheiner, E., et al. "Incidence, Obstetric Risk Factors and Pregnancy Outcome of Preterm Placental Abruption: A Retrospective Analysis," *Journal of Maternal and Fetal Neonatal Medicine* 11(1):34-39, January 2002.

Simpson, K.R., and Creehan, P.A. *AWHONN's Perinatal Nursing,* 2nd ed., Philadelphia: Lippincott Williams & Wilkins, 2001; co-published with AWHONN.

Speroff, L. and Darney, P. *A Clinical Guide for Contraception,* 3rd ed. Philadelphia: Lippincott Williams & Wilkins, 2000.

Index

i refers to an illustration; t refers to a table.

i refers to an illustration; t refers to a table.

i refers to an illustration; t refers to a table.

---

i refers to an illustration; t refers to a table.

i refers to an illustration; t refers to a table.

i refers to an illustration; t refers to a table.

i refers to an illustration; t refers to a table.